Abdomen and OB/GYN

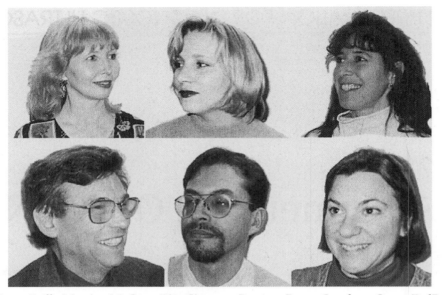

The Authors. *Top:* Jann Dolk, Monica McCrea, Lisa Simons. *Bottom:* Roger Sanders, Oscar DelBarco, Nancy Miner.

EXAM PREPARATION FOR DIAGNOSTIC ULTRASOUND

Abdomen and OB/GYN

Roger C. Sanders, MA, BM, Bch (Oxen), MRCP, FRCR, FACR, FAIUM
Research Professor of Radiology
Thomas Jefferson University School of Medicine
Philadelphia, Pennsylvania
Consultant
Los Alamos Woman Clinic
Los Alamos, New Mexico

Janice Dolk, MA, RT(R), RDMS
Adjunct Faculty, George Washington University
Former Program Director, University of Maryland
Former Faculty, Advanced Ultrasound Seminars
Baltimore, Maryland

Nancy Smith Miner, RT(R), RDMS
Adjunct Faculty in Diagnostic Ultrasound
New Hampshire Technical Institute
Concord, New Hampshire

ASSISTED BY:

Oscar DelBarco, BSRT, RDMS
Chief Sonographer
University of Maryland Hospital
Department of Radiology, Division of Ultrasound
Baltimore, Maryland

Monica McCrea, RDMS, RVT
Senior Sonographer
Formerly, Johns Hopkins Medical Institution
Department of Radiology, Division of Ultrasound
Baltimore, Maryland

Lisa Simons, RT(R), RDMS, RDCS, RVT
Freelance Sonographer, Hanover Hospital
Formerly, University of Maryland Hospital
Baltimore, Maryland

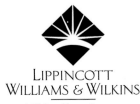

LIPPINCOTT
WILLIAMS & WILKINS
A **Wolters Kluwer** Company

Development Editor: Rosanne Hallowell and Lisa Bolger
Managing Editor: Marette Magargle-Smith
Design Coordinator: Doug Smock
Marketing Manager: Debby Hartman

Copyright © 2002 Lippincott Williams & Wilkins

351 West Camden Street
Baltimore, Maryland 21201-2436 USA

530 Walnut Street
Philadelphia, Pennsylvania 19106 USA

Printed in China

The publishers have made every effort to trace the copyright holders for borrowed material. If they have inadvertently overlooked any, they will be pleased to make the necessary arrangements at the first opportunity.

We'd like to hear from you! If you have comments or suggestions regarding this Lippincott Williams & Wilkins title, please contact us at the appropriate customer service number listed below, or send correspondence to **book_comments@lww.com**. If possible, please remember to include your mailing address, phone number, and a reference to the book title and author in your message. To purchase additional copies of this book call our customer service department at **(800) 638–3030** or fax orders to **(301) 824–7390**. International customers should call **(301) 714–2324.**

12 13 14 15

DEDICATION

To all who strive to become professional sonographers. Without my sonographer friends I could never have become a competent sonologist.
RCS

To Hank, my significant other, for his patience as I spent hours at my computer. For Antigone, our precious feline, for spending hours sitting next to me at my keyboard.
JDD

To my past, present, and future students: remember to set your standards high.
NSM

CONTENTS

PREFACE

Test taking is a harrowing experience. *Exam Preparation for Diagnostic Ultrasound: Abdomen and OB/GYN* offers both text for review and multiple-choice questions to sharpen readers' skills for taking the national registry examinations, specifically in the areas of Abdomen and Obstetrics & Gynecology. Test questions are provided in both paper and computer formats. The scope of this book does not include physics, except as it is relevant to obtaining abdominal, obstetric, and gynecologic images.

Part I: Abdomen and **Part II: Obstetrics and Gynecology** consist of brief, outline-format text which is intended for review rather than beginning study. The outline text is organized in accordance with the guidelines currently used by the American Registry of Diagnostic Medical Sonographers (ARDMS) for their abdomen and obstetrics & gynecology registries. (As these specifications change with time, updated versions of the question distribution are available from the ARDMS.)

Part III: Comprehensive Examinations consists of two separate mock registry exams, one for Abdomen and one for Obstetrics & Gynecology. Each test includes more than twice as many questions as the actual exam. Most of the question contributors have been item writers for the national registry exams. (We are not affiliated with the ARDMS; we have simply chosen their format to help familiarize students with the most comprehensive test available. Our intent is to prepare students well enough to succeed on any ultrasound certification exam.)

All ARDMS exams will be taken as computerized tests; this is a trend that other examination boards are following. While questions about prenatal ultrasound may feel like familiar territory, testing on a computer may not. The **accompanying CD** (attached to the inside back cover of this book) allows the reader to take our mock exams on the computer and to focus on specific topics for study once areas of weakness have been identified.

The questions in the book and on the CD-ROM are identical. Both the book and the CD provide the correct answer for each question, along with a brief explanation. Usually there is also an explanation of why the other choices are wrong. Those taking the test on paper will find the correct answers and explanations in the **Answers and Explanations** section at the end of the book. A number of the explanations include **"Test Noteworthy Tips"** (indicated by ⊞) that are designed to take the reader inside the mind of the beleaguered test writer for a better understanding of why questions are written the way they are.

As mentioned above, the CD version of the mock exam will automatically pinpoint your areas of weakness. Readers taking the paper version of the mock test can determine their areas of weakness by using the Self-Evaluation Charts at the end of the **Answers and Explanations** section. Each explanation begins with a code that is keyed to the Self-Evaluation Charts. The charts indicate which topic is being tested in each question; for example, the code "1,I" in an Abdomen test answer lets the reader know that the question and explanation deal with liver (Chapter 1) anatomy (roman numeral heading I). The blank answer sheets provided also contain the self-evaluation codes, making it easy for readers to grade themselves on the self-evaluation charts and determine at a glance which topics need more study.

We have tried to be concise but still include all of the essential concepts to help the reader make sense of anything encountered on a test that is not understood. **Appendix A** is a table of **laboratory values** that shows what increases and what decreases in various conditions, complete with actual values in the few instances when they're needed. **Appendix B** provides translations of the **Latin and Greek roots of medical terms** to help the reader understand terminology. **Appendix C: Suggested Readings** refers the user to more comprehensive texts that may be helpful for review of weak areas.

It is worth pointing out that there are some differences between the questions in this book and those on the actual exams. For example, we often ask several questions about the same image. While the ARDMS exam occasionally uses an image more than once, it does not group questions about an image together as we have done; instead, it repeats the image. Our reason for grouping multiple questions about one image is simple—we wanted to keep the cost of this book manageable for students. Even so, there are over 200 sonograms in this book, allowing for plenty of practice in answering image questions. (Note: Like the actual exam, our CD version of the test does repeat the image with each related question.)

As for our questions, some of them seem more complex than you would expect to see on the actual registry exam. There are reasons for this:

- We are interested in packing as much teaching information into each item as we can. We may never mention the entity being discussed in the question or the answer list; you might have to make the diagnosis and then dig into your store of knowledge to get the answer. That way, the explanation can go more in depth to cover a topic.
- The time factor is not as crucial here as on the actual exam. This way you can figure out the best and most efficient way to approach complex questions, and practice.
- Figuring out tough questions is like swinging two bats before your turn at the plate. Once you've done that, the real thing seems easier, and that is our goal.

Roger C. Sanders

Janice Dolk

Nancy Smith Miner

HOW TO USE THIS BOOK

STOP! DON'T SKIP THIS PAGE!

We've worked hard to figure out good strategies for both studying and test taking (see *How to Take a Test*, which follows). This section explains how to get the most out of this book. You will find that after completing our practice exams (Part III, Comprehensive Examinations), it will be easy to figure out the areas in which you are proficient and those that need more work.

BRIEF TEXT

Actually, there is not much text because this book is not intended for those just beginning their studies. Rather, this is a concise review text based on the content guidelines from the ARDMS. When you see a term you don't recognize, that is the time to review it in a more comprehensive text. (We have provided a list of suggested texts in Appendix C.)

EXAM CONTENT

This book is essentially a mock registry exam; the questions are strictly based on the content of the American Registry of Diagnostic Medical Sonographers (ARDMS). The ARDMS publishes the distribution of questions on the internet (www.ardms.org) and updates it annually; for example, the latest content outline states that 2%–6% of the obstetrics & gynecology exam will be questions about assessment of gestational age. Not only have we provided the right ratio of questions, but we've made sure that they include all of the subdivisions of this category (e.g., biparietal diameter, fetal lung maturity, femur length, transcerebellar measurements). These percentages can be found in the table of contents, at the beginning of each chapter, and on the self-evaluation charts.

LABORATORY VALUES (APPENDIX A)

Although it may seem important to memorize lots of numbers before the exam, we have not provided you with many on our laboratory values chart. Interpretations of what constitutes normal and what unit of measurement is correct can vary from place to place. Mostly, this table is to help you remember what increases and what decreases in various medical conditions, and to what extent they change (mildly, moderately, or markedly.)

WORD ORIGINS (APPENDIX B)

Now, we know you've studied and used medical terminology. You may even have studied Latin. However, you will still find the table in Appendix B helpful. It provides French, Greek, and Latin origins for prefixes, suffixes, and parts of words that can be melded together so you can figure out the meaning of many medical words, especially those that induce panic ("But I've never heard of that before!"). Don't neglect this appendix.

NOW, THE TEST

ANSWER SHEETS

In the back of the book are two blank, numbered answer sheets. They are fenestrated (see Appendix B if you don't know what that means) so they can be torn out easily. Copy the blank sheets if you wish—no copying anything else, please—and use them to mark your answers.

ANSWERS AND EXPLANATIONS

Reading the explanations may be the most satisfying part of a mock registry exam. Once you've done your best, you can find out not only *what* is the right answer, but also *why* it is the right answer. The explanations may be the best review of all, so don't just look for the correct answers and skip the explanations.

Note: Within the explanations, the **correct answers** are in bold and the *incorrect choices* are in italics. Occasionally, a word or phrase is <u>underlined</u> in the explanation. This is usually because there was no mention of the actual disease process in the question or answer choices. Sometimes we did this to force you to think ahead to the logical conclusion, just as you must do when scanning. By underlining the name of the condition in the explanation, it draws your eye to the "why" of your correct answer.

There is a bonus for those willing to read the explanations—we will take you into the mind of the test writer to show you what they were thinking by giving you **"Test Noteworthy Tips"**:

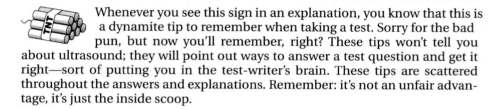 Whenever you see this sign in an explanation, you know that this is a dynamite tip to remember when taking a test. Sorry for the bad pun, but now you'll remember, right? These tips won't tell you about ultrasound; they will point out ways to answer a test question and get it right—sort of putting you in the test-writer's brain. These tips are scattered throughout the answers and explanations. Remember: it's not an unfair advantage, it's just the inside scoop.

CODES AND SELF-EVALUATION CHARTS

In the book version of the Answers and Explanations, each explanation begins with a code in brackets (e.g., "[2,IV]"). This code is based on the table of contents, which is based on the ARDMS guidelines. The Arabic numeral is the chapter number, or the main topic, and the Roman numeral is the heading in that chapter, or the subtopic. These codes let you know what topic that particular question and explanation covers. For example, the code "4,II" tells you that the question is about the technique (heading II) for scanning the urinary tract (Chapter 4). When you look at the Self-Evaluation Chart, find the II on one axis and the 4 on the other; the box where they meet will be labeled "urinary tract/technique" and will give you the percentage of questions that cover this topic on the exam. See the Sample Question and Explanation and the Sample Self-Evaluation Chart (pp xiv–xv).

The Self-Evaluation Charts that correspond with these codes are located at the back of the book. You may wish to keep track of wrong answers only on these charts so that when you complete an exam you can see your weak areas mapped out for you. To use these charts, first determine which questions you got wrong. Then, put a hash mark in the box of the chart that corresponds with the code of the question you got wrong. Then, for example, if you missed four "22,IV" questions, you should probably go back and review fetal anomalies (Chapter 22), and specifically spinal abnormalities (outline heading IV). (The CD-ROM version of the tests included with this book automatically pinpoints your "weak" areas and allows you to select questions specific to those areas for further practice.)

ADDITIONAL SUGGESTIONS

- **Time yourself.** The ARDMS abdomen and obstetrics & gynecology exams each have approximately 170 questions. You will have 3 hours to complete each test. In the book we have more than twice as many questions as there are on the actual registry exams, so remember that you only need to complete about 56 questions per hour.
- **Use the self-evaluation charts.** On the answer sheets there are codes provided next to each answer space that you can plug into the self-evaluation charts. You may wish to keep track of wrong answers only on the charts so that when you are finished you can see your weak areas at a glance.
- **Use a pencil.** Test takers have been known to change their minds. Also, after reviewing your weak areas, you may want to erase the self-evaluation charts and try the exams again.

If you haven't read *How To Take a Test* yet, this would be the time (see p xvii).

Refer to the obstetric sonogram below:

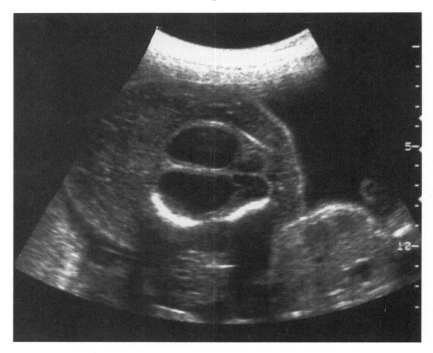

9. Which of the following conditions does this image MOST likely represent?
   A. Stuck twin syndrome
   B. Twin-to-twin transfusion syndrome
   C. A normal twin and a twin with intrauterine growth retardation (IUGR)
   D. An acardiac twin with a "pump" twin
   E. A rudimentary twin and a normal-sized twin

Correct answer

Outline heading

Chapter number

Correct answer

Incorrect answers

19-D [18, II]. A fetus with grossly thickened skin is anterior and a smaller, normal fetus is posterior and to the right. The intersac membrane is visible posterior to the abnormal head. This severe skin thickening is virtually specific for **acardiac twins.** It is too severe for the hydrops sometimes seen in *twin-to-twin transfusion syndrome* and *stuck twin syndrome.* Skin thickening is not seen in the other types of twins mentioned.

Test Noteworthy Tip

Looking at the image before you skim the options can waste time. For example, in question #19 the options all tell you that these are twins, putting you on the right track and preventing you from thinking of incorrect possibilties.

SAMPLE QUESTION AND EXPLANATION. *Important to note:* We have assigned only one code to each question and explanation to make sure that all areas have been adequately covered. Many, if not most, questions can be coded two or three ways. For instance, the above example is coded as a multiple gestation complication (18, II). Well, it certainly is that, but you could also code it as "19, IV" (polyhydramnios), even if it's just to remind you that you aren't comfortable with that area. This is your personalized study plan; use it to suit your needs.

SAMPLE SELF-EVALUATION CHART					
	14 **FIRST TRIMESTER** **(6–8%)**	**15** **SECOND AND THIRD TRIMESTER** **(8–12%)**	**16** **PLACENTA** **(1–5%)**	**17** **ASSESSMENT OF GESTATIONAL AGE** **(2–6%)**	**18** **COMPLICATIONS** **(6–10%)**	**19** **AMNIOTIC FLUID** **(1–5%)**
I	Gestational Sac	Basic Guidelines for Obstetric Sonograms	Development	Gestational Sac	Intrauterine Growth Retardation	Characteristics
II	Yolk Sac	Evaluation of Anatomy A. Cranium /// B. Spine C. Heart D. Thorax E. Abdomen F. Extremities G. Fetal Position	Position	Embryonic size/ Crown Rump Length	Multiple Gestation	Functions
III	Embryo		Anatomy /	Biparietal Diameter	Maternal Illness A. Diabetes Mellitus B. Pregnancy-Induced Hypertension	Assessment
IV	Ovaries		Membranes ₪	Femur Length	Antepartum A. Preterm Labor, Cervical Incompetence, and PROM B. Rh Isoimmunization	Polyhydramnios

Your incorrect answers

HOW TO TAKE THE TEST

ABOUT THE TEST

Most sonography students in the United States become registered in abdominal and obstetric & gynecologic ultrasound by the American Registry of Diagnostic Medical Sonographers (ARDMS). Consequently, the format and allocation of questions in this book mirror the ARDMS exam. An exam sponsored by the American Registry of Radiologic Technologists (ARRT) is now available. We have no doubt that the information and test-taking concepts presented in this book are a valid source to study for any multiple-choice ultrasound exam in obstetrics and gynecology and the abdomen.

The ARDMS examination can be taken at any time using a computer system and is typically administered through Assessment Systems, Inc. (ASI) [www.asisvcs.com]; the ARDMS will send you a check-in code to use when selecting a testing center on-line at ASI, or the phone numbers and instructions with your verification letter. Each ARDMS exam consists of approximately 170 questions taken over a 3-hour period. All questions are multiple choice, usually with five options, although occasionally four or even three options are used. Two question formats used in the past have been dropped—there are no true/false questions or matching questions. The option "all of the above" has been eliminated from the ARDMS exams, presumably because it biases the test by pointing to the correct answer. At least one third of the questions are associated with images. On the registry, the format is one question per image. To cut book costs down, in our mock exams we have written several questions per image.

Each exam question is allocated a minimum pass level (MPL) by the ARDMS, which is the examiner's estimate of how many candidates should get the answer correct. A very basic but important question that is required knowledge for anybody practicing sonography would be given an MPL of 0.90, implying that 90% of the candidates who pass would get it right. A more difficult question that only a superior candidate could answer correctly might be given an MPL of 0.50, so only 50% of successful candidates would get it right. Inevitably, questions vary greatly in difficulty. Just because you do not know about Klippel-Trénaunay-Weber syndrome, all is not lost. Only a few candidates are expected to know this esoteric answer.

The fields of abdominal, obstetric, and gynecologic ultrasound cover a daunting amount of information, and it's hard to draw the line on how much to learn. **Don't panic**. By definition, the Registry is only supposed to ask you about topics that are "current practice in ultrasound," meaning that the newest laser technique for obliterating the cord that is approved for use in only a single site won't be on the exam. It also means that aspects of obstetrics that don't relate to ultrasound, such as the medical management of toxemia, are not appropriate topics for questions. Of course, that doesn't mean they won't ask about hyperluminoid casastophalitis (don't worry; we made that up). One way to prepare for this possibility is to familiarize yourself with several different takes on the same subject—perhaps review in a different text than you used in school.

STUDYING PRIORITIES

Reminder: On the abdomen exam, the liver, biliary tract, pancreas, and genitourinary tract between them comprise 48%–80% of the questions. On the obstetrics & gynecology exam, the normal anatomy of the first and second trimesters and normal pelvic anatomy comprise 24%–25% of the test; fetal anomalies comprise only 10%–15%. The exam is biased toward anatomy and technique because these two areas are considered the forte of the sonographer. With this in mind:

- Your first priority should be topics that have a **high concentration** of questions on the test and are **difficult for you.**
- Next, look at topics with a **low priority** on the test that are **difficult for you.**
- Only then should you spend time on those topics that are **easy for you** and that have a **high concentration** on the test. Basically, don't waste time on memorizing obscure details about rare pathology.

STUDYING STYLE

How do you learn best? Figure out what topics to work on as discussed above, then try some of these ideas.

Are you a *visual* person who learns best by seeing things in print or diagrams? If you are, write down information that is hard or complex. If highlighting your notes or a textbook helps you remember, do so, but don't highlight facts you already know. One week before the test, reread your highlighted notes. One good method of study is to make up questions about your difficult topics (the authors know how useful *that* is . . .) and read up to get answers. Reword the question and answer and **write it down** to reinforce and make sure you understand. Only then should you go on to the next question.

Perhaps you are an *auditory* learner who is especially good at remembering information explained in a seminar or heard while listening to tapes. If you are one of these people, find someone—preferably a sonographer—and describe a difficult topic to them. An alternative suggestion is to make yourself a study tape based on what is important for you to learn, and listen to it in your car. The very act of making the tape is helpful in itself.

THE NIGHT BEFORE THE EXAM

- Don't cram. Memory retention is patchy and ineffective with this system (despite the number of tests you aced that way in school).
- Don't drink too much alcohol or caffeine or smoke too many cigarettes. You'll be sorry—the loss of oxygenated blood to your brain will be detrimental and will affect your performance. However, don't vary your routine too much if you are already dependent on these substances, especially caffeine. An intractable headache is too distracting while you are taking an exam.

THE DAY OF THE EXAM

- Eat breakfast, even if it's not part of your usual routine. Eat a lot of fruit for energy, and you might want to lighten up on the ham, biscuits, and gravy (there is no scheduled naptime).
- Again, pay attention to your caffeine intake—not so little you are feeling befuddled, but not so much that your hands are shaking. What is your body accustomed to?
- In the case of a 1 pm test, follow the same rules regarding lunch. It's not a good idea to consume massive quantities of water; fluid rebalancing is not in the game plan and you may, of necessity, waste critical exam time!

THE HOUR BEFORE THE EXAM

Remember to bring two forms of identification, one bearing your photograph, and your verification number. Don't take personal belongings, especially books—this is not the time to cram. ASI doesn't allow any food or drink in the test site. You must report to the test site a half an hour before your exam is scheduled; those arriving late will not be allowed to enter and will not get a refund. Within that half an hour you will register and go through a tutorial so that you understand the system.

EXAM-TAKING TECHNIQUES

- Relax, take a few breaths, and **don't panic.**
- **Don't leave any answers blank.** Even a guess is better. Mark items if you want to come back to a question during the computer exam.
- Read the questions carefully—are you to exclude the one **wrong answer** or find the one **right answer?** Look for words in the question stem (the sentence or two at the beginning of the question that prefaces the options) like "not" or "except."
- Eliminate wrong choices first; some will be obvious. Typically, you will be able to narrow it down to two choices. Pick the most logical one.
- Read the question for possible clues (e.g., fever, pain in a certain area, age of the patient). The ARDMS exam does not contain long-winded, confusing questions; everything in the stem is pertinent to the answer.
- Watch your time, but try not to worry about it the first time through. When you are finished, look at the remaining time, and go back only if you feel you really need to.
- **Never change** your answer **unless you know** you blew it—most often your first hunch was right.

AFTER THE EXAM IS DONE

When you are finished, your test scores will be printed out and handed to you on the spot. This is perhaps the best advantage computer testing has to offer—no suspense. The ARDMS will send you a final copy when you pass. Then celebrate! We no longer mind *what* you eat or drink.

PART I

Abdomen

CHAPTER 1

LIVER (16%–24%)

I. ANATOMY

A. Structure

1. The liver is the largest organ in the body, measuring approximately 13–15 cm in length and weighing approximately 1500 g in an adult. It lies beneath the diaphragm in the right upper quadrant.

2. The liver is composed of **biliary epithelial cells, hepatocytes,** and **Kupffer cells.**

3. With the exception of the **bare area** in the posterosuperior region, the liver is covered with a fibrous layer of connective tissue called **Glisson's capsule.**

B. Lobar arrangement (Figure 1–1)

– The liver is divided into three lobes: the **right, left,** and **caudate lobes.** The right and left lobes are separated by the middle hepatic vein and the **main lobar fissure,** which extends from the right portal vein to the neck of the gallbladder.

1. The **right lobe** is the largest lobe. It has anterior and posterior segments, which are separated by the **right hepatic vein. Riedel's lobe,** a normal variant that is more common in women, is an enlarged right lobe that may extend to the level of the iliac crest.

2. The **left lobe** usually lies in the epigastrium and left hypochondrium. It varies in size and shape, although it is always smaller than the right lobe. The left lobe is divided into medial (formerly known as the quadrate lobe) and lateral segments. The **ligamentum teres** (obliterated umbilical vein), **falciform ligament** (conducted the umbilical vein to the liver in the fetus), and **left hepatic vein** separate the two segments.

3. The **caudate lobe** is the smallest lobe. It is situated on the posterosuperior surface of the right lobe and is bordered by the inferior vena cava posteriorly. The caudate lobe is separated from the left lobe by the **ligamentum venosum,** which was the fetal ductus venosus. The caudate lobe has its own perfusion and drainage systems.

C. Vascular supply

– **The blood supply to the liver is derived from the hepatic artery and portal vein.**

– The **portal triad** includes the **hepatic artery, portal vein,** and **common bile duct.** This group of structures is surrounded by Glisson's capsule, which accounts for the echogenicity of this region.

1. The **hepatic artery,** a branch of the celiac axis, supplies 20%–30% of oxygenated blood.

2. The **portal vein** supplies the remaining 70%–80% of the blood. It supplies nutrients and other substances derived from the intestine.

   a. The portal veins have echogenic, well-defined borders and branch toward the diaphragm. Glisson's capsule gives the walls of the portal veins their echogenic appearance.

   b. The **main portal vein** is formed by the confluence of the **splenic** and **superior mesenteric veins.** It divides into right and left branches at the porta hepatis.

   c. The **right portal vein** has anterior and posterior branches that supply the segments of the right lobe.

   d. The **left portal vein** branch feeds the left lobe.

3. The hepatic and portal blood mix together in the **sinusoids,** capillaries that connect hepatic arterioles, hepatic venules, and terminal portal venules. The **hepatic venules** unite to form the hepatic veins.

4. Blood leaves the liver via the three **hepatic veins** (right, middle, and left). The hepatic

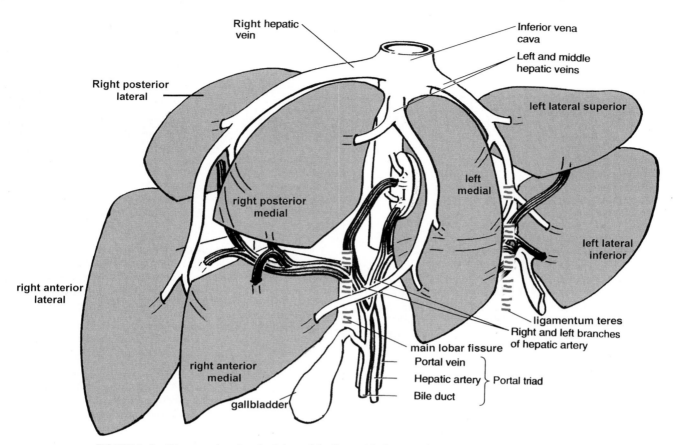

FIGURE 1-1   Diagram showing the lobes of the liver with the vascular structures that separate them.

veins drain toward the right atrium, increasing in diameter as they approach the diaphragm. They enter the inferior vena cava, which almost immediately drains into the right atrium of the heart. Hepatic veins do not have echogenic walls, and they branch toward the feet.

D. Functions
  – The liver has **excretory, metabolic, storage,** and **synthetic** functions.
  1. A single liver cell performs 500 different metabolic functions, including the formation of fats, carbohydrates, proteins, and bile.
  2. The liver secretes approximately 1–2 L of bile daily.
  3. The liver metabolizes fats (lipids) to produce cholesterol and ketones; amino acids are the by-products of proteins, and glucose is manufactured from the conversion of simple sugars that enter the liver. The liver converts glucose into glycogen.
  4. The liver detoxifies drugs and phagocytizes bacteria.

II. TECHNIQUE
  – Scanning is performed on full inspiration. Both sagittal and transverse views are obtained. A sagittal view of the liver for length is obtained at the midclavicular line. Other standard views include sagittal and transverse views through the gallbladder and porta hepatis and sagittal views of the inferior vena cava and aorta to include the liver.
  – In addition to demonstrating the common bile duct and the various vascular landmarks in the liver, it is important to document the parenchyma carefully to exclude small lesions. A texture comparison is made with the right kidney and, if possible, the pancreas.

III. LABORATORY VALUES

  A. **Aspartate aminotransferase (AST, formerly SGOT)** is an enzyme normally found in the liver, in the muscles, and in tissues with high metabolic rates; therefore, increases do not necessarily indicate liver disease.
    1. Liver abnormalities that cause an **increase** in AST levels include

– acute hepatitis.
– cirrhosis.
– hepatic necrosis.
– injury to the liver.
– metastases to the liver.
– fatty changes.
2. Significant causes of increased AST levels **not associated with the liver** include
– mononucleosis.
– myocardial infarction.

B. **Alanine aminotransferase (ALT, formerly SGPT)** is an enzyme produced in the hepatocytes; therefore, it is more specific to the liver than AST.
1. All forms of hepatitis show elevations in ALT.
2. Moderately increased levels of ALT occur in obstructive jaundice and hepatocellular disease.
3. Shock and drug toxicity can cause liver cell death and a subsequent rise in ALT levels.

C. **Alkaline phosphatase** is an enzyme produced in the liver, kidneys, bones, intestines, and placenta.
1. An **increase** in alkaline phosphatase with normal ALT and AST levels occurs in diseases of the bile duct, including
– bile duct obstruction.
– primary biliary cirrhosis.
– sclerosing cholangitis.
2. **Nonbiliary causes** of increased alkaline phosphatase levels include
– abscesses.
– liver carcinoma.
– cirrhosis.

D. **Lactate dehydrogenase (LDH)** is found in multiple organ systems. It is used primarily in the detection of myocardial and pulmonary infarction.
1. LDH increases mildly in
– hepatitis.
– cirrhosis.
– hepatic congestion.
– obstructive jaundice.
2. LDH increases moderately in infectious mononucleosis.

E. **Albumin** is a protein that is a component of blood. It is synthesized by the liver and is largely responsible for the maintenance of osmotic pressure in the blood. **Decreased** albumin levels are seen in liver dysfunction, malnutrition, and certain renal diseases.

F. **Prothrombin,** an enzyme produced in the liver, is a clotting factor that is affected by the level of vitamin K. Prothrombin time (PT) is a test administered before invasive proce-

dures to evaluate the patient's ability to withstand excessive bleeding.
1. A **prolonged PT** suggests compromised liver function and usually carries a poor prognosis; however, it can revert to normal when liver damage resolves. A prolonged PT with hepatocellular disease is seen in metastases to the liver and cirrhosis.
2. A **shortened PT** is seen in extrahepatic duct obstruction, gallbladder carcinoma, and cholecystitis.
3. Normal PT values vary from institution to institution, so it is more common to see PT given in terms of an **international normalized ratio (INR)** [see III G].

G. The **INR** is a ratio determined by dividing the patient's PT by a controlled standard.
1. A normal INR is obtained when the patient's PT is the same as the control (i.e., a ratio of 1).
2. An elevated INR could render a patient ineligible for an invasive procedure. For example, a ratio of 1.5 is often the cutoff point for a large-bore biopsy. However, a patient with a ratio up to 2.0 could still be considered for a skinny-needle procedure.

H. **γ-Globulins** are enzymes produced in the liver. Although γ-globulins are extremely sensitive indicators of liver dysfunction, elevation can be seen in almost any liver disease as well as in normal patients.

I. **Bilirubin** is bile pigment resulting from the breakdown of old red blood cells. It is formed by Kupffer cells and excreted by hepatocytes. **Serum bilirubin** is a protein that increases with any chronic inflammatory disease. It is reported by the laboratory as total, unconjugated, or conjugated.
1. **Total bilirubin** is a mixture of conjugated and unconjugated bilirubin. Elevation of total bilirubin is seen in chronic liver cell disease (e.g., cirrhosis).
2. **Unconjugated** or **indirect bilirubin** increases in isolated acute hepatocellular disease.
3. **Conjugated** or **direct bilirubin** increases in biliary duct obstruction.

IV. INDICATIONS

– Typical indications for scanning the liver include:
1. Suspected metastatic disease
2. Abnormal liver function tests
3. Evaluation of parenchymal liver disease (e.g., cirrhosis, hepatitis)
4. Evaluation of autosomal dominant polycystic disease
5. Jaundice
6. Portal hypertension

V. PARENCHYMAL DISEASE

A. **Fatty infiltration** is a benign, reversible disorder that occurs when fat is deposited in the liver, predominantly in the right lobe.

1. **Causes** include
   - alcoholic liver disease.
   - obesity.
   - pregnancy.
   - severe hepatitis.
   - starvation.
   - glycogen storage disease.
   - corticosteroid therapy.
   - diabetes mellitus.
   - massive tetracycline therapy.

2. **Clinical features** may include hepatomegaly and right upper quadrant discomfort; however, the patient is often asymptomatic.

3. **Laboratory values** in patients with fatty liver changes may be normal or may show an increase in AST, ALT, and conjugated bilirubin levels.

4. **Sonographic findings** vary depending on whether there is focal or diffuse infiltration. The following characteristics may appear only in the region of the liver that is affected.
   a. The liver is typically enlarged and echogenic (i.e., much more echogenic than the kidneys). The vessel borders cannot be seen.
   b. In severe cases, there is such poor penetration that the kidneys and diaphragm cannot be seen.
   c. In focal infiltration, much of the liver has increased echogenicity along with areas of normal liver tissue that are relatively echopenic and may be mistaken for localized masses. A typical location for one of these fat-spared areas is anterior to the right portal vein.

B. **Cirrhosis** is an irreversible disease that leads to the loss of normal liver function and structure with death of the hepatocytes. Fibrosis of the liver cells replaces the normal parenchyma. In the long term, liver failure and portal hypertension occur.

1. **Causes** include
   - alcohol abuse.
   - hepatitis B and C.
   - poor nutrition.
   - certain drugs.
   - biliary obstruction.
   - idiopathic factors.

2. **Clinical features** include
   - malaise.
   - weight loss.
   - abdominal pain with distention.
   - skin changes.
   - jaundice.
   - portal hypertension.
   - splenomegaly.
   - hypoalbuminemia.
   - edema.
   - ascites.

3. **Sonographic findings**
   a. In the early stages, the liver is usually enlarged by hepatitis.
   b. In later stages, fatty infiltration occurs.
   c. In the final regenerative stage, there is a small or normal-sized liver with a lobulated contour that is often outlined by secondary ascites. The liver texture shows increased echogenicity. There is inhomogeneous parenchyma and poor visualization of the vessels because of sound attenuation.
   d. Focal, less echogenic areas representing areas of regeneration are a common finding before the patient reaches end-stage cirrhosis.
   e. Portal hypertension develops as the disease becomes more severe.

C. **Portal hypertension** occurs when intrahepatic processes such as fibrosis or metastases lead to increased portal vein pressure, which has many secondary manifestations.

1. **Underlying mechanism**
   - Normal portal vein flow toward the liver is known as **hepatopetal** flow.
   - Reversed flow through the portal vein is known as **hepatofugal** flow.
   a. Pressure increases in the portal vein if it is narrowed by a thrombus or is compressed (e.g., by fibrotic changes in the liver that occur with cirrhosis).
   b. Additional venous pathways develop to bypass the narrowed area and are known as collaterals or varices. For example, the umbilical vein in the ligamentum teres may reopen (i.e., recanalized paraumbilical veins). If the portal vein is thrombosed, collaterals develop in the porta hepatis (i.e., cavernous transformation).
   c. As pressure increases, portal vein blood flow decreases, impairing liver function.
   d. Decreased albumin production results in less osmotic pressure in the arteries and veins, and ascites forms.
   e. Liver resistance increases until it is greater than the portal vein blood pressure. Blood flow reverses and moves backward through the portal vein (i.e., hepatofugal flow).
   - Note: hepatofugal flow occurs naturally in the hepatic veins.
   f. Splenomegaly occurs as the spleen

takes over some of the functions of the liver and becomes engorged with blood.

2. Causes include
- cirrhosis.
- portal vein thrombosis.
- hepatocellular disease.
- Budd-Chiari syndrome.
- metastases.
- trauma (rare).

3. Sonographic findings

  a. The portal vein is usually enlarged. An enlarged portal vein with hepatofugal flow and collaterals leads to gastrointestinal bleeding, splenomegaly, and ascites. Portal vein thrombosis is also a common complication.

  b. Collaterals (or varices) may be visible
- around the gastroesophageal junction (i.e., around the fundus of the stomach).
- in the bed of the pancreas.
- in the porta hepatis.
- in the hilum of the spleen (splenorenal).
- in a recanalized ligamentum teres (paraumbilical vein).
- in the porta hepatis. If the portal vein is thrombosed, multiple collaterals form with the development of **cavernous transformation.**

D. Hepatitis is an inflammation of the liver. It can be a self-limiting process, as in **acute viral hepatitis,** or it can lead to **cirrhosis** and **liver failure.** If the condition has been present for at least 3–6 months, it is called **chronic hepatitis.**

1. Causes include
- intravenous drugs.
- alcohol.
- viruses (e.g., hepatitis A, B, C, D, E, and G are all caused by viruses).

  a. Hepatitis A is transmitted through infected food or water.

  b. Hepatitis B is conveyed by blood, body fluids, and mother-to-infant transmission; it is seen in intravenous drug abusers and health care workers.

  c. Hepatitis C (formerly known as non-A, non-B hepatitis) is transmitted by blood transfusions or sexual contact.

2. Clinical features include
- fatigue.
- dark urine.
- light-colored stool.
- nausea.
- fever.
- skin rashes.
- jaundice.
- hepatosplenomegaly.

3. Laboratory values include
- increased ALT.
- increased AST.
- increased conjugated and unconjugated bilirubin.
- increased PT.

4. Sonographic findings are subtle and are primarily seen in cases of acute hepatitis. Possible findings include
- an apparent increase in the portal vein echogenicity caused by a decrease in liver echogenicity (i.e., the "starry night" appearance).
- thickening of the gallbladder wall.
- hepatosplenomegaly.

E. Budd-Chiari syndrome
- Occlusion of the hepatic veins with or without occlusion of the inferior vena cava leads to liver failure.

1. Causes include
- polycythemia rubra vera.
- chronic leukemia.
- paroxysmal nocturnal hemoglobinuria.
- trauma.
- pregnancy.
- congenital membranes.
- oral contraceptive use.

2. Clinical features include
- ascites (always seen).
- hepatomegaly.
- right upper quadrant pain.

3. Sonographic findings

  a. Ascites and hepatosplenomegaly may be seen.

  b. Infarcted liver areas become fibrotic and echogenic.

  c. The caudate lobe is often spared because it has a separate blood supply and venous drainage.

  d. Color flow Doppler of the hepatic veins will show apparent absence of veins, intravenous thrombi, intrahepatic collaterals, and variable vein size.

VI. MASSES

A. Benign masses

1. Cavernous hemangiomas are the most common benign liver tumor. These vascular lesions are seen more frequently in women.

  a. Clinical features
- Cavernous hemangiomas are usually asymptomatic.

  b. Sonographic findings

    (1) Cavernous hemangiomas usually occur in the right lobe.

    (2) There is typically a small echogenic lesion that may display posterior enhancement. The hyperechoic appearance is caused by the numerous interfaces of the vessel walls.

(3) There are usually well-defined borders with a slightly less echogenic center.

(4) Larger hemangiomas may have a coarser pattern.

2. **Adenomas** are benign epithelial liver tumors seen more frequently in women. Adenomas are often surgically removed because they occasionally progress to hepatocellular carcinoma.

   a. Causes
   - Adenomas are linked to the use of oral contraceptives.

   b. Clinical features

(1) Although adenomas are asymptomatic, they can sometimes be palpated.

(2) The lesion may bleed or rupture, causing pain.

   c. Sonographic findings are nonspecific. The mass can be hypoechoic or hyperechoic.

3. **Focal nodular hyperplasia** is a rare, benign tumor.

   a. Clinical features
   - Focal nodular hyperplasia is asymptomatic.

   b. Sonographic findings

(1) The tumor may be hypoechoic or hyperechoic.

(2) The tumor has a well-defined border and a central scar.

B. Malignant masses

1. **Hepatocellular carcinoma (hepatoma)** is more common in men.

   a. Causes

(1) Hepatocellular carcinoma is common in the Far East, Greece, and southern Africa because of the prevalence of chronic hepatitis B infection and exposure to aflatoxin, a fungus found in certain foods.

(2) In the United States, hepatocellular carcinoma is usually associated with macronodular liver **cirrhosis** (80%) and alcoholism.

   b. Clinical features include
   - right upper quadrant pain.
   - weight loss.
   - abdominal swelling (if ascites is present).
   - fatigue.

   c. Sonographic findings

(1) Either solitary or multiple nodules or diffuse infiltration may be seen.

(2) Hepatocellular carcinoma can be echogenic or complex in appearance.

(3) Hepatocellular carcinoma may invade the portal vein and mimic a portal vein thrombosis.

2. **Hepatoblastoma** is a rare malignant liver tumor. However, it is the most common liver mass in infants.

   a. Clinical features include
   - a palpable mass.
   - hepatomegaly.

   b. Laboratory values
   - α-Fetoprotein levels are increased.

   c. Sonographic findings include
   - a highly vascular, solitary mass.
   - calcifications (not always present).

3. **Metastases** are very common in the liver.

   a. Primary sites include the
   - gastrointestinal tract.
   - lungs.
   - pancreas.
   - breasts.

   b. Clinical features include
   - abnormal liver function tests.
   - weight loss.
   - abdominal distention.
   - jaundice.
   - hepatomegaly.
   - ascites.

   c. Sonographic findings include
   - hypoechoic masses (from lymphoma, breast, lung).
   - echogenic masses (kidneys, pancreas).
   - calcified masses (colon, pancreas, stomach, neuroblastoma).
   - masses with a "bull's eye" or "target" appearance (i.e., an echogenic center surrounded by a hypoechoic halo) [colon, lung].

VII. CYSTS

   - in the liver may be congenital or acquired.

A. Clinical features
   - Patients with cysts are asymptomatic.

B. Laboratory values
   - will be normal in the presence of liver cysts with no underlying liver or biliary disease.
   - Very severe dominant polycystic kidney disease involving the liver may cause elevated liver function tests.

C. Sonographic findings

1. Liver cysts may be single or multiple, and unusual shapes are common.

2. Aside from shape, liver cysts have the same features as cysts elsewhere in the body (i.e., smooth walls, anechoic con-

tents, and good through transmission and posterior enhancement).

3. Overall liver echogenicity may be increased if polycystic liver disease is present. Multiple tiny cysts that cannot be resolved as cysts are seen as echoes.

VIII. ABSCESSES

A. **Hydatid (echinococcal) cysts** are usually related to tapeworms in dogs. They are seen more frequently in sheep- and cattle-raising areas.
   1. **Clinical features** include
      - pain.
      - fever.
      - jaundice.
      - anaphylactic shock (if cyst ruptures).
   2. **Laboratory values** include
      - a slight rise in alkaline phosphatase (can be a biochemical marker).
      - an increased white blood cell count.
   3. **Sonographic findings**
      a. Hydatid cysts usually involve the right lobe.
      b. Although the cyst may appear to be simple, a cyst within a cyst is often seen (i.e., the **daughter cyst** or "water lily" sign from the collapse of the germinal layer with a resultant membrane within the cyst).
      c. The cyst may have a mass-like appearance with internal echoes or it may become calcified as it ages.

B. **Pyogenic abscesses** may be secondary to diverticulitis, appendicitis, cholecystitis, or surgery. Aerobic and anaerobic organisms (e.g., *Escherichia coli, Staphylococcus* species) are found in the abscess.
   1. **Clinical features** indicating the need for a sonogram include
      - fever and malaise.
      - an elevated white blood cell count.
      - elevated alkaline phosphatase levels.
      - right upper quadrant pain.
      - chills.
      - a palpable mass.
   2. **Sonographic findings** include
      - a complex fluid collection with good through transmission.
      - an irregular, thick wall.

C. **Amebic abscesses** occur more frequently in tropical regions.
   1. **Causes** include
      - the protozoa *Entamoeba.*
      - poor sanitary conditions.
   2. **Clinical features** include
      - diarrhea.
      - abdominal discomfort.
      - elevated liver function tests.
   3. **Sonographic findings** include
      - a round, hypoechoic or hyperechoic mass when compared to the liver.

D. **Fungal abscesses** occur most often in immunocompromised patients.
   1. **Causes**
      - Fungal abscesses are usually caused by the fungus *Candida albicans.*
   2. **Sonographic findings**
      a. Small lesions with echogenic centers are typically seen.
      b. A hypoechoic center is seen in the early stages.
      c. Echogenic or calcified centers may be present in the healing stages.

E. ***Pneumocystis carinii*** is seen in AIDS patients. Lesions appear as multiple, small, nonshadowing, echogenic foci. In more severe cases, the lesions may become large calcified areas.

F. ***Schistosomiasis*** is a parasitic infection predominantly seen in the Middle East that affects the porta hepatis. It causes periportal fibrosis and echogenicity. Portal vein thrombosis may be a complication.

IX. HEMATOMAS

   - are blood collections in or around the liver.

A. **Indications** include
   - blunt or penetrating trauma.
   - postoperative hematocrit drop.

B. **Sonographic findings**
   1. **Intrahepatic hematomas** may be hyperechoic or hypoechoic, depending on the time since the injury. They have an irregular shape and may be difficult to distinguish from liver tissue.
   2. **Subscapular hematomas** are curvilinear in appearance and displace the liver centrally or inferiorly. The contents may be hypoechoic or echogenic, depending on age.

CHAPTER 2

BILIARY TREE (10%-18%)

I. ANATOMY (Figure 2–1)

  A. The gallbladder
- is a pear-shaped sac that is approximately 7–10 cm in length and 3–4 cm in transverse diameter with a wall less than 3 mm thick (when normal).
- may be extrahepatic or intrahepatic and is usually located on the inferoposterior surface of the liver.
- The regions of the gallbladder consist of the neck, body, and fundus.
- **Rokitansky-Aschoff sinuses** are multiple folds along the inner border of the gallbladder that are coated with epithelial mucosa.
- Blood supply to the gallbladder is from the cystic artery, a branch of the right hepatic artery.

  B. Bile ducts
1. The **common hepatic duct** is formed by the union of the right and left hepatic ducts near the porta hepatis.
2. The **common bile duct** is formed in the porta hepatis by the union of the common hepatic duct and the cystic duct.
3. The common bile duct, an extrahepatic duct, joins the **duct of Wirsung** (pancreatic duct) in the pancreas at the **ampulla of Vater,** the opening where the common bile duct and pancreatic duct enter the duodenum.
4. The **cystic duct** arises from the superior aspect of the neck of the gallbladder and contains the spiral valves of Heister.
5. The peripheral branches of the biliary system are known as biliary radicles.

  C. Bile
- is a waste product formed by the hepatic parenchymal cells and released into the biliary tree.
- is composed of water, bile salts, cholesterol, and bilirubin.
- is alkaline, unlike the contents of the stomach.
1. The gallbladder stores and concentrates approximately 30–60 ml of bile in a fasting state.
2. Bile is transported to the duodenum to aid in digestion.
   - **a.** When bile is needed, the duodenum releases an enzyme called **cholecystokinin,** which travels via the bloodstream to the gallbladder.
   - **b.** Cholecystokinin stimulates the gallbladder to contract, sending bile through the common bile duct to the duodenum.
3. The **sphincter of Oddi** controls bile and pancreatic juice flow.
   - **a.** With gallbladder removal, the sphincter of Oddi loses tone and the pressure in the common bile duct lowers to equal intra-abdominal pressure.
   - **b.** Bile flows into the duodenum during fasting and nonfasting states because it is no longer held in the gallbladder.
   - **c.** Some bile can also remain in the ducts.

  D. Normal anatomical variants
1. A **junctional fold** normally located close to the gallbladder neck can look similar to a septation.
2. A **phrygian cap** occurs when the junctional fold is found at the fundus of the gallbladder.
3. The segment between the cystic duct and the junctional fold is called **Hartmann's pouch.**
4. **Pneumobilia** is air in the biliary system that can be caused by a surgical anastomosis between the bowel and biliary tree, sphincterotomy, or gallstone ileus.
   - **a.** Patients with pneumobilia are asymptomatic.
   - **b.** Sonographic findings include multiple,

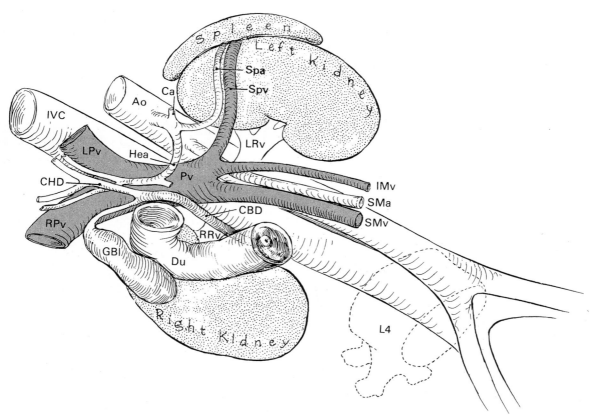

FIGURE 2–1 An oblique view showing the relationship of the portal vein (*Pv*), inferior vena cava (*IVC*), and aorta (*Ao*) to the kidneys and gallbladder (*GBl*). The major branches of the portal vein, hepatic artery (*Hea*), and common hepatic duct (*CHD*) in relationship to the porta hepatis are shown. *Ca* = celiac artery; *CBD* = common bile duct; *Du* = duodenum; *IMv* = inferior mesenteric vein; *LPv* = left portal vein; *LRv* = left renal vein; *RPv* = right portal vein; *RRv* = right renal vein; *SMa* = superior mesenteric artery; *SMv* = superior mesenteric vein; *Spa* = splenic artery; *Spv* = splenic vein. (Reprinted with permission from Sanders RC: *Clinical Sonography: A Practical Guide*, 3rd ed. Philadelphia, Lippincott, 1998, p 209.)

linear, echogenic foci with weak acoustic shadowing and ring down artifact caused by the gas in the biliary tree.

II. TECHNIQUE

A. Gallbladder

1. The gallbladder is best scanned with the patient in a fasting state to ensure an adequate size because the normal gallbladder contracts after eating.
2. The gallbladder should be scanned in at least two positions. Scanning with the patient supine on deep inspiration is complemented with oblique, left lateral decubitus, and possibly upright and semiprone patient positions. Wall thickness is measured on the anterior surface with the transducer perpendicular to the wall.
3. Average-sized adults are usually scanned with a 3.5 MHz transducer. A 5.0 MHz transducer is used for better resolution and to verify the presence or absence of stones.

B. Bile ducts

1. An oblique right axis view is required to see the common bile duct.
2. The distal common bile duct in the head of the pancreas is examined at an axis parallel to the inferior vena cava.
3. On transverse view, the common bile duct is seen on the posterolateral margin of the pancreatic head, adjacent to the duodenum.
4. The hepatic artery can be confused for a dilated duct, so examination with color flow helps to exclude a dilated hepatic artery masquerading as a dilated bile duct.

III. LABORATORY VALUES

– The biochemical markers used in gallbladder and biliary diseases are the same as those used to determine liver problems (see Chapter 1, III and Appendix A).

A. The standard test for hyperbilirubinemia is **serum bilirubin.**

B. **Unconjugated (indirect) bilirubin** is elevated in hepatocellular disease and hemolytic anemia because the hepatocytes are unable to conjugate bilirubin.

C. **Conjugated (direct) bilirubin** is elevated in extrahepatic obstruction.

D. **Alanine aminotransferase, aspartate aminotransferase,** and **lactate dehydrogenase** levels increase in biliary obstruction.

E. Elevated **serum alkaline phosphatase** is an early indication of biliary obstruction.

IV. INDICATIONS

A. **Gallbladder disease** is indicated by
   – acute or chronic right upper quadrant pain.
   – fatty food intolerance.

B. Common indications for scanning the **bile ducts** include
   – jaundice.
   – abnormal liver function tests (if the ducts are blocked in one lobe).
   – unexplained acute pancreatitis.

V. DILATION

A. **Types of jaundice**
   – Jaundice is yellowing of the skin and eyes from excessive bilirubin. It can be classified as prehepatic (hemolytic), hepatic, or obstructive.
   1. **Hemolytic** jaundice results from the breakdown of red blood cells with a consequent increase in bilirubin. This condition is treated medically.
   2. **Hepatic** jaundice relates to defective liver function (e.g., severe cirrhosis, hepatitis). It is treated medically.
   3. **Obstructive** jaundice results from obstruction of the bile ducts. It is treated with surgery or percutaneous drainage.

B. **Causes of bile duct obstruction**
   1. **Choledochal cysts**
      – are usually congenital, focal dilations of the common bile duct.
      – are more common in children and women.
      a. **Clinical features** include
         – intermittent jaundice.
         – a palpable right upper quadrant mass.
         – colicky pain.
      b. **Sonographic findings** include
         – a cyst in the porta hepatis separate from the gallbladder.
         – a dilated common bile duct entering the cyst.

   2. **Biliary atresia**
      – is a rare obstructive disease seen in infants.
      a. **Causes**
         – Biliary atresia is thought to result from a viral infection after birth.
      b. **Clinical features** include
         – jaundice.
         – cirrhosis.
         – portal hypertension.
      c. **Sonographic findings**
         – To a varying extent, the distal bile ducts and gallbladder are atretic.
      d. **Treatment**
         – Biliary atresia is fatal if not treated by performing a liver transplant or a Kasai procedure in which a segment of bowel is anastomosed to an exposed area of the liver.

   3. **Hydrops of the gallbladder**
      a. **Causes** include
         – a traumatic event (e.g., recent surgery, myocardial infarction).
         – an infection (e.g., Kawasaki's disease).
         – biliary obstruction.
      b. **Sonographic findings** include
         – a massively enlarged gallbladder (i.e., at least 4 cm by 12 cm).
         – a locally tender gallbladder.

   4. **Caroli's disease**
      – is a congenital anomaly.
      a. **Clinical features,** if the disease is extensive, can include
         – abscesses.
         – intrahepatic biliary obstruction.
         – cholangitis.
         – stones.
      b. **Sonographic findings** include
         – focal saccular dilation of the intrahepatic ducts.

   5. **Sclerosing cholangitis**
      – is a chronic inflammatory process.
      – is associated with ulcerative colitis (25%).
      a. **Clinical features** include
         – pain.
         – fever.
      b. **Laboratory values** include
         – an elevated white blood cell count.
      c. **Sonographic findings** include
         – narrowed bile ducts.
         – bile ducts with thick, scarred walls.

   6. **Biliary calculi**
      – form in the gallbladder but can be located in the hepatic ducts.
      – can cause obstruction at any level.
      – are typically located in the common hepatic duct and distal common bile duct at the sphincter of Oddi.

   7. **AIDS cholangitis**

– Smooth or irregular thickening of the bile duct walls occurs.

8. **Masses** (see VI)

C. Clinical features of obstruction

1. **Jaundice** with itching is the principle symptom.
2. Pain in the right upper quadrant may be present; however, some jaundice presents without pain.
3. The patient will have clay-colored stools.
4. If obstruction is limited to the left or right duct, clinical features will include
   – pain.
   – nausea.
   – abnormal liver function tests, but not an elevated bilirubin.

D. Sonographic findings of obstruction

1. With obstruction, paired tubular structures (i.e., the bile ducts and portal veins) are seen throughout the liver (the "parallel channel" sign).
   – Bile ducts typically run anterior to portal veins.
   – Bile ducts branch more, have more irregular borders, and better through transmission than portal veins.
2. Obstruction is most easily detected in the common bile duct as it runs anterior to the crossing hepatic arteries and the portal vein, provided the obstruction is distal to the common bile duct.
3. The common bile duct is considered dilated if it is larger than 6–8 mm in an adult. Duct size increases by approximately 1 mm per decade; therefore, a 6-mm duct in a 35 year old is dilated whereas it is normal in a 70 year old.
4. After cholecystectomy, the common bile duct may remain enlarged even though it is not obstructed. A provocative test (i.e., giving fat by mouth) will cause an obstructed duct to dilate, whereas an unobstructed duct will stay the same size or decrease in width.

VI. MASSES

A. Klatskin's tumor

– is an uncommon carcinoma of the bile duct that originates at the junction of the right and left hepatic ducts.
– is small at the time of presentation and metastasizes late.
– has a poor prognosis.

1. **Clinical features** include
   – slowly worsening jaundice.
2. **Sonographic findings** include
   – no common bile duct dilation.
   – dilation of the peripheral ducts.

– Note: the tumor is small and difficult to see.

B. Pancreatic cancer

1. **Pancreatic cancer** is indicated by a mass in the head of the pancreas that obstructs the common bile and pancreatic ducts. The patient may present with a palpable gallbladder and painless jaundice (i.e., **Courvoisier's sign**).
2. An **ampulla of Vater tumor** is indicated by dilation of the common bile and pancreatic ducts with no obvious stones or masses.

C. Gallbladder polyps

– are small, benign growths arising from the gallbladder wall.
– may be inflammatory, adenomatous, or composed of cholesterol.

1. **Clinical features**
   – Polyps are usually asymptomatic and discovered serendipitously.
2. **Sonographic findings** include
   – an immobile, small, intraluminal mass.

D. Adenomyomatosis

– is a benign, hyperplastic change in the wall of the gallbladder.

1. **Pathologic findings** include
   – thickening of the mucosa.
   – cholesterol crystal deposits in the Rokitansky-Aschoff sinuses.
2. **Sonographic findings** include
   – bright reflections with **comet tail artifacts** from the gallbladder wall.
   – multiple septations.
   – cholesterolosis (i.e., strawberry gallbladder) [the gallbladder is filled with cholesterol polyps].

E. Gallbladder cancer

– is uncommon.

1. The cause of gallbladder cancer is unknown. **Associations** include
   – gallstones.
   – a porcelain gallbladder.
2. **Sonographic findings** include
   – focal gallbladder wall thickening.
   – a mass in the gallbladder.
   – gallstones (usually present).
   – metastasis to the liver and lymph nodes.

F. Metastasis

– **Malignant melanoma** is the most common tumor to metastasize to the gallbladder.

VII. CHOLELITHIASIS

A. Sludge

– Sludge consists of bile crystals. Stasis of bile induces the formation of bile crystals (sludge), which consist of calcium bilirubinate and cholesterol crystals.

1. **Causes** include
   – fasting.
   – hyperalimentation and total parenteral nutrition.
   – extrahepatic biliary obstruction.
   – hepatocellular disease.
2. **Clinical features**
   – The condition is asymptomatic, but is a precursor to gallstone formation.
3. **Sonographic findings**
   a. A homogeneous, nonshadowing, dependent group of echoes is seen that moves very slowly if the patient's position is changed.
   b. Tumefactive sludge (i.e., a sludge ball) may not layer in the gallbladder. It may look similar to a mass; however, it does not shadow and may roll with a change in the patient's position.

B. **Cholelithiasis (gallstones)**
   – is a common disease of the gallbladder.
   – is more frequently seen in middle-aged, obese women (remember: **fat, fertile, fair, 40-year-old female**).
   – When stones form in the ducts or pass into the ducts from the gallbladder the condition is called **choledocholithiasis.**
1. **Types of calculi**
   a. **Cholesterol** gallstones are the most common type of calculi in the United States.
   b. **Pigment** gallstones are seen in patients with hemolytic anemia and are caused by excess destruction of red blood cells.
   c. **Mixed** gallstones consisting of cholesterol and pigment may be seen.
2. **Causes** include
   – bile stasis with increased concentration of bile.
   – gallbladder inflammation.
   – metabolic factors (e.g., obesity, diabetes, pregnancy, pancreatitis, hypercholesterolemia, hyperlipidemia, hemolytic anemia).
3. **Clinical features** of gallbladder pathology include
   – midepigastric or right upper quadrant pain.
   – nausea and vomiting.
   – fatty food intolerance.
   – fever.
   – focal tenderness over the gallbladder on full inspiration (i.e., Murphy's sign).
4. **Sonographic findings**
   a. An echogenic, mobile mass with posterior shadowing may be seen.
   b. When the gallbladder is packed with stones and no bile is present, the **WES sign** (**w**all, **e**cho of stone, **s**hadowing) is seen.

c. Small stones may not shadow unless very high-frequency transducers are used.
d. Floating and adherent stones are unusual variants.

VIII. CHOLECYSTITIS

A. **Acute cholecystitis**
   – is inflammation of the gallbladder secondary to an obstruction of the cystic duct.
   – is seen more frequently in women.
1. **Causes** include
   – gallstones.
   – acalculous cholecystitis.
2. **Clinical features** include
   – acute, intermittent pain.
   – local tenderness over the gallbladder (i.e., positive Murphy's sign).
   – fever.
   – fatty food intolerance.
3. **Laboratory values** include
   – leukocytosis.
   – elevated serum amylase.
4. **Sonographic findings** can include
   – gallstones with local tenderness over the gallbladder (i.e., sonographic Murphy's sign).
   – wall thickening (i.e., 3 mm or greater).
   – perforation of the gallbladder.
   – a pericholecystic pus collection.

B. **Emphysematous cholecystitis**
   – is a rare variant of cholecystitis.
   – is more common in men.
   – occurs when gas develops in the gallbladder wall.
   – Approximately one third of these patients have diabetes.
1. **Clinical features** include
   – acute right upper quadrant pain.
   – fever.
2. **Sonographic findings**
   – A ring down artifact from the gas in the wall obscures the gallbladder contents.

C. **Chronic cholecystitis**
   – is a result of recurrent acute cholecystitis.
1. **Causes** include
   – gallstones.
2. **Clinical features** include
   – intermittent right upper quadrant pain.
3. **Sonographic findings** include
   – a thick, fibrotic gallbladder wall.
   – a small gallbladder.
   – gallstones.

D. **Acalculous cholecystitis**
1. **Causes** include
   – trauma.
   – surgery.
   – burns.

– sepsis.
– dehydration.
– total parenteral nutrition.
– Crohn's disease.
– shock.

2. **Sonographic findings** include
– a thickened gallbladder wall.
– a locally tender gallbladder (sonographic Murphy's sign).
– absence of gallstones.

E. **Porcelain gallbladder**
– is a rare condition that results in an increased risk of carcinoma.
1. **Causes** are unknown.
2. **Sonographic findings**
a. There is fibrosis and calcification of the wall of a nonfunctioning gallbladder.
b. The calcification and consequent shadowing makes porcelain gallbladders difficult to examine.

F. **Mirizzi's syndrome**
– is a rare complication of acute cholecystitis.
– A stone impacted in the cystic duct or neck of the gallbladder inflames the surrounding structures, including the common hepatic duct, causing biliary obstruction above the level of the common bile duct.
– **Sonographic findings**
1. There will be dilated bile ducts and a dilated gallbladder with a normal common bile duct.
2. A stone will be seen in the common bile duct area.
3. The cystic duct may be visibly dilated.

CHAPTER 3

PANCREAS (6%–14%)

I. ANATOMY (Figure 3–1)

- The pancreas lies in the retroperitoneum, located obliquely between the **duodenal C-loop** and **splenic hilum.**
- It is approximately 12–15 cm in length.
- The pancreas is a pinkish yellow gland that is unencapsulated.

A. Subdivisions
- The pancreas is divided into the **head, uncinate process, neck, body,** and **tail.**
  1. The **head** has an anteroposterior diameter of 2–3 cm.
     a. The head is partially encircled by the duodenal C-loop and lies inferior and to the right of the body and tail.
     b. The head is anterior to the **inferior vena cava** and caudal to the portal vein.
     c. The **common bile duct** runs through or lateral to the right posterior aspect of the head.
     d. The **gastroduodenal artery,** a branch of the common hepatic artery, is in the anterior aspect of the head.
  2. The **uncinate process** is a medial and posterior extension of the head. It lies between the superior mesenteric vein and the inferior vena cava.
  3. The **neck** has an anteroposterior diameter of 1–2 cm.
     a. The neck lies between the head and body and is anterior to the **superior mesenteric vein.**
     b. The **portal confluence,** formed by the union of the splenic vein and superior mesenteric vein, is posterior to the neck.
  4. The **body** is the largest area of the pancreas.
     a. The body is the most anterior aspect of the pancreas.
     b. The body is located anterior to the **splenic vein** and the superior mesenteric artery.
     c. The **splenic artery** lies just superior to the body.
  5. The **tail** lies anterior to the upper pole of the left kidney and cephalad to the body of the pancreas.

B. Pancreatic ducts
  1. The **duct of Wirsung** is the main pancreatic duct.
  2. The **duct of Santorini** is an accessory pancreatic duct.

C. Blood supply
  1. Arterial blood supply to the head of the pancreas is derived from branches of the **gastroduodenal artery.**
  2. The **splenic artery** and **superior mesenteric artery** supply blood to the body and tail of the pancreas.
  3. The splenic, superior mesenteric, inferior mesenteric, and portal veins drain the pancreas.

D. Functions
  1. **Exocrine system (acinar cells)**
     a. Acinar cells in the pancreas produce digestive enzymes in pancreatic juice.
     b. The enzymes produced by the pancreas include
        - **amylase** for the digestion of starch (carbohydrates).
        - **lipase** for the digestion of lipids.
        - **peptidases** (e.g., **trypsin, chymotrypsin, carboxypolypeptidase, ribonuclease,** and **dioxyribonuclease**) for protein digestion.
        - **sodium bicarbonate** to neutralize gastric acid.
  2. **Endocrine system (islet cells)**
     a. **Glucagon** and **insulin** are secreted by the **islets of Langerhans.**
     b. Failure to adequately produce insulin results in diabetes mellitus.

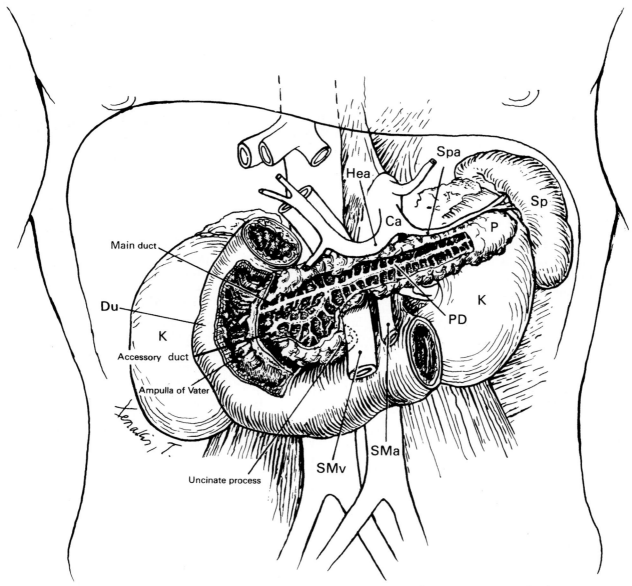

FIGURE 3-1 Diagram showing the relationship of the pancreas (*P*) to the celiac artery (*Ca*), duodenum (*Du*), kidneys (*K*), and spleen (*Sp*). Note that the pancreatic duct (*PD*) runs through the center of the pancreas to the papilla (ampulla) of Vater. The splenic artery (*Spa*) lies superior to the pancreas. *Hea* = hepatic artery; *SMa* = superior mesenteric artery; *SMv* = superior mesenteric vein. (Adapted with permission from Sanders RC: *Clinical Sonography: A Practical Guide,* 3rd ed. Philadelphia, Lippincott, 1998, p 220.)

II. TECHNIQUE

A. Examination of the patient in a **fasting state** is desirable to see the relationship to the gallbladder.

B. Obtain oblique transverse views through the head, body, and tail.

C. Obtain the standard sagittal views through the head, through the body, and along the axis of the inferior vena cava and aorta. Obtain a sagittal view of the tail, if possible.

D. If the pancreas is obscured by gas, filling the stomach with water or sitting the patient up may help show the pancreas. This approach is particularly useful when viewing the tail.

E. Turning the patient on his side and using the left kidney as an acoustic window can also demonstrate the tail.

III. LABORATORY VALUES

A. Serum amylase

– increases within the first 24 hours in acute pancreatitis and then slowly reverts to normal.

– increases in chronic pancreatitis, obstruction of the pancreatic duct, perforation of a peptic ulcer, and acute cholecystitis.

B. Urine amylase
– increases in pancreatitis.

C. Lipase
– increases in pancreatitis, pancreatic duct obstruction, carcinoma of the pancreas, cirrhosis, and acute cholecystitis.

IV. INDICATIONS

– Typical indications for scanning the pancreas include:

A. Evaluation of acute or chronic pancreatitis

B. Suspected pancreatic tumor (e.g., Courvoisier's sign)

C. Possible endocrine tumor (e.g., islet cell tumor)

V. PARENCHYMAL DISEASE (PANCREATITIS)

A. Acute pancreatitis
– is an inflammation of the pancreas that results in edema of the pancreas and release of pancreatic enzymes into pancreatic tissue.
1. **Causes** include
   – alcoholic damage to the acinar cells.
   – gallstones obstructing the pancreatic duct.
   – obstruction at the ampulla.
   – trauma.
   – viral infection.
   – drugs (e.g., steroids).
2. **Clinical features** include
   – sudden onset of pain that can radiate to the back.
   – paralytic ileus.
   – a rigid abdomen.
   – nausea and vomiting.
   – fever.
   – elevated pancreatic enzymes.
   – decreased hematocrit (if hemorrhagic).
   – increased white blood cell count.
3. **Sonographic findings** include
   – an edematous and enlarged gland.
   – an isoechoic or hypoechoic texture (compared to the liver).
   – possible fluid collections surrounding the pancreas.
   – possible ascites.
4. **Complications**
   a. Phlegmon is a serious and sometimes fatal complication of acute pancreatitis. Inflammation spreads across fascial pathways and creates a hemorrhagic, edematous mass.
   b. Other complications of acute pancreatitis include
   – pseudocysts.
   – chronic pancreatitis.
   – hemorrhagic necrosis.
   – biliary obstruction.
   – pulmonary edema.

B. Chronic pancreatitis
– is a progressive, irreversible process seen more frequently in men.
– leads to fibrous scarring and is associated with an increased risk of cancer.
1. **Causes** of repeated episodes of acute pancreatitis include
   – alcoholism.
   – trauma.
   – chronic gallbladder disease.
2. **Clinical features** include
   – severe abdominal pain.
   – diabetes mellitus (if the pancreatic cells are severely damaged).
   – weight loss.
   – normal laboratory values or mild increases in amylase and lipase levels.
3. **Sonographic findings** can include
   – a shrunken pancreas with an irregular contour.
   – pseudocysts.
   – an echogenic texture with diffuse calcifications.
   – Multiple calcifications may develop along the course of a dilated pancreatic duct.
   – Pancreatic duct dilation is seen when a stricture is present or when there is a stone in the duct.
4. **Complications** include
   – pseudocysts.
   – dilation of the common bile duct.
   – portal vein thrombosis.

C. Cystic fibrosis
– involves the pancreas.
– There is an increase in echogenicity of the gland secondary to fatty infiltration and fibrotic atrophy.

VI. MASSES

A. Endocrine tumors
– develop from **islet cells** and usually have a good prognosis.
– are more common in the tail and body.
– are benign, but may become malignant (rare). Malignant endocrine tumors are indistinguishable from benign tumors.
1. **Insulinomas** are the most common endocrine tumor. They secrete insulin and present as small, hypoechoic, solid areas that are difficult to visualize.

2. **Gastrinomas** cause the **Zollinger-Ellison syndrome** and are associated with diarrhea and **peptic ulcer disease.** These tumors are also very small.

B. **Adenocarcinoma**
   – is almost always fatal.
   – is the most common type of cancer of the pancreas.
   1. **Clinical features** are seldom noticed until the disease is already too far advanced to treat and include
      – loss of appetite.
      – loss of weight.
      – jaundice.
      – upper abdominal pain.
   2. **Sonographic findings**
      a. Tumors are poorly defined, hypoechoic masses.
      b. Invasion of the neighboring vessels can occur; assess carefully for this because vessel involvement renders the tumor inoperable.
      c. Metastases to the lymph nodes, liver, lungs, bone, duodenum, peritoneum, and adrenal glands may occur.
   3. **Complications** include
      – biliary duct dilation.
      – obstruction of the pancreatic duct.
      – secondary pancreatitis.

C. **Metastases** to the pancreas
   – are uncommon.
   – come from primaries such as melanoma, breast cancer, and lung cancer.

D. **Lymphoma**
   – can infiltrate the pancreas focally or diffusely.
   – causes echopenic masses.

VII. CYSTS AND PSEUDOCYSTS

A. **True cysts** of the pancreas
   – are typically single and are lined by mucous epithelium.
   – can be congenital or acquired.
   – have the typical characteristics of all cysts (see Chapter 4, VII A 1–5).

B. **Pseudocysts**
   – are walled-off collections of fluid from extravasated pancreatic secretions.
   – occur in 10%–20% of patients after an episode of acute pancreatitis.
   – can be single or multiple and are usually round or oval in shape.
   – can develop in any of the spaces and organs in and around the pancreas, but most occur within the borders of the pancreas.
   1. **Sonographic findings**
      a. Pseudocysts are usually echo-free masses with good through transmission, but some contain internal debris.
      b. Multiloculation and calcified walls may occur.
      c. No epithelial lining or capsule is present.
   2. **Treatment**
      a. Pseudocysts usually resolve spontaneously.
      b. For pseudocysts that do not resolve spontaneously, decompression may be necessary.
   3. **Complications** include
      – gastrointestinal obstruction.
      – biliary duct obstruction.

C. **Cystic neoplasms**
   – may be similar in appearance to pseudocysts.
   – comprise 5% of pancreatic tumors and a small percentage of pancreatic cancers.
   1. **Macrocystic (mucinous) cystadenomas** are rare, slow-growing tumors seen more frequently in women and occurring more often in the tail. They may be large, well circumscribed, and either unilocular or multilocular. Sonographically, a benign cystadenoma cannot be distinguished from a malignant cystadenoma.
   2. **Microcystic cystadenomas** are well defined, echogenic, and solid in appearance. Tiny cysts may be seen.

D. **Adult polycystic kidney disease**
   – is autosomal dominant.
   – can occasionally involve the pancreas.
   – Single or multiple cysts are scattered throughout the pancreas.

I. Postrenal transplant assessment

J. Prior to renal transplant donation

V. RENAL PARENCHYMAL DISEASE

– is the term used to describe poorly functioning but unobstructed kidneys.

A. Causes include
- acute or chronic glomerulonephritis.
⊥ diabetes.
- lupus and sclerodermatous nephritis.
- nephrotic syndrome.
- heroin-induced nephropathy.
- acute tubular necrosis.
- leukemia.
- chronic renal vein thrombosis.
- amyloidosis.

B. Sonographic findings
1. In most forms of renal parenchymal disease, the kidney parenchyma is echogenic.
2. When the disease is of recent onset, the kidneys enlarge.
3. As the disease becomes chronic, the kidneys contract.
4. Atrophic, small kidneys with a thin cortex represent end-stage renal disease.
5. Enlarged, densely echogenic kidneys are seen in AIDS nephropathy.

VI. MASSES

A. Benign masses
1. **Angiomyolipoma**
   - is a common benign neoplasm composed of vessels, fat, and muscle.
   - is seen most often in middle-aged women.
   - is usually an incidental finding; however, it may bleed and cause a hematoma.
   - A well-defined, highly echogenic, cortical mass is seen.
2. **Mesoblastic nephroma**
   - is a benign mass that occurs in infants.
   - The mass is usually solid, but may contain cystic areas.

B. Malignant masses
1. **Renal cell carcinoma** (also called **hypernephroma** and **Grawitz' tumor**)
   - is the most common malignant renal mass in adults.
   a. **Risk factors** include
      - elderly men.
      - smoking.
      - von Hippel-Lindau syndrome.
      - long-term dialysis.
   b. **Clinical features** include
      - hematuria.
      - anemia.
      - weight loss.
      - fatigue.
      - flank pain.
   c. **Sonographic findings**
      (1) A unilateral focal mass will be present, which may be hyperechoic or isoechoic. The mass is occasionally calcified or partially cystic.
      (2) Scanning of the affected main renal vein or inferior vena cava may show tumor invasion.
      (3) Renal cell carcinoma typically metastasizes to local lymph nodes, the lungs, bone, and the liver.
2. **Oncocytomas**
   - account for 5% of renal neoplasms.
   - may be benign.
   - have a similar appearance to renal cell carcinoma.
   - are well-defined, homogenous masses usually isoechoic to the renal parenchyma.
3. **Von Hippel-Lindau syndrome**
   - is an autosomal dominant genetic disorder seen between the third and fifth decades of life.
   - is associated with a greatly increased risk of renal carcinoma.
   - **Clinical features** include retinal angiomas, pancreatic cystic neoplasms, and cerebral aneurysm.
4. **Transitional cell carcinoma (TCC)**
   - is a **urothelial tumor** that typically spreads from an origin in the urinary bladder.
   - may be multiple and is usually small; therefore, it is usually not detected by sonography unless the tumor is large.
   - An intrapelvic, echopenic mass may be seen. This mass may be mistaken for a peripelvic cyst or sinus lipomatosis.
5. **Metastases** to the kidney
   - are common at autopsy but are rarely seen in life.
   - often originate in the lungs, breasts, and colon.
6. **Renal lymphoma**
   - usually involves the kidneys late in the disease.
   - is typically bilateral.
   - Enlarged kidneys with multiple hypoechoic areas are usually seen.
7. **Wilms' tumor** (nephroblastoma)
   - is the second most common solid tumor in children.
   - usually affects boys 3–5 years of age.
   a. **Clinical features** include
      - a palpable mass.
      - hypertension.
      - pain.
      - weight loss.

b. Sonographic findings
(1) The mass appears large with an even, high-level echogenicity.
(2) Cystic spaces representing necrosis may be seen.
(3) The tumor is bilateral approximately 10% of the time.
(4) Wilms' tumor metastasizes to the lymph nodes, lungs, liver, and bone.

VII. CYSTS

A. Simple renal cysts
  – are common, especially in patients older than 50 years.
  – have the typical components inherent in all cysts:
  1. Round or oval in shape
  2. Smooth walls
  3. No internal echoes
  4. Well-defined back walls
  5. Acoustic enhancement
  – One to approximately five cysts may be present in a kidney.

B. Parapelvic cysts
  – are not true cysts.
  – are derived from lymphatic tissue.
  – are irregular in shape and outline.
  – may be confused with hydronephrosis because of their location in the renal hilum.
  – do not communicate with the collecting system.
  – Atypical cysts contain low-level echoes or septations.

C. Acquired cystic disease
  – occurs in patients who have been on dialysis for more than 3 years.
  – is associated with an increased risk of malignancy.
  – Spontaneous hemorrhage often occurs.

D. Tuberous sclerosis
  – is an autosomal dominant genetic disorder that often affects the kidneys.
  1. Clinical features include
    – epilepsy.
    – skin lesions on the face.
  2. Sonographic findings
    a. The kidney size is normal to enlarged.
    b. Multiple renal cysts and **angiomyolipoma** may be present.

E. Autosomal recessive (infantile) polycystic kidney disease (IPKD)
  – is a fatal disorder.
  – Enlarged, echogenic kidneys without visible cysts are seen in the neonate and small child.
  – In the later stages, an echogenic liver related to hepatic fibrosis may be seen.

F. Multicystic dysplastic kidney disease (see Chapter 22, VII D)
  – is usually a nonhereditary condition.
  – may be unilateral or bilateral. If bilateral, it is fatal.
  – No renal parenchyma can be seen.
  – Large, noncommunicating cysts are interspersed with echogenic areas.

G. Autosomal dominant (adult) polycystic kidney disease (APKD)
  – is a genetic disorder.
  1. Clinical features
    – Patients are usually hypertensive.
  2. Sonographic findings
    a. Multiple irregularly shaped cysts are present bilaterally in massively enlarged kidneys.
    b. Cysts may also appear in the liver, spleen, and pancreas.
    c. A **berry aneurysm** (i.e., an aneurysm in the circle of Willis) occurs in 20% of affected cases.

VIII. ABSCESSES

A. Renal abscesses
  1. Causes include
    – localized pyelonephritis.
    – renal calculi.
    – trauma.
    – intravenous drug abuse.
  2. Clinical features include
    – fever.
    – abdominal pain.
    – local tenderness.
    – an increased white blood cell count.
  3. Sonographic findings
    a. The abscess has a thick, echogenic border.
    b. There may be cystic or echogenic contents with acoustic enhancement.
    c. Intra-abscess gas and fluid debris levels are unusual variants.
    d. Perirenal abscesses are extensions of infective conditions that appear as hypoechoic masses around the kidney.

B. Pyelonephritis (lobar nephronia)
  – is an infection of a portion of or a complete kidney.
  – may be unilateral or bilateral.
  1. Causes
    a. Retrograde flow of bacteria up the ureter results in parenchymal inflammation.
    b. Pyelonephritis is more common in women because of vesicoureteral reflux.
  2. Clinical features include
    – flank pain.

- fever.
- pyuria.
- bacteremia.
- dysuria (i.e., painful urination).
- urinary frequency.
   3. **Sonographic findings**
      a. Either a small area or the entire kidney may be enlarged and hypoechoic.
      b. With chronic infection, focal scarring is seen and the kidneys become small and echogenic.

C. **Xanthogranulomatous pyelonephritis**
   - is a form of chronic pyelonephritis.
   - The renal pelvis contracts around a stone but the calyces are dilated and the cortex is narrowed.

D. **Emphysematous pyelonephritis**
   - typically occurs in diabetics.
   - Gas develops in the renal parenchyma.
   - Enlarged kidneys with areas of high-level echoes and acoustic shadowing are seen.

E. **Renal fungal disease**
   - is seen particularly in infants.
   - Echogenic fungus balls develop in the dilated renal pelvis.

F. **Pyonephrosis**
   - Pus develops in the dilated renal pelvis of an obstructed kidney after long-standing infection and urinary stasis.
   - Fluid debris levels and low-level echoes in the fluid in the pelvis are seen.
   - This is a deadly disease unless the obstructed pelvis is drained on an emergency basis.

IX. HEMATOMAS

A. **Causes** include
   - surgery.
   - trauma.
   - lithotripsy.
   - biopsy.

B. **Sonographic findings**
   1. Diminishing in size over time, the sonographic appearance changes from cystic to echogenic in the acute phase and then to complex or anechoic later.
   2. Although focal intrarenal hematomas may be present, hematomas frequently occur around the kidneys (see Chapter 8, VI).

X. CALCULI

A. **Urinary calculi**
   - affect up to 12% of the population.
   1. **Causes** include
      - infection.
      - elevated serum calcium levels.

- familial predisposition (e.g., cysteinuria).
- gout.
- iatrogenic factors.
   2. **Clinical features** include
      - flank pain.
      - hematuria.
      - signs of infection.
   3. **Sonographic findings**
      a. Stones, regardless of their composition, are highly echogenic.
      b. Stones greater than about 3 mm in diameter exhibit shadowing; the smaller the stone, the higher the frequency of the transducer required to make it shadow.
      c. Stones less than 5 mm in diameter can drop into the ureter, but may be held up at the narrowest points (i.e. the ureteropelvic junction or the entrance of the ureters into the bladder).

B. **Staghorn calculi**
   - are large and fill the pelvis and calyces.
   - usually result from infection.

C. **Nephrocalcinosis**
   1. **Causes** include
      - medullary sponge kidney.
      - hypercalcemia related to hyperparathyroidism.
      - renal tubular acidosis.
      - long-term furosemide administration.
      - hypervitaminosis.
   2. **Sonographic findings**
      a. In the usual form, small calculi develop only in the renal pyramids.
      b. In **cortical nephrocalcinosis,** there are echogenic foci in the cortex with loss of the corticomedullary junction.

XI. OBSTRUCTIVE DISEASE

A. **Hydronephrosis**
   - is a dilation of the renal collecting system caused by obstruction.
   - can be unilateral or bilateral.
   1. **Causes** include
      - pregnancy.
      - ureteral or urethral stricture.
      - calculi.
      - ureteral or extrinsic masses.
      - bladder outlet obstruction.
      - surgery.
      - congenital conditions (e.g., ureteropelvic junction obstruction).
      - ureterocele.
   2. **Clinical features** include
      - back or flank pain.
      - a palpable mass (i.e., the dilated kidney).
      - increased BUN and creatinine.
   3. **Sonographic findings**

a. The renal pelvis and calyces will be dilated.

b. Dilated ureters will be seen if the obstruction is in the bladder neck or ureters.

c. Cortical thinning and renal atrophy occur if hydronephrosis is long-standing.

d. Several normal variants can mimic hydronephrosis.

   (1) An overdistended bladder can cause pelvocalyceal dilation, particularly in children and patients with a renal transplant.

   (2) A dilated renal vein may be mistaken for a dilated renal pelvis if Doppler imaging is not used to prove otherwise.

   (3) Peripelvic cysts can mimic hydronephrosis. Sinus echoes are separated by true hydronephrosis, not just displaced.

B. Ureteropelvic junction obstruction
   – Congenitally, there is narrowing of the ureter just below the kidney, sometimes related to the presence of an aberrant vessel.
   – The renal pelvis becomes very large as the dilation gradually increases over time.

C. Posterior urethral valves
   – is a condition seen only in males.
   – A congenital membrane forming a valve partially obstructs the posterior urethra.
   – Secondary dilation of the posterior urethra, bladder, ureters, and pelvicalyceal system occurs.

   1. Clinical features include
      – renal failure.
      – a pelvic mass due to the distended bladder.

   2. Sonographic findings include
      – a massively distended bladder and posterior urethra in an infant or child.
      – tortuous dilated ureters.
      – a dilated renal pelvicalyceal system.
      – Dysplastic changes in the kidneys are common.
      – There may be echogenic parenchyma with peripherally placed small cysts.

D. Prune-belly syndrome (Eagle-Barrett syndrome)
   – occurs in male children only.
   – There is dilation of the posterior urethra, bladder, ureters, and pelvicalyceal system with no obstruction in the posterior urethra.
   – The abdominal muscles are lax and there are undescended testicles.

E. Ureterocele
   – is a congenital obstruction of the distal ureter.

   1. Clinical features
      – Ureteroceles are usually asymptomatic until a palpable kidney mass due to secondary hydronephrosis is found.

   2. Sonographic findings
      – There is a cobra-headed expansion of the distal ureter as it enters the bladder.
      – Secondary ureteral and pelvicalyceal dilation is common.
      – The condition is often bilateral and is strongly associated with double (duplex) collecting systems.
      – The lower of the two ureters supplies the upper collecting system and is obstructed by the ureterocele.
      – The upper ureter is often affected by reflux and supplies the lower collecting system.

XII. INFARCTIONS

A. Renal artery occlusion
   – results from the occlusion of the main arteries supplying the kidney.

   1. Causes include
      – trauma.
      – vascular disease.

   2. Clinical features include
      – acute flank pain.
      – hematuria.

   3. Sonographic findings
      a. If the main renal artery is occluded, the kidney briefly enlarges and then slowly contracts to a small size.
      b. With focal infarctions, a wedge-shaped area becomes hypoechoic in the acute phase and later contracts and becomes echogenic. A scar is formed.
      c. No flow will be seen in the renal artery with color flow Doppler.

B. Renal vein thrombosis

   1. Clinical features include
      – flank pain.
      – proteinuria.
      – hematuria.
      – a palpable mass.

   2. Sonographic findings
      – Hematuria causes initial swelling and prominence of the sinus echoes.
      – Later, the kidney contracts.
      – The renal artery has a biphasic flow in the presence of renal vein thrombosis.

XIII. ANOMALIES

A. Renal agenesis (unilateral)
   – is the absence of one kidney.
   – is a common malformation, occurring in 1 of every 100 adults.
   – is more common in men.

– may be familial.
– is associated with genital malformations (e.g., congenital uterine anomalies).
– The existing kidney is enlarged because of compensatory hypertrophy.
– **Note:** bilateral renal agenesis can occur *in utero;* this condition is fatal at birth.

B. Ectopic kidney
– One kidney is located in an atypical location.
1. The ectopic kidney can be located in the true pelvis or thoracic region.
2. In a variant, both kidneys are on the same side and are usually fused (i.e., **crossed renal ectopia**).

C. Horseshoe kidney
– is an abnormal congenital variant in which an isthmus of renal parenchyma connects either the lower or the upper poles of the right and left kidneys. Both kidneys lie closer to the midline than usual.
– is usually an incidental finding.
– is associated with an increased risk of obstruction and infection.
– is also associated with Turner's syndrome.

D. Renal sinus lipomatosis
– is present when there is additional fat in the renal sinus.
1. **Causes** include
– obesity.
– chronic infection.
– old age.
2. **Sonographic findings**
a. The renal parenchyma becomes narrowed and the renal sinus becomes enlarged and more prominent.
b. Most of the fat is echogenic, but portions may look hypoechoic.

XIV. RENAL TRANSPLANTS

A. Donor kidney origin
1. The donor kidney may be taken from
– a recently deceased cadaver.
– a compatible donor.
2. The donor should
– have a compatible immunologic system.
– be free of disease.
– have good renal function.

B. Anatomy
1. The donor kidney is surgically placed in the right or left iliac fossa of a patient with chronic renal failure. The right side is more frequently used because the iliac vessels are more superficial on the right.
2. Placement of the donor kidney in the iliac fossa of the recipient allows for

– easy assessment of changes in size.
– good access for biopsy.
– use of a short segment of the ureter.
– ability to connect vessels.

C. Sonography
– Baseline sonography is performed 2 days after surgery to establish renal and renal pelvic size and to check for fluid collections.
1. A slight distention of the renal pelvis is a normal finding.
2. Fluid collections often occur in or around transplanted kidneys.

D. Fluid collections
1. A **urinoma**
– is usually related to a leak from the ureterovesical anastomosis site.
– usually occurs within the first 2 weeks after surgery.
– is usually located between the lower pole of the kidney and the urinary bladder.
a. **Clinical features** include
– decreased urine output.
– fever.
– tenderness.
b. **Sonographic findings** include
– an echo-free fluid collection.
2. **Lymphoceles**
– usually occur 2–8 weeks after the transplant.
– The lymph collection is located between the bladder and the transplant.
a. **Clinical features** include
– painless swelling over the transplant.
– decreased renal function.
– lower leg swelling.
b. **Sonographic findings** include
– a cystic area that often contains septa.
3. **Hematomas**
– are common within a few days of surgery.
a. **Clinical features** include
– decreased hematocrit.
– fever.
b. **Sonographic findings**
(1) The hematoma will vary from echo-free to echogenic, depending on how organized it is.
(2) The hematoma is usually located around the kidney or at the surgical incision.
4. **Abscesses**
– occur 1 week to 4 months after the transplant.
a. **Clinical features** include
– fever.
– local tenderness.
– Symptoms may be unimpressive because the patient is immunosuppressed.

b. Sonographic findings
  (1) Internal echoes are seen.
  (2) The abscess may be indistinguishable from a hematoma.
    – Percutaneous aspiration is used to distinguish an abscess from a hematoma after a urinoma has been excluded by nuclear medicine techniques.

E. Post-transplant renal failure
  1. Acute tubular necrosis
    – occurs 1–2 days after the transplant.
    – is the most common cause of acute post-transplant failure.
    a. Clinical features include
      – low urinary output.
    b. Laboratory values include
      – increased creatinine levels.
    c. Sonographic findings include
      – renal enlargement.
      – a high-resistance Doppler pattern.
  2. Rejection
    a. Acute rejection
      – is the most common cause of renal transplant failure in the initial weeks after surgery.
      – **Sonographic findings** include an enlarged kidney, decreased absent end-diastolic flow, or reversal of flow on pulsed Doppler.
    b. Chronic rejection
      – occurs months to years after the transplant.
      – A small kidney with increased parenchymal echogenicity will be seen.
  3. Cyclosporine toxicity
    – Cyclosporine is a drug used to treat rejection.
    – Sonographic findings are indistinguishable from those seen with rejection (see XIV E 2).

F. Vascular complications
  1. Renal vein thrombosis
    – is uncommon.
    – presents with renal failure.
    – is usually in the peripheral veins.
    – results in an enlarged kidney.
    – Doppler results include a high-resistance arterial waveform in the renal artery; reversed diastole may occur.
    – No venous flow is detected.
  2. Renal artery stenosis
    – occurs at the anastomosis site.
    – results in a high-resistance pattern with markedly elevated systolic flow at the stenotic site.
    – Damping with poststenotic turbulence distal to the stenosis may be seen.
  3. Renal artery thrombosis

    – The arterial signal will be absent in the main renal artery and intrarenal vessels.
  4. Postbiopsy complications
    – Arteriovenous fistulas and pseudoaneurysms are usually caused by percutaneous biopsy of the renal parenchyma.
    – Color flow Doppler shows an arteriovenous communication or an aneurysm.
    – Pulsed Doppler will show both arterial and venous signals.

XV. URINARY BLADDER

A. Neurologic bladder
  1. Detrusor arreflexia
    – The bladder is enlarged, inert, and does not empty completely with urination (i.e., overflow incontinence).
    – There is a thin bladder wall but no trabeculae.
  2. Detrusor hyperreflexia
    – Sonographic findings vary.
    a. The bladder may be enlarged with a thick wall and multiple trabeculae (i.e., small indentations on the wall).
    b. The bladder may be small and spastic with a thick, irregular wall and multiple trabeculae.

B. Diverticula
  – are either congenital or associated with urethral obstruction.
  – There is a predisposition to bladder cancer within the diverticula.
  – There are local areas of eventration of the bladder wall.

C. Urethral obstruction
  1. Causes include
    – an enlarged prostate.
    – urethral stricture.
    – urethral neoplasm.
    – posterior urethral valves.
  2. Sonographic findings include
    – an enlarged, thick-walled bladder.
    – trabeculae and possibly diverticula in the bladder wall.

D. Cystitis
  – is an inflammation of the bladder wall seen more frequently in women.
  1. Clinical features include
    – urinary frequency.
    – pain on urination.
  2. Sonographic findings
    – The bladder wall is focally or generally thickened and irregular.

E. Blood clots
  1. Causes include
    – neoplasms.
    – infection.

– calculi.

– trauma.

2. Sonographic findings

a. Blood clots usually appear as echogenic masses on the posterior wall.

b. A blood clot will move when the patient is turned; a neoplasm will not move.

c. When the bleed is recent, a fluid level may be seen with the hypoechoic blood clot located posteriorly.

F. Masses

1. Papillomas

– are benign, superficial neoplasms of the bladder wall that may be multiple.

– are also seen in the ureters and renal pelvis.

a. Clinical features include

– hematuria.

b. Sonographic findings include

– superficial masses arising from the bladder wall.

– masses that do not move with patient movement.

2. TCC (see VI B 4)

– is the most common primary malignant bladder neoplasm.

a. Clinical features include

– hematuria.

b. Sonographic findings

(1) TCC appears as a focal thickening of the wall or a discrete mass.

(2) When the mass can be seen to extend through the bladder wall, it is unresectable.

(3) A mass is difficult to see on the anterior wall because of reverberation artifacts. Endovaginal scanning may help with this.

CHAPTER 5

SCROTUM (3%–7%)

I. ANATOMY (Figure 5–1)

A. The **scrotum**
- is a musculocutaneous sac containing the **cremaster muscle.**
- is divided into two parts by the **median raphe.**
- Housed within the two sacs are the testicles, epididymides, blood vessels, spermatic cords, and fluid.

B. Scrotal walls
1. The **tunica vaginalis** is a peritoneal sac that covers the inner aspect of the scrotal walls and testicles.
2. The tunica vaginalis encloses a potential space (i.e., the cavity of the tunica vaginalis).

C. The **testes**
- are the paired male reproductive glands where spermatozoa are produced.
- are oval in shape and measure approximately $5 \times 3 \times 3$ cm.
1. The capsule of each testicle is known as the **tunica albuginea.**
2. Multiple tortuous seminiferous tubules become the **rete testis** at the hilum, where the mediastinum is located.
3. From the rete testis, the sperm passes into the efferent ducts, which join the **epididymis,** a long tubular structure on the posterior aspect of each testicle.
4. The upper pole of the epididymis is the **head** or **globus major.** Arising from the head is the **appendix epididymis.**
5. The epididymis connects to the spermatic cord and **vas deferens.** It carries the semen superior and anterior to the pubic symphysis.
6. The vas deferens then turns posteriorly and passes posterior to the bladder to connect to the **seminal vesicles** and the **ejaculatory ducts of the prostate.**

D. Blood supply
1. **Arterial supply**
   a. The **testicular artery** that supplies the testes arises from the aorta.
   b. The **deferential artery** is a branch of the vesical artery. It supplies the vas deferens and epididymis.
   c. The **cremasteric artery,** a branch of the inferior epigastric artery, supplies the paratesticular tissue.
2. **Venous supply**
   a. The **pampiniform plexus** is a network of veins that drains the spermatic cord and epididymis.
   b. The pampiniform plexus divides into three veins—the testicular, deferential, and cremasteric veins.
      (1) The right testicular vein drains into the inferior vena cava.
      (2) The left testicular vein drains into the left renal vein.

II. TECHNIQUE

A. A high-frequency transducer is required to see superficial detail, such as the scrotal wall thickness.

B. The testicles should be immobilized as much as possible.

C. It is desirable to examine both testicles simultaneously so that textural differences can be seen.

D. Sagittal, transverse, and coronal views may be obtained.

E. Trace the epididymis inferiorly from the prominent head. The body of the epididymis may lie lateral or posterior to the testicle.

F. Doppler imaging, especially color flow, is an efficient way to assess the extent of infarction or torsion.

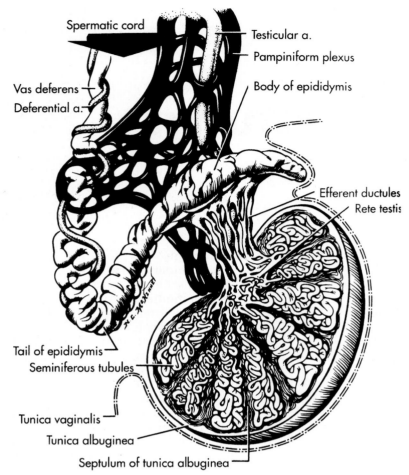

Spermatic cord

Testicular a.

Pampiniform plexus

Vas deferens

Deferential a.

Body of epididymis

Efferent ductules

Rete testis

Tail of epididymis

Seminiferous tubules

Tunica vaginalis

Tunica albuginea

Septulum of tunica albuginea

FIGURE 5-1 A diagram of the scrotum showing the testis, epididymis, and spermatic cord with their blood supply. (Reproduced with permission from Rumack C, Wilson S, Charbonneau W: *Diagnostic Ultrasound.* Philadelphia, Mosby, 1998, p 792.)

III. LABORATORY VALUES

– Human chorionic gonadotropin (HCG) levels are elevated in choriocarcinoma, a rare tumor of the testicle.
– The sperm count is diminished and the sperm are hypomotile with some varicoceles.

IV. INDICATIONS

– Scrotal ultrasound is performed if any one of the following conditions is present:

A. A palpable mass in the scrotum

B. Acute or chronic scrotal pain

C. Male infertility (to rule out a varicocele) [see VII B]

D. Scrotal enlargement

E. Apparent undescended testicles

V. PARENCHYMAL DISEASE

A. Cryptorchism
– is a congenital condition in which the testicles fail to descend into the scrotum.

They normally descend *in utero* at 28 weeks' gestation.
– can be unilateral or bilateral.

1. Sonographic findings

a. The malpositioned testicle appears similar to the normal testicle, but is located above the normal site in the inguinal canal.

b. In a minority of cases, the testicle is located in the abdomen and cannot be seen with ultrasound.

2. Complications include
– an increased risk of testicular cancer.
– infertility.

B. Microlithiasis
– Multiple small calcifications are scattered throughout the testicles.
– Microlithiasis has no clinical significance, except that it may be a precursor to a malignancy, such as seminoma (see VI A).

C. Testicular torsion
– results from twisting of the testicle and spermatic cord.
– The resulting infarction may be complete

or incomplete, depending on the severity of the twist.

– A congenital variant position of the testicle known as **bell clapper deformity** predisposes to testicular torsion.

1. **Clinical features** include
   – acute onset of severe testicular pain.
2. **Sonographic findings**
   a. If the sonogram is performed within the first 4 hours, the testicle is enlarged with decreased echogenicity.
   b. There is thickening of the scrotal wall, a possible hydrocele, and enlargement of the related epididymis.
   c. There is absent or decreased flow with color flow Doppler imaging.
3. **Treatment**
   a. Testicular torsion is a surgical emergency.
   b. If the torsion is not urgently treated, the testicle contracts and becomes avascular and atrophic.

VI. MASSES

– Most intratesticular masses are malignant.
– Cysts and small benign adenomas may also be seen.

A. Seminoma

– is the most common germ cell tumor, accounting for 40%–50% of testicular tumors.
– usually occurs between 30 and 50 years of age.
– has a good prognosis, providing it is recognized before extensive spread.
– **Sonographic findings**
1. A hypoechoic lesion in the testicle with smooth, well-defined borders is seen.
2. The mass can occupy the entire testicle.

B. Embryonal cell carcinoma

– is the second most common germ cell tumor.
– typically occurs between 20 and 30 years of age and before 2 years of age.
– **Sonographic findings** include a heterogeneous mass with necrotic areas containing cystic spaces and echogenic foci.

C. Teratomas

– are the second most common tumor in infants.
– are considered malignant when seen in adults.
– **Sonographic findings**
1. A well-defined, heterogeneous mass will be seen.
2. Cystic and echogenic areas with shadowing may be present.

D. Choriocarcinoma

– is highly malignant and rare.

– has a poor prognosis.
– **Sonographic findings** include an irregularly shaped tumor with cystic and calcified regions.

E. Testicular metastases

– usually originate from leukemia or non-Hodgkin's lymphoma.
– Sonographic appearances are varied, but the mass is usually hypoechoic.

VII. CYSTS AND FLUID COLLECTIONS

A. Hydroceles

– occur when fluid accumulates between the two layers of the tunica vaginalis.
– can be congenital or acquired.
– are considered a normal variant if small.
1. **Causes** include
   – trauma.
   – epididymo-orchitis.
   – testicular (spermatic cord) torsion.
   – iatrogenic factors.
2. **Clinical features** include
   – painless scrotal swelling.
3. **Sonographic findings**
   a. In a typical hydrocele, an echo-free fluid collection surrounds the testicle. Internal echoes caused by proteinaceous contents may be seen.
   b. After trauma, the contents may be blood (**hematocele**). Internal echoes will be seen.
   c. In association with epididymitis, the contents may be pus (**pyocele**). Internal echoes will be seen.

B. Varicoceles

– are an enlargement of the veins of the spermatic cord resulting from incompetent valves in the internal spermatic vein.
– usually occur on the left side. The left gonadal vein drains into the left renal vein, which passes between the aorta and the superior mesenteric artery. These can compress the vein, causing the "nutcracker" effect.
– When a varicocele is only seen on the right, a renal mass may be present.
1. **Sonographic findings**
   a. Tortuous, enlarged veins (i.e., greater than 3 mm) are seen superior and posterior to the testicle.
   b. When the patient stands and performs the Valsalva maneuver, the veins distend.
   c. Pulsed Doppler imaging shows flow reversal during the Valsalva maneuver.
2. **Complications**
   – Varicoceles are a common cause of infertility; they are associated with hypomotile sperms and a low sperm count.

C. Epididymal cysts
– occur anywhere in the epididymis.
– have the typical echo-free cyst appearance.

D. Spermatoceles
– are single or multiple cystic masses at the head of the epididymis.
– are filled with nonviable sperm, fat, cellular debris, and lymphocytes.
– are indistinguishable from epididymal cysts.

E. Scrotal hernia
– occurs when bowel protrudes through the **processus vaginalis,** a congenital remnant in the inguinal canal, into the scrotum.
– Peristalsis of the bowel confirms the diagnosis.
– The normal testicle can usually be distinguished within the mass, which can be very large with heterogeneous contents.

VIII. INFLAMMATION

A. Orchitis
– is an inflammation of the testicles, usually resulting from epididymitis.
1. Clinical features
– The scrotum containing the testicle will be tender, reddened, and hot.
2. Sonographic findings
   a. Orchitis may be focal or diffuse, appearing as hypoechoic areas.
   b. Color flow will show increased vascularity.
   c. Untreated epididymo-orchitis often results in testicular **infarction.**
     (1) Hypoechoic, avascular areas are seen that look similar to orchitis, except that they exhibit no flow on Doppler.
     (2) If the infarction is generalized and long-standing, the testicle shrinks and becomes atrophic.

B. Epididymitis
– is inflammation of the epididymis.

– may be unilateral or bilateral (less common).
1. Clinical features
   a. The posterior aspect of the testicle is tender and hot; however, it is not as tender as with torsion and the onset is not as abrupt.
   b. The patient may be febrile.
2. Sonographic findings
   a. In the acute stage, there is an enlarged epididymis that appears hypoechoic.
   b. As the disease becomes chronic, more internal echoes and even calcification are seen in the enlarged epididymis.
   c. Secondary orchitis is common.

C. Abscesses
– usually result from epididymo-orchitis.
– are most often located in the epididymis, but can occur in the testes.
– A tender, fluid-filled mass with a capsule and internal echoes is present.

IX. HEMATOMA

A. Sonographic findings
1. The outline of the testicle is irregular, and a visible fracture line through the testicle may be seen.
2. A hematocele is usually present surrounding the fractured testicle. The internal echoes in the hematocele may resemble testicular tissue.
3. Blood supply to the testicle is often absent on Doppler imaging.

B. Treatment
– Trauma to the scrotum is a surgical emergency.
1. If the testicle is fractured (i.e., the tunica albuginea is disrupted), the tubules and contents leave the testicle and the testicle ceases to produce sperm.
2. However, if the testicular wall is repaired within a few hours, testicular function can be preserved.

CHAPTER 6

PROSTATE (0%–2%)

I. ANATOMY

A. Prostate

1. **Structure**
   a. The prostate is a chestnut-shaped gland measuring approximately $4 \times 3 \times 4$ cm with a weight of 16–25 g.
   b. The base is the superior aspect and the apex is the inferior aspect.
   c. The prostate contains four zones (Figure 6–1).
      (1) The **peripheral zone,** the largest zone, is posterolateral and occupies most of the apex. The majority of cancers are seen in this zone.
      (2) The **central zone** surrounds the ejaculatory ducts. It houses 20% of the glandular tissue and 10% of prostate cancers.
      (3) The **transitional zone** is a bilobed area composed of glandular and stromal elements. Benign prostatic hypertrophy (BPH) develops from this zone but spreads to other areas.
      (4) The anterior surface of the prostate is the **anterior fibromuscular stroma.** It is typically free of disease.
2. **Function**
   – The prostate secretes fluid to assist sperm mobility.

B. The **seminal vesicles** and **vas deferens**
   – lie superior to the prostate.
1. The vas deferens unites with the seminal vesicle to become the **ejaculatory duct** (see Figure 6–1B).
2. The ejaculatory duct runs through the prostate and joins the urethra at the **verumontanum** (see Figure 6–1B).

II. TECHNIQUE

   – The prostate can be scanned using a transabdominal or endorectal approach.

A. The **transabdominal** approach requires a fully distended urinary bladder and a caudal approach with the transducer. This scanning technique is only useful for determining gland size and radiotherapy planning.

B. The **endorectal** approach is necessary to document disease and to guide biopsy. When performing a biopsy, the transducer is inserted in the rectum and a needle is inserted alongside in a predetermined path.

III. LABORATORY VALUES

   – Two biochemical markers are commonly used to detect prostate disease.

A. Prostate-specific antigen (PSA) is an enzyme produced only in the prostate.
1. A level of 4 or greater prompts investigation.
2. Normal levels gradually increase as a patient ages.
3. PSA is elevated in
   – prostate cancer.
   – preinvasive neoplasm (a precancerous condition).
   – BPH.
   – prostatitis.

B. Acid phosphatase is increased in prostate cancer with bone metastases.

IV. INDICATIONS

   – The prostate is scanned in the following situations:

A. To assist with biopsy in patients with elevated PSA levels or a possible mass on rectal examination

B. To evaluate the size of the prostate in patients with an enlarged prostate

C. Possible infection of the prostate

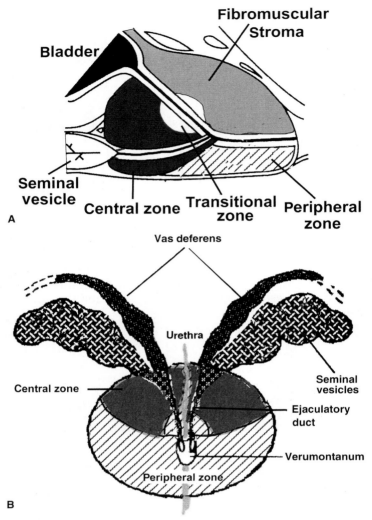

FIGURE 6-1 (*A*) Sagittal view of the prostate showing the zonal arrangement. (*B*) Coronal view of the prostate and seminal vesicles showing the ejaculatory ducts and zonal arrangement.

D. Male infertility (if there is azoospermia)

V. PARENCHYMAL DISEASE—BENIGN PROSTATIC HYPERTROPHY

– is a disease seen in elderly men.
– The gland enlarges, usually starting in the transitional zone.

A. Clinical features include
– frequency and difficulty in starting or stopping urination.
– nocturia.
– hematuria.

B. Sonographic findings
1. The prostate is enlarged with a compressed peripheral zone (i.e., the surgical capsule). The central portion of the prostate has an even, moderately echogenic texture.
2. Occasionally, deposits of BPH bulge out of

the prostate in an eccentric fashion (e.g., toward the bladder).
3. Focal hypoechoic deposits of BPH may develop in the peripheral zone.

VI. MASSES—PROSTATE CANCER

– is the most commonly diagnosed cancer in men, and is the second leading cause of cancer death in men.
– is familial, with an increased risk in African-American men.
– can metastasize to lymph nodes and bone, preventing surgical treatment; both sites are poorly seen with ultrasound.

A. Clinical features
1. There are no symptoms until metastases occur.
2. A small proportion of cancers can be felt on

a rectal digital examination; however, most are found because the PSA level is elevated.

B. Sonographic findings
- Biopsy of possible cancerous lesions in the prostate is often performed under ultrasound guidance through an attachment on the transrectal transducer.
1. Most lesions appear hypoechoic, although some are isoechoic and there are occasional hyperechoic cancers. Remember that other lesions (e.g., focal prostatitis, focal deposits of BPH) can also appear hypoechoic.
2. Most are located in the peripheral zone.
3. Invasion with extension through the capsule may be seen.

VII. CYSTS

A. Utricles
- are congenital midline cysts connected to the verumontanum by a small duct.
- can be associated with unilateral renal agenesis.

B. Müllerian duct cysts
- develop from remnants of the müllerian duct.
- lie in the midline at the base of the prostate.

C. Retention cysts
- result from BPH.

- often occur in the central zone.
- contain mucus.

VIII. ABSCESSES

A. Prostatitis
1. **Clinical features** include
   - rectal pain.
   - dysuria.
   - fever.
2. **Sonographic findings**
   a. In the acute form, hypoechoic areas are seen, particularly in the peripheral zone.
   b. In the chronic form, echogenic areas are present, sometimes with calcification.
   c. **Granulomatous prostatitis,** a rare form, causes focal hypoechoic areas that closely resemble cancerous lesions.

B. Abscesses
- may be a sequel to acute prostatitis.
1. **Clinical features**
   - Fever may be the only symptom.
   - Tenderness on rectal examination is present.
2. **Sonographic findings**
   - Abscesses will be seen on the transrectal sonogram as hypoechoic areas in the prostate that usually contain some debris.

CHAPTER 7

SPLEEN (1%-5%)

I. ANATOMY

A. Spleen

1. **Structure**
   a. The spleen is located in the left upper quadrant and is predominately a vascular, **intraperitoneal** organ.
   b. The spleen is part of the reticuloendothelial system, composed of **lymphoid tissue** and containing **white pulp** and red pulp.
   c. It is approximately 12 cm in length, 6 cm in width, and has a convex superior surface and a concave inferior surface.
   d. With the exception of the hilum, the spleen is covered with peritoneum.

2. **Blood supply**
   a. The splenic artery enters at the hilum.
   b. The splenic vein leaves at the hilum.

3. **Functions** include
   - defense against disease (especially in children).
   - production of lymphocytes.
   - storage of iron.
   - maturation, storage, and removal of erythrocytes.

B. An **accessory spleen (splenule)**

- is a normal variant seen in 10% of the population.
- is usually located around or near the hilum of the spleen or along the major vessels.
- is typically small in size and appears round or oval in shape with the same texture as the spleen.

II. TECHNIQUE

- The spleen is scanned intercostally with the patient in a left-side-up position. Longitudinal and transverse views are obtained. If the patient must remain supine, coronal scans are taken through the left side.

III. LABORATORY VALUES

- Most diseases that involve the spleen affect the red and white blood cell counts.

IV. INDICATIONS

- Ultrasound of the spleen is ordered in the following situations:

   A. Possible splenomegaly in **portal hypertension, connective tissue disorders,** and **infections**

   B. Possible site for metastatic disease (particularly **lymphoma**)

V. PARENCHYMAL DISEASE

A. Splenomegaly is an enlargement of the spleen.

B. Causes include
   - connective tissue disorders (e.g., rheumatoid arthritis).
   - portal hypertension.
   - infectious diseases (e.g., abscess, tuberculosis, mononucleosis, AIDS, malaria).
   - hematologic disorders (e.g., sickle cell anemia, polycythemia, thalassemia).
   - lymphoma.
   - leukemia.

VI. MASSES

A. Benign primary neoplasms
   - are uncommon.
   - include **cavernous hemangiomas, hamartomas,** and cystic **lymphangiomas.**

B. Lymphoma
   - is a malignant process with **Hodgkin** or **non-Hodgkin's** variants.
   - The spleen is usually enlarged.
   - Solitary or multiple focal masses that are

IV. INDICATIONS

- The retroperitoneal area is scanned in the following situations:

- is a malignant tumor involving the smooth muscle.
- usually resides in the uterus or gastrointestinal tract.

anechoic or hypoechoic may be seen in the spleen.

C. Malignant primary neoplasms
- are very rare.
- Metastases occur late in the disease and are

- bacterial endocarditis associated with drug abuse.
- trauma with hematoma development.
  2. Sonographic findings
  a. Abscesses appear as ill-defined, complex masses.

- grows rapidly as it metastasizes to the lungs.
  3. Benign lipomas
  - are evenly echogenic masses.
  4. Retroperitoneal fibrosis
  - is a condition in which a fibrous sheath envelops the distal aorta, inferior vena cava, and sacrum.
    a. Causes include
    - idiopathic factors.
    - low-grade infections.
    - ergot medication for migraine headaches.
    - metastatic spread.
    b. Sonographic findings
    - Smooth-bordered, echopenic tissue coats the distal aorta and inferior vena cava and extends down to the sacrum.

VI. HEMATOMAS

- may occur in the retroperitoneum.

A. Typical locations include
- the psoas muscles (most common, especially in hemophiliacs).
- around the kidney.

B. Causes include
- trauma.
- surgery.
- anticoagulant therapy.
- bleeding problems, such as hemophilia.

C. Clinical features include
- local pain.
- transient fever.
- hematocrit drop.

D. Sonographic findings
- Hematomas can be hypoechoic or echogenic.

VII. ADRENAL GLANDS

A. Anatomy
1. The adrenals are paired endocrine glands located in the retroperitoneum, superior to the kidneys. They are enclosed in **Gerota's fascia.**
   a. The left adrenal gland is lateral to the aorta and posterior to the pancreatic tail.
   b. The right adrenal gland is medial to the right lobe of the liver, anterior to the right crus of the diaphragm, and superior to the medial aspect of the kidney.
2. The normal size of an adrenal gland is approximately 3 × 1 × 3 cm. However, the left adrenal gland is somewhat larger than the right.

3. Both adrenal glands have an emaciated triangular shape.
4. The outer portion of the adrenal glands, the **cortex,** is composed of the
   - **zona glomerulosa** [produces mineralocorticoids (**aldosterone**)].
   - **zona fasciculata** (produces **glucocorticoids**).
   - **zona reticularis** (produces **androgens, estrogens,** and **glucocorticoids**).
5. The inner portion of the adrenal glands is the **medulla.** Its endocrine functions include the production of
   - **epinephrine** (adrenaline).
   - **norepinephrine** (noradrenaline).
6. The **anterior pituitary gland** produces **adrenocorticotropic hormone (ACTH),** which is responsible for the release of hormones from the adrenal cortex.

B. Pathology
1. **Adrenal cysts**
   - have the typical appearance of a cyst (see Chapter 4, VII A 1–5).
2. **Adrenal adenomas**
   - are small, solid, hypoechoic masses.
   - are often found on an incidental basis.
3. **Hemorrhage,** or **hematoma,**
   - is often seen in neonates.
   - is usually bilateral.
   - has either a cystic or complex appearance.
   - becomes cystic over the course of time and often eventually calcifies.
4. **Pheochromocytomas**
   - are uncommon adrenaline-secreting tumors.
   - may cause episodic hypertension.
   a. Laboratory values include
   - an increase in epinephrine levels.
   - an increase in norepinephrine levels.
   b. Sonographic findings
   (1) Unless the pheochromocytoma is malignant, it is too small to be seen with sonography.
   (2) If the pheochromocytoma is malignant, a small, echopenic mass will be present.
5. **Cushing's disease**
   a. Causes include
   - adrenal hyperplasia (most common).
   - adenoma.
   - malignancy (rare).
   b. Clinical features include
   - hirsutism.
   - hypertension.
   - abnormal fat distribution.
   c. Sonographic findings
   - almost all masses are too small to see
6. **Myolipoma**

– is a rare, benign, nonfunctioning tumor containing fat and bone marrow elements.
– With echogenic masses, the speed of sound through the mass, which is mostly fat, is slower than through surrounding tissues. As a result, the posterior borders of the mass and the diaphragm distal to the mass appear to lie posterior to the diaphragm and liver adjacent to the mass.

7. **Neuroblastoma**
   – is a common malignancy found in small children between 0 and 5 years of age.
   – is a sympathetic nervous system tumor.
   a. **Laboratory values**
      – Vanilmandelic acid (VMA) levels are elevated.
   b. **Sonographic findings**
      (1) There is usually a hypoechoic, or heterogeneous, large, solid mass.
      (2) Calcifications often occur in the tumor.
      (3) The mass spreads locally around the aorta and vena cava.
      (4) It metastasizes to the liver and brain rapidly.

8. **Metastases**
   a. The adrenal glands are the fourth most common site for metastases, after the lungs, liver, and bone.
   b. Bronchogenic lung carcinoma may metastasize to both adrenal glands, forming large, bilateral, hypoechoic masses (i.e., the "headlight" sign).
   c. Metastases are solid masses that may be unilateral or bilateral.

CHAPTER 9

ABDOMINAL VASCULATURE (INCLUDING DOPPLER) (7%-15%)

I. ANATOMY

A. Arteries (Figure 9–1)
– The largest artery in the body is the **abdominal aorta,** which has several branches.
1. The **celiac axis** divides into the
   – **splenic** artery.
   – **hepatic** artery.
   – **left gastric** artery.
2. The **superior mesenteric artery (SMA)** divides into
   – the **inferior pancreaticoduodenal** artery.
   – **branches to the colon.**
   – **ileal branches.**
3. The **renal arteries** branch off at the level of L1–2.
4. The **inferior mesenteric artery** comes off the distal aorta and supplies the left colon.
5. At the level of the umbilicus, the abdominal aorta bifurcates into the right and left **common iliac arteries.**

B. Veins
1. The **inferior vena cava (IVC)**
   – is formed from the union of the right and left common iliac veins and ascends to enter the right atrium of the heart.
   – has several major tributaries.
   a. The **renal veins enter the IVC laterally, near the renal arteries.**
      (1) The left renal vein takes a long course between the SMA and the aorta, where it can be pinched between the two vessels (i.e., the "nutcracker" effect).
      (2) A normal variant course for the left renal vein is posterior to the aorta.
   b. **Three hepatic veins** drain the liver as they converge into the IVC.
   c. The **left gonadal vein** enters directly into the left renal vein.
2. The **portal vein**
   – is formed from the confluence of the splenic vein and superior mesenteric vein.
   – is normally less than 13 mm in diameter during quiet respiration.
   – branches into a right and left portal vein in the porta hepatis.
   – Normally, the portal vein and hepatic artery flow in the same direction (i.e., hepatopetal flow).

II. TECHNIQUE

A. Gas, which often obscures the abdominal aorta, can be displaced by compression with a linear array transducer.

B. Each iliac artery is traced obliquely from the aortic bifurcation toward the groin.

C. Doppler signals from the abdominal vessels are obtained by placing the Doppler gate in the vessel after localizing the vessel using color flow. The beam should be at a 60° angle to the flow for a valid Doppler signal to be obtained.

D. Venous signals in the IVC are best elicited as the patient performs the Valsalva maneuver.

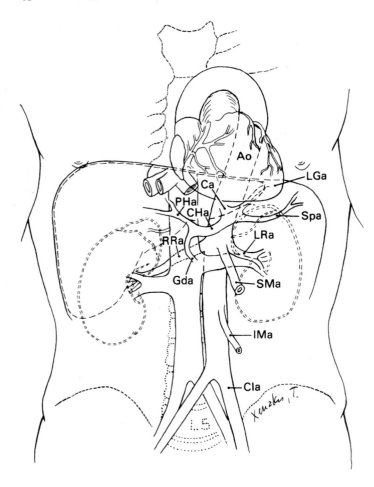

FIGURE 9-1 Commonly visualized vessels arising from the aorta (*Ao*) are the celiac artery (*Ca*), splenic artery (*Spa*), left gastric artery (*LGa*), common hepatic artery (*CHa*), proper hepatic artery (*PHa*), gastroduodenal artery (*Gda*), right and left renal arteries (*RRa* and *LRa*), superior mesenteric artery (*SMa*), inferior mesenteric artery (*IMa*), and below the bifurcation at the level of the fourth lumbar vertebra, the right and left iliac arteries. Only the portion of the aorta below the diaphragm is visualized on an abdominal study. *CIa* = common iliac artery. (Reprinted with permission from Sanders RC: *Clinical Sonography: A Practical Guide,* 3rd ed. Philadelphia, Lippincott, 1998, p 207.)

III. LABORATORY VALUES (not relevant to this topic)

IV. INDICATIONS

– Examination of the abdominal vasculature is requested in the following situations:

A. Suspected aortic aneurysm by palpation or abdominal bruit (detection and follow up)

B. Possible arteriovenous fistula after biopsy or femoral artery catheterization

C. Possible mesenteric ischemia (indigestion)

D. Leg swelling (to rule out a thrombus in the IVC)

E. Portal hypertension (to see if flow reversal has occurred)

V. ANEURYSMS

– A true aneurysm is a dilation of an artery as the result of wall weakness. It is lined by the three components of an arterial wall: intima, media, and adventitia.

– False or pseudoaneurysms (see VIII) are lined by the outer layers of the aortic wall or by clot.

– Dissecting aneurysms (see V E) occur when blood forms a passage through a hole in the intima and reenters the main lumen at a distance.

– Aneurysms can rupture, leading to sudden death.

– Rarely do aneurysms dissect.

– An aneurysm is usually an incidental finding on palpation or a radiograph.

– Although most common in the aorta, aneurysms can be seen in any major artery.

A. Causes include
– atherosclerosis (most common).
– trauma.
– syphilis.
– Marfan's syndrome.
– mycotic (infective).

B. Clinical features include
– abdominal or back pain.
– abdominal bruit.
– pulsatile abdominal mass.
– impaired arterial supply to the lower limbs.

C. Sonographic findings
1. A localized bulge (**saccular aneurysm**) or extended area of widening (**fusiform aneurysm**) may be seen.
2. An abdominal aneurysm may involve the major branches of the aorta, especially the renal arteries. Determining what arteries are involved is important for surgical planning.
3. Thrombus formation is common. The ex-

tent of the thrombus may be obscured by wall calcification.

D. Treatment
1. Aneurysms 3–5 cm in width are usually followed.
2. Aneurysms that are greater than 5 cm in width are operative candidates.

E. Dissecting aneurysm of the aorta
- is damage to the internal arterial wall.
- results from a break in the **intima.**
- is a rare intra-abdominal process that usually extends from the thoracic aorta to the abdomen.
- Blood will flow between the layers of the wall and in the true aorta, creating true and false lumens.

VI. THROMBI

A. IVC thrombus
- The IVC may be the site of a clot or tumor, either primary or metastatic.
- Low-level echoes may be seen in the clot, and are more obvious with the aid of color flow Doppler imaging.
- A fresh clot can be nearly sonolucent.
- Filters may be placed in the IVC to prevent the clot from embolizing. Echogenic structures with shadowing will be seen when filters are in position.

B. Hepatic vein thrombus
- In **Budd-Chiari syndrome,** the hepatic veins are partially or completely filled with clot.

C. Renal vein thrombus
1. **Causes** include
   - renal transplant (post-transplant complication).
   - nephrotic syndrome.
   - renal tumors.
   - trauma.
2. **Clinical features** include
   - hematuria.
   - flank pain.
3. **Sonographic findings**
   a. A hypoechoic thrombus will be seen in a distended vein.
   b. The thrombus may be seen to extend into the vena cava.
   c. No venous Doppler signal is present because of complete occlusion of the renal vein.

VII. ARTERIOVENOUS SHUNTS AND FISTULAS

- are communications between the arterial and venous systems.

A. Possible locations include the
- kidneys (after biopsy).

- groin (at the site of femoral artery puncture).

B. Causes include
- biopsy.
- trauma.
- surgery.
- malignancy.
- congenital.

C. Clinical features include
- painful swelling.
- a bruit.

D. Sonographic findings
1. On color flow Doppler imaging, a pool of blood will light up, which shows a turbulent pattern.
2. Pulsed Doppler imaging will show a to-and-fro pattern because there is a combination of arterial and venous signals.

VIII. PSEUDOANEURYSMS

- are contained ruptures of a blood vessel.
- are most commonly seen after catheterization via femoral artery puncture.

A. Causes include
- trauma.
- infection.
- surgery.
- biopsy trauma.

B. Sonographic findings include
- a swirling blood collection adjacent to the injury site.
- a narrow neck connecting the pseudoaneurysm to the vessel lumen.

C. Treatment
- Pseudoaneurysms are usually successfully treated using prolonged ultrasound-guided compression. Compression can require up to 1 hour before the neck is clotted off.

IX. DOPPLER WAVEFORMS

A. Arterial Doppler waveforms
1. The **aorta** changes its **Doppler signal** from low to high resistance as it travels from the renal artery level to the **bifurcation** and lower **abdomen.**
2. A **low-resistance** signal with a high flow in diastole is seen in the **organ systems** perfused by the proximal branches of the aorta.
3. The **renal arteries** receive 15%–30% of the cardiac output. The right renal artery is longer than the left; however, both have a low-resistance signal because they feed an organ.
4. **High-resistance signals** with little or re-

versed diastolic flow are seen in the **distal aorta, distal limbs,** and **muscular beds.**

B. **Venous Doppler waveforms**
   1. The normal IVC has a multicomponent waveform (i.e., sawtooth appearance).
   2. The portal vein has a low-velocity, consistent signal on Doppler that is not influenced by respiration.
   3. The hepatic veins are close to the right atrium of the heart. They display a pulsatile triphasic flow pattern. In right heart failure, the pattern will be exaggerated.
   4. The normal renal vein has a low-velocity, continuous signal.

C. **Arterial pathology on Doppler**
   1. **Superior mesenteric artery (SMA) ischemia**
      – The SMA can be scanned in patients with abdominal pain of unknown origin to rule out **small bowel ischemia.**
      a. In the normal patient, the Doppler signal will change from high to low resistance when the patient goes from a fasting to nonfasting state.
      b. When small bowel ischemia is present, the change from high to low resistance does not occur.
      c. To diagnose bowel ischemia, obstruction must be present in two of the three following arteries:
         (1) Celiac axis
         (2) SMA
         (3) Inferior mesenteric artery
   2. **Renal artery stenosis**
      a. **Causes** include
         – arteriosclerosis.
         – fibromuscular disease (in younger individuals, predominantly women).
      b. **Clinical features** include
         – hypertension (treatable).
      c. **Sonographic findings**
         (1) The renal arteries are best examined in the decubitus or oblique position with color flow Doppler.
         (2) A high-resistance waveform with a slow acceleration phase is abnormal and indicative of stenosis. The ratio of peak velocities in the aorta and stenotic renal artery segment is helpful. A 3.5 ratio indicates a greater than 60% chance of stenosis.

CHAPTER 10

GASTROINTESTINAL TRACT (1%–5%)

I. ANATOMY

A. The **peritoneum**
– is a thin membrane consisting of two layers.
1. The parietal layer lines the abdominal cavity wall.
2. The visceral layer lines the organs.
– A posterior portion of the liver known as the **bare area** is not covered by peritoneum.

B. The **peritoneal cavity**
– is the space between the layers of the peritoneum that contains a small amount of serous fluid to prevent friction.
1. The peritoneal cavity is divided into a **greater sac** and a **lesser sac.**
a. The cavity is an enclosed sac in males.
b. The sac has an opening for the fallopian tubes in females.
2. Spaces in the peritoneal cavity for potential fluid collection include the
– **subhepatic** region (**Morison's pouch**).
– right and left **subphrenic** areas (beneath the diaphragm).
– **lesser sac.**
– **paracolic** gutters.
– **cul-de-sac.**

C. **Intraperitoneal organs** include the
– liver.
– gallbladder.
– spleen.
– stomach.
– intestines.
– ovaries.

II. TECHNIQUE

A. Filling the **stomach** with water facilitates examination of the wall.

B. An inflamed **appendix** is examined with graded compression. The landmarks—the terminal ileum, cecum, and psoas muscle—should be identified.

C. To detect an **inguinal hernia,** place the transducer in the groin, align it sagittally, and identify the inferior epigastric artery. Have the patient lift his head and perform the Valsalva maneuver so that intra-abdominal pressure is increased. If present, the hernia will move into the inguinal canal.

D. A **water enema** is a rarely used technique in which water is placed in the rectum and sigmoid colon to determine whether an apparent mass is actually normal gut.

III. LABORATORY VALUES

A. A stool guaiac test can be performed to determine the presence or absence of blood in the stool.

B. The white blood cell count increases in inflammatory conditions (e.g., appendicitis).

IV. INDICATIONS

– Examination of the gastrointestinal tract is helpful in the following situations:

A. Presence of an intermittent abdominal mass that could be a hernia

B. Possible appendicitis

C. Abdominal size increase that could be caused by ascites

D. Possible intraperitoneal bleed after trauma

V. INFLAMMATORY DISEASE

A. **Appendicitis**
– The appendix is a long, narrow tube.
– When the appendix becomes inflamed, rupture with peritonitis is a risk, and surgical removal is necessary.

1. **Clinical features** include
   – severe abdominal pain that starts at the umbilicus and moves to the right iliac fossa.
   – fever.
   – nausea and vomiting.
   – altered bowel habit.
   – rebound tenderness at McBurney's point.
2. **Laboratory values** include
   – an increased white blood cell count.
3. **Sonographic findings** include
   – a **noncompressible** appendix (recognized by relationship to blood vessels and ileum).
   – thickened appendix walls (i.e., greater than **6 mm**).
   – local tenderness.
   – **appendicolith** (i.e., echogenic shadowing structure in the lumen).

B. **Crohn's disease (regional enteritis)**
   1. **Clinical features** include
      – ileitis.
      – abdominal pain.
      – anemia.
      – weight loss.
      – altered bowel habit.
      – rectal bleeding.
   2. **Sonographic findings**
      a. The bowel wall will be more than 4 mm thick with an echogenic center (i.e., "donut" sign).
      b. There will be an inert length of bowel with a thickened wall.
   3. **Complications** include
      – fistulas.
      – abscesses.

C. **Abscesses**
   – form in the potential spaces in the peritoneal cavity (see I B 2) and at surgical sites.
   1. **Clinical features** include
      – fever.
      – local tenderness.
   2. **Laboratory values** include
      – an increased white blood cell count.
   3. **Sonographic findings**
      a. Abscesses generally have low-level echoes within, but may appear cystic.
      b. They expand into adjacent tissues.

D. **Gossyphiboma**
   – If a sponge is left in the peritoneal cavity at surgery, a sterile abscess forms around it.
   – A tender linear echo with acoustic shadowing will be seen.

E. **Diverticulitis**
   – Diverticula are small outpouchings through the wall of the colon.
   1. **Clinical features** include
      – abdominal pain.

– constipation.
– mucus in stools.
2. **Sonographic findings**
   a. Circumferential or asymmetrical thickening of the bowel wall will be seen.
   b. Edematous fat surrounding diverticula has a similar appearance to thyroid tissue.
3. **Complications**
   – Inflammation in a diverticulum leads to obstruction and abscess formation.

VI. MASSES—GUT CANCER

– is most common in the stomach and colon.
– Thickened bowel wall (i.e., greater than 4 mm) with an echogenic center gives a kidney-like appearance.

VII. OBSTRUCTION

A. **Bowel obstruction**
   – Multiple tubular, dilated, fluid-filled bowel loops are seen in **gut obstruction** and **paralytic ileus.**
   – If peristalsis is seen, mechanical obstruction is present.

B. **Hypertrophic pyloric stenosis**
   – presents in the first 6 weeks of life.
   – Congenital narrowing of the pylorus is seen more frequently in male infants.
   1. **Clinical features** include
      – projectile vomiting.
      – a palpable mass felt at the site of the hypertrophied muscle (the "olive" sign).
   2. **Sonographic findings**
      a. Hypertrophied, circular muscle of the pylorus will measure more than 13–17 mm in length and 3–4 mm in thickness.
      b. A large amount of fluid will be seen in the stomach.

C. **Intussusception**
   – occurs when a loop of small or large bowel invaginates into a more distal loop of bowel and causes obstruction.
   – is principally a disease of children.
   1. **Clinical features** include
      – vomiting.
      – a palpable mass.
   2. **Sonographic findings**
      a. A mass with a series of linear components to its wall will be seen.
      b. The mass can be reduced under ultrasound using a water enema.

VIII. HERNIA

A. **Typical locations** include
   – at the umbilicus (**umbilical** or **ventral** hernia).

– in the groin (**inguinal** hernia) or medial to the femoral vein (**femoral** hernia).
– a more superolateral location (**spigelian** hernia; rare).

B. Sonographic findings
– Bowel possibly showing peristalsis protrudes through the echogenic fascial lining of the abdominal wall.

IX. PERITONEAL FLUID—ASCITES

– is fluid accumulation in the peritoneal cavity.
– can be differentiated from abscess formation by the way it outlines bowel and moves if the patient is repositioned.
– can be a transudate or an exudate.

A. Transudate ascites
– is the accumulation of fluid resulting from insufficient osmotic pressure to keep fluid in blood vessels.

1. Causes include
– cirrhosis and liver failure.
– renal failure with the nephrotic syndrome.
– congestive heart failure.
– hypoproteinemia.

2. Sonographic findings
– Echo-free fluid surrounds the gut.

3. Treatment
– Transudate ascites is treated with a low-sodium diet, diuretics, and removal under ultrasound guidance (i.e., **therapeutic paracentesis**).

B. Exudate ascites
– is a reaction to an abnormality involving the peritoneum.

1. Causes include
– hemorrhage.
– infection.
– peritoneal malignancy (e.g., ovarian cancer).

2. Sonographic findings
a. If peritonitis is present, multiple septa with a cobweb-like appearance will be seen.
b. If malignancy is present, a tethered bowel with peritoneal metastases will be seen.

CHAPTER 11

NECK (1%-5%)

I. ANATOMY

A. Thyroid
1. The thyroid is a highly vascular organ that consists of a right and left lobe connected by an **isthmus.** It is located just anterior to the trachea.
2. The thyroid measures approximately 3–5 cm in length and 2–3 cm in depth and width; the right lobe is typically longer than the left.
3. The anterior border of the thyroid is bordered by the **strap muscles,** such as the **sternohyoid** and **sternothyroid** muscles, and the **sternocleidomastoid muscles,** which are more superficial and lateral.
4. The **longus colli** muscles lie posterior to the thyroid, in contact with the prevertebral space.
5. The carotid arteries lie posterolateral to the thyroid. The jugular veins are lateral to the carotid arteries.

B. Parathyroid glands
1. The two pairs of parathyroid glands are posterolateral at midlevel and inferior to the thyroid.
2. The parathyroid glands are round, hypoechoic structures normally less than 0.5 cm in size.
3. Variant normal sites include in the thyroid and in the mediastinum.
4. Parathyroid glands secrete parathyroid hormone, which regulates calcium and phosphorus metabolism.

II. TECHNIQUE

A. A high-frequency transducer of 7.5 MHz or greater, preferably a linear array transducer, is needed for quality images of the thyroid.

B. A low-frequency transducer with a standoff pad is a less desirable option.

C. The patient is examined in the supine position with the head extended.

III. LABORATORY VALUES

A. The **thyroid** is an **endocrine gland** important in the regulation of body growth and metabolism. The growth and basal metabolic rates are controlled by two hormones produced in the thyroid, which are
  – **triiodothyronine (T_3).**
  – **thyroxine (T_4).**

B. **Thyroid-stimulating hormone (TSH),** which is excreted by the pituitary gland, regulates the thyroid. T_3 and T_4 are either increased or decreased by the level of TSH.

C. Serum calcium and parathormone levels are assayed to rule out a parathyroid mass.

IV. INDICATIONS

– The neck is scanned in the following situations:

A. Evaluation of a cold nodule found on nuclear medicine scan

B. Evaluation of a questionable palpable nodule

C. Aid in biopsy of a thyroid nodule

D. Rule out recurrence of an excised thyroid neoplasm

E. Possible parathyroid mass

F. Possible inflammatory mass in the neck

G. Carotid vascular lesions

V. THYROID PARENCHYMAL DISEASE

A. Multinodular goiters
  – appear as an enlarged thyroid containing many nodules, cystic areas, and calcifications.

– may be isoechoic with the remaining thyroid tissue.
– There can be normal thyroid function (euthyroid) or, more often, hypothyroidism.

B. Subacute thyroiditis
– is a painful inflammatory disease of the thyroid that is self-limiting.
– The thyroid is enlarged and hypoechoic.

C. Hashimoto's thyroiditis
– is a chronic, progressive, autoimmune disease seen more frequently in women.
– Hypothyroidism is present.
– The thyroid is diffusely, asymmetrically enlarged and has a coarsened texture.
– Fibrotic septations may produce a pseudolobulated appearance.

D. Graves' disease
– is the cause of thyrotoxicosis (i.e., hyperthyroidism).
  1. Clinical features include
   – weight loss.
   – increased heart rate.
   – **exophthalmos** (i.e., protruding eyes).
   – excess energy and anxiety.
  2. Sonographic findings
   a. The gland is diffusely enlarged and hypoechoic, sometimes with a heterogeneous texture.
   b. There is increased gland vascularity.

VI. THYROID MASSES

A. Adenomas
– are benign neoplasms found in many adults, particularly in elderly women.
– can be multiple and can contain functioning thyroid tissue.
– A hyperechoic, hypoechoic, or isoechoic mass with a hypoechoic halo is the typical finding.
– "Popcorn" calcification and cystic changes may be seen.

B. Carcinoma
– in the thyroid is rare, considering the number of benign masses.
– is more common in women.
  1. The cell type of the tumor controls the metastatic behavior. There are four **main types of thyroid carcinoma.**
   a. Papillary carcinoma
    – represents most thyroid cancers and is the least aggressive.
    – has a good prognosis if treated early.
    – is often multifocal with lymph node metastases present early in the course of the disease.
   b. Follicular carcinoma

– is the second most common type of thyroid cancer.
– occurs later in life, especially in women.
– spreads via the bloodstream rather than through nodes, so distant metastases to the bone, lungs, brain, and liver are more common than local spread.
   c. Medullary carcinoma
    – is uncommon.
    – typically exhibits microcalcifications.
   d. Anaplastic carcinoma
    – is highly malignant and grows rapidly.
    – is typically a disease of the elderly.
  2. Metastases to the thyroid
   – may occur with lymphoma.
   – may be from the breasts, lungs, and colon.
  3. General **sonographic findings of thyroid carcinoma**
   a. Most thyroid malignancies are hypoechoic.
   b. Thyroid malignancies typically have an irregular border.
   c. Microcalcifications may be seen.
   d. As with benign masses, there is increased vascularity compared to the remaining thyroid tissue.
   e. Metastatic cervical lymph nodes, which do not effect the prognosis, may be present.

VII. THYROID CYSTS

– account for 20% of all cold lesions on nuclear medicine studies. True thyroid cysts are rare.
– are typically benign.
– usually result from hemorrhage or cystic degeneration of an **adenoma.**
– A **thyroglossal duct cyst** is a congenital cyst arising from an embryological remnant. It is located in the midline above the thyroid and is usually tubular in shape.

VIII. PARATHYROID MASSES (PARATHYROID ADENOMAS)

– are benign masses. Carcinoma of the parathyroid gland is very rare.
– cause primary **hyperparathyroidism.**

A. Clinical features include
– mood swings.
– muscle weakness.
– malaise.

B. Laboratory values include
– an increase in serum calcium.
– a decrease in phosphorus, which accompanies hyperparathyroidism.

C. **Sonographic findings**
1. A hypoechoic mass larger than 0.5 cm with rounded borders occupies the parathyroid glands.
2. Most parathyroid adenomas involve only one gland, but in **multiple endocrine neoplasia, type II** more than one gland may be enlarged.

D. **Complications**
– of hypercalcemia (e.g., renal calculi) may occur.

IX. ABSCESSES

– in the neck are uncommon.

A. **Causes** include
– tonsillitis.
– upper respiratory tract infection.

B. **Sonographic findings**
– A complex, cystic mass will be seen lateral to the thyroid.

X. LYMPH NODES

A. **Causes of enlarged lymph nodes** include
– local infection.
– mononucleosis.
– metastatic disease.

B. **Sonographic findings of enlarged lymph nodes**
1. Enlarged lymph nodes will appear as oval, hypoechoic, well-circumscribed, solitary or multiple masses.
2. Benign nodes have a central echogenic hilum.

XI. CAROTID ARTERIES AND JUGULAR VEINS

A. The carotid artery may contain plaque and show abnormal flow on pulsed Doppler examination.

B. The carotid artery and jugular vein may show focal enlargement and may become aneurysmal.

CHAPTER 12

SUPERFICIAL STRUCTURES (BREAST, MUSCULOSKELETAL, NONCARDIAC CHEST) (1%-5%)

BREAST

I. ANATOMY

A. The breast is an **endocrine gland** that is affected by changes in hormone levels. Its primary function is milk secretion during lactation.

B. **Regions** of the breast include
- the skin.
- the nipple (creates posterior shadowing).
- a subcutaneous layer composed of fatty tissue and divided by connective tissue.
- **mammary** and **parenchymal layers.**
  1. In the mammary and parenchymal layers, there are 15–20 lobes separated by **Cooper's ligaments,** which appear as thin, echogenic, linear structures.
  2. **Lactiferous ducts,** which are visible as tiny tubular structures, drain these lobes to the nipple.
- a **retromammary layer.**
  1. The retromammary layer contains loose areolar tissue, the pectoralis major muscle, ribs, and intercostal cartilage.
  2. The ribs are seen as oval, hypoechoic, shadowing structures behind the hypoechoic pectoralis muscles.

C. The composition of the breast changes with the menstrual stage.
  1. During menstrual years, the breast is predominately composed of **glandular tissue** interspersed with occasional hypoechoic fat lobules. Glandular tissue is homogeneously echogenic.
  2. During menopause, there is an equal amount of glandular and fatty tissue.
  3. In the postmenopausal patient, the breast is composed of **fatty** and **fibrous tissue** and is relatively homogeneous and hypoechoic.

II. TECHNIQUE

A. Before scanning the patient, the sonographer should palpate any masses, review the mammogram report, and obtain a medical history, including
- age.
- previous breast cancer history.
- family history of cancer.
- age at first pregnancy.
- number of pregnancies.
- age at menopause.
- previous breast biopsies.
- mammographic findings.
- nipple discharge.
- breast pain or tenderness.

B. Place the patient in a supine oblique position with the side that is being examined mildly elevated. The arm on the same side is placed above the patient's head.

C. To scan the breast in its entirety, take images in a clockwise fashion, radiating around the nipple. Take views at right angles to any suspect area and use compression on these areas.

D. Angle under the nipple to visualize the region posterior, which may have been obscured by the normal shadowing from the nipple.

E. Take views of the axilla to exclude enlarged nodes.

III. LABORATORY VALUES (not relevant to this topic)

IV. INDICATIONS

– Breast sonography is performed in the following situations:

A. Dense glandular breast tissue prevents a satisfactory mammogram (e.g., in young women with a possible mass)

B. Evaluation of a questionable mass seen on mammography

C. Evaluation of a palpable mass not seen on mammography

D. To differentiate between cystic and solid lesions

E. To guide biopsy or aspiration

F. To perform a follow-up examination

V. MASSES

A. Criteria for determining the **nature of a mass** include
  – skin changes.
  – shape and position of the mass.
  – echogenicity.
  – boundary echoes.
  – asymmetry.
  – prominent ductal pattern.
  – calcifications.

B. Benign masses
  1. Fibroadenomas
    – are the most common benign mass in young women.
    – are slow growing and stimulated by estrogen.
    – can be multiple and bilateral.
    – On ultrasound, a solid, smooth-bordered, ovoid, hypoechoic mass with edge shadowing will be seen.
  2. Lipomas and fat deposits
    – are composed of fat.

  – are hypoechoic.

C. Malignant masses
  1. Infiltrating ductal carcinoma
    – is the most common neoplasm (80%).
    – **Sonographic findings**
    a. It is poorly circumscribed with irregular borders.
    b. It has a stellate pattern.
    c. It is hypoechoic.
    d. There is shadowing.
    e. It is taller than it is wide—a criteria for all breast malignancies.
    f. Detection of axillary metastatic lymph nodes (i.e., hypoechoic without an echogenic center) alters the staging and management.
  2. Medullary carcinoma
    – is less common than infiltrating ductal carcinoma.
    – is highly cellular and mainly composed of epithelial tissue.
    – is not easily differentiated from fibroadenoma.
    – On ultrasound, the mass is hypoechoic with smooth, well-defined borders.
  3. Infiltrating lobular carcinoma
    – originates in the ductules of lobules.
    – is usually located in the upper, outer quadrant.
    – There are decreased echoes, no posterior walls, and irregular central shadows.
  4. Diffuse carcinoma
    – is an inflammatory process that results from infiltrative types of breast cancer.
    – There is capillary invasion with skin and lymphatic involvement.
    – The breast is enlarged and the skin is reddened, blotchy, and thickened.

VI. CYSTS AND FLUID COLLECTIONS

A. Cysts
  – are the most common type of lesion in women 35–50 years of age.
  – are echo-free with well-defined borders, strong back wall, and posterior enhancement.
  – Post-traumatic cysts may contain internal echoes related to blood.

B. Galactoceles
  – are milk-filled cysts more commonly seen in lactating women.
  – have well-defined walls and are usually anechoic.

VII. ABSCESSES

A. Clinical features include
  – local tenderness and warmth.
  – reddened skin.

B. Sonographic findings include
  - poorly defined borders (if not fully formed).
  - sharp borders with posterior enhancement (if mature).
  - internal echoes.

MUSCULOSKELETAL

I. ANATOMY

A. Muscles
  - are hypoechoic with parallel, linear, echogenic strands.
  - change shape with limb movement.

B. Tendons
  - are linear and well defined with an echogenic, fibrillar structure.
  - are only seen well if the transducer is parallel to the tendon.

C. Bone
  - The superficial border of the bone can be seen, but the shaft is shadowed out.

D. Joints
  - Ultrasonic access is limited, but joint effusions and cartilage tears may be seen.

E. Soft tissues (e.g., muscle and skin)
  - are easily demonstrated by ultrasound if no bone or air is blocking access.

II. TECHNIQUE

A. Use a high-frequency linear array transducer for most soft tissue examinations.
  - Scan with the highest frequency that is practical for the site to demonstrate a **foreign body.**
  - Evaluation of skin may require some form of standoff pad.

B. To examine rotator cuff tears with the patient in a sitting position, place the patient's arm behind the back and examine the shoulder from an anterolateral approach. Moving the arm may make recognition of the muscles of the rotator cuff more obvious.

III. LABORATORY VALUES (not relevant to this topic)

IV. INDICATIONS

  - Musculoskeletal ultrasound can be helpful in the following situations:

A. Trauma to the ankle with a possible Achilles tendon tear

B. Painful shoulder with inability to lift the arm normally (to exclude rotator cuff tear)

C. Soft tissue mass (to define extent and structures involved)

D. Swollen, red, tender limb or joint with possible abscess or osteomyelitis

E. Abrupt onset of lower leg pain with possible deep venous thrombosis or Baker's cyst

V. MASSES—SOFT TISSUE OR BONE TUMORS

  - The extent of the tumor and vascularity are well seen.
  - Defining the extent and structures involved can alter the surgical approach.

VI. CYSTS AND FLUID COLLECTIONS

A. Baker's cysts
  - are synovial fluid collections in the calf related to a break in the synovial membrane around the joint.
  #### 1. Clinical features
    - Local tenderness may mimic deep venous thrombosis.
  #### 2. Sonographic findings
    a. A collection that consists of synovial fluid develops posterior to the knee joint and/or in the calf.
    b. A connection to the knee joint may be seen.

B. Joint effusions
  - are fluid collections that directly surround joints.
  - may be related to repeated trauma or infection.
  - can be aspirated under ultrasound guidance.

C. Bursae
  - are fibrous pockets of synovial fluid that lie between tendons and bones to reduce friction.
  - can become inflamed after repeated traumatic episodes.
  - have a typical cystic appearance.

VII. ABSCESSES

A. Cellulitis
  - is an infection of the skin and subcutaneous tissue.
  - The skin is tender and warm; if untreated, abscess formation results.
  - On ultrasound, the muscles become less echogenic and are swollen.

B. Muscle and soft tissue abscesses

– have the same complex but basically cystic appearance seen elsewhere.

VIII. HEMATOMAS AND OTHER TRAUMA-RELATED INJURIES

A. Tendon problems
1. Breaks or trauma to the tendons, particularly the Achilles tendon, are well demonstrated as gaps in the tendon or tendon disruption.
2. Breaks in the rotator cuff tendon in the shoulder joint can be seen provided the tendon is observed from several different approaches and with several different arm positions.

B. Bone fractures
– are usually visible as breaks in the outline of the bone.

C. Muscle and soft tissue hematomas
– are seen as fluid collections of varying echogenicity, depending on the age of the bleed.
1. An actively bleeding hematoma is echogenic.
2. As the blood coagulates, the hematoma becomes so homogeneous as to be echopenic, or echo-free.
3. The hematoma then begins to lyse, and scattered echogenicity occurs due to increased acoustic interfaces.
– If a muscle is torn, the separation between two segments of the muscle may be visible.

NONCARDIAC CHEST

I. NORMAL CHEST APPEARANCE

– Alternating bands of shadowing related to ribs and reverberation artifact caused by gas are seen.

II. PLEURAL EFFUSION

A. Fluid accumulates around the lungs. Usually the fluid is freely mobile, but it can become loculated.
1. When the fluid is mobile, it accumulates around the inferior and posterior margin of the lungs and changes shape with respiration. The fluid falls to a dependent position when the patient is sitting.
2. A loculated, immobile fluid collection may be hard to differentiate from **pleural**

fibrosis, a common sequela to chronic inflammation.
a. Fibrosis appears as a straight, thickened border to the lung or effusion.
b. Loculated fluid collections usually have a rounder border.

B. The **lungs** can be seen as echogenic structures with a smooth border angulated at their inferior lateral margin.

C. If the fluid contains echogenic material or septa, there is probably blood or pus in the effusion.

D. Thoracentesis (i.e., removal of the fluid) is generally performed under ultrasound guidance with the patient supported in a sitting position. Thoracentesis may be complicated by pneumothorax. If the patient becomes breathless and complains of pain on breathing, an expiration posteroanterior chest radiograph helps in the diagnosis of pneumothorax.

III. PERIPHERAL LUNG MASSES

A. Masses can be seen as long as they abut on the pleura and are not obscured by air in the lungs.

B. It may be difficult to judge whether a mass is solid or a fluid collection because the very strong posterior interface caused by lung air makes assessment of through transmission difficult.

C. Masses can be biopsied under ultrasound guidance.

D. Masses that can be detected with ultrasound include
– peripherally placed lung cancer.
– metastatic lesions.
– cystadenomatoid malformations of the lung (CAM) in children.
– pulmonary sequestration in children.

IV. LUNG CONSOLIDATION

A. Normal lung does not transmit sound because the air reflects the beam.

B. Consolidated lung is full of fluid and allows sound penetration. Linear, bright echoes related to air-filled bronchi can be seen within the area of consolidation.

C. The fluid often contains low-level, homogeneous echoes, which can be mistaken for spleen on the left; therefore, the diaphragm must be clearly demonstrated.

CHAPTER 13

INSTRUMENTATION (1%-3%)

I. TECHNIQUE

  A. Patients should have nothing to eat and only water to drink for at least 6 hours before any study that requires a look at the gallbladder.

  B. The bladder should be full before a bladder sonogram.

  C. The bladder should be empty if the kidneys are being assessed for hydronephrosis.

  D. The rectum should be empty before a transrectal sonogram.

  E. Needle guidance
  1. Needle guidance is performed by inserting the needle at an approximately 45° angle to the transducer beam.
  2. Using a transducer guide located alongside the transducer, the path of the needle can be predetermined.

II. TRANSDUCERS

  – are devices that convert electrical energy into sound waves and sound waves back into electrical impulses.

  A. The key element in a transducer is a piezo-electric material, which converts a shape change caused by a sound wave into an electrical impulse, and vice versa. The piezoelectric material is now a ceramic-based material rather than the quartz crystals used in early devices.

  B. Transducer images are displayed in a linear, sector, or curved linear format. Currently, almost all images are created by a series of transducer elements arranged in an array. Electronic delays allow echoes from the more peripheral elements to be integrated into a two-dimensional image that is focused over a considerable distance.

  C. Transducers vary in frequency (2–12.5 MHz when used in the abdomen).

III. IMAGE RECORDING

  – The image on the monitor can be saved in various formats.

  A. Videotape
  – is convenient and continuous.
  – Image quality decays with time.

  B. Thermal paper
  – is expensive to use but is a cheap device.
  – Image quality rapidly fades.

  C. X-ray film or paper
  – is of high quality.
  – is space- and time-consuming.
  – is expensive (i.e., the film and equipment).

  D. Laser imaging
  – gives a faithful reproduction of the image.
  – The equipment is expensive and cumbersome.

  E. PACs system
  – gives a faithful, permanent reproduction of the image.
  – is very expensive.

IV. ARTIFACTS

  – are spurious echoes created by the interaction of sound with tissues or by instrumentation.

  A. Mirror artifacts
  1. Sound waves may bounce around the borders of a curved object (e.g., the bladder) so they take a long time to return to the transducer.

2. An apparent structure is created at depth (e.g., an apparent cyst posterior to the bladder or spurious structure beyond the diaphragm in the lung).

B. Shadowing
– from dense structures (e.g., calculi) prevents visualization of structures deep to the shadowing object.

C. Enhancement
1. Sound travels through fluid-filled structures unimpeded by interfaces and reflections.
2. Structures distal to the fluid may be lost in excessive echoes.

D. Reverberation artifacts
1. When the sound wave strikes a strong interface, so much sound is reflected back to the transducer that a secondary echo is sent into tissue, creating a series of ever-deepening, duplicate, parallel interfaces at a depth related to the time since the signal was emitted.
2. Reverberation artifacts are most common at the interface between the transducer and the skin, forming the "main bang" artifact.

E. Comet tail artifact
1. This artifact is derived from very strong interfaces (e.g., metallic objects).
2. A thin series of strong, parallel interfaces is seen beyond the interface with a shape resembling a comet.

F. Grating lobe artifact
– is a form of side lobe artifact.
– is predominantly seen with linear array transducers.
1. A curved linear echo is created when sound beams are deflected off of a strong interface (e.g., the bladder border).
2. The echoes are at a distance from the interface.

G. Slice thickness artifact
1. If the interface between a fluid-filled space and soft tissue is sharply angled, spurious echoes may be created in the fluid-filled area.
2. This artifact is related to the width of the ultrasound beam and is seen when sound is partially passing through fluid and soft tissue.

H. Split-image artifact
1. A duplicate image is created when the transducer is placed in the midline in the pelvis.
2. The curved rectus muscles cause the refraction of the sound beam, creating a double image of structures (e.g., intrauterine contraceptive devices, gestational sacs).

V. QUALITY ASSURANCE

A. Checks on the function of the ultrasound system are required at intervals. Modern systems are relatively stable, so a 6-month interval may be adequate.

B. The time elapsed for sound to reach marker objects and the sensitivity of detection of subtle objects are both checked using a phantom, which has pins and structures inside.
1. The depth and width of the known structures are checked.
2. System sensitivity, penetration, and distance accuracy are checked.

VI. INVASIVE PROCEDURES

– Ultrasound can be used to guide invasive procedures.

A. Typical procedures in which ultrasound guidance is used include
– drainage of pleural effusions.
– biopsy of chest masses.
– aspiration of ascites.
– prostate mass biopsy.
– liver and pancreatic mass biopsy.
– abscess drainage.

B. Ultrasound guidance can be performed freehand or using a needle guide.
1. Guidance can be performed in a freehand fashion by putting the needle in at a 45° angle to the ultrasound beam. This technique is best used when there is fluid around the target.
2. Needles can be inserted into needle guides located alongside the transducer, allowing the needle to follow a predetermined tract. This technique is often used in the prostate and liver.

C. Various techniques exist to improve needle visualization (e.g., roughening the needle). The greater the angle of the needle to the beam, the easier it is to see.

PART II

Obstetrics and Gynecology

SECTION A • OBSTETRICS

CHAPTER 14

FIRST TRIMESTER (6%–8%)

I. GESTATIONAL SAC

A. Embryology of the gestational sac (Figure 14–1)

– The formation of an embryo is the result of the union of the sperm and the mature ovum.

1. The **oocyte,** or mature ovum, is released from the follicle on approximately day 14 of the menstrual cycle.

2. The oocyte is swept by the fimbria into the fallopian tube, where union of the **sperm and ovum** (i.e., **fertilization**) takes place. The sperm and the ovum each have **23 chromosomes.**

3. Approximately 24–36 hours postovulation, the sperm penetrates the zona pellucida of the ovum.

4. The genetic components of the sperm and ovum unite to form a single fertilized cell called the **zygote,** which is a diploid cell with 46 chromosomes.

5. The process of **mitosis,** or cell division, begins 24–36 hours later. Cleavage occurs in the fallopian tube and two **blastomeres** form.

6. Cleavage continues (i.e., from a 2-part, to an 8-part, to a 16-part, to a 32-part division) with the creation of more blastomeres. Eventually, a solid ball of 16–32 cells called the **morula** forms.

7. The morula travels through the fallopian tube over 3 days until it comes to rest in the uterine cavity, where it changes into a hollow ball of cells called the **blastocyst.**

8. The blastocyst develops an outer layer of cells from which is derived the **trophoblast.** The trophoblast, which eventually becomes the chorionic membrane, surrounds a fluid-filled inner cell mass, the blastocyst, from which the embryo develops.

9. The trophoblast attaches to and invades the endometrium; the blastocyst becomes implanted. Implantation occurs approximately 7 days' postfertilization (or day 20–21 of the menstrual cycle).

10. The **corpus luteum,** which is located in the ovary, begins to produce human chorionic gonadotropin (HCG), as do the chorionic villi developing from the invasion of the endometrium.

11. The endometrium thickens as the three layers of the decidua form (i.e., it becomes decidualized) and become visible as a gestational sac. The three layers of the decidua include the

   – **decidua capsularis,** which surrounds the blastocyst.

   – **decidua vera** or **parietalis,** which lines the remainder of the endometrial cavity.

   – **decidua basalis,** which develops at the point of attachment by the blastocyst to support the trophoblastic implantation.

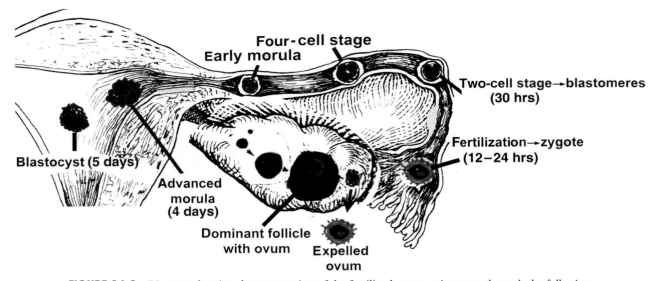

FIGURE 14-1 Diagram showing the progression of the fertilized ovum as it moves through the fallopian tube to become an embryo.

B. Sonographic findings of gestational sac development

1. At **4 weeks**
   - there is thickening of the decidua.
2. Between **4 and 5 weeks** (Figure 14–2)
   - the **blastocyst** develops into a 3- to 5-mm cyst with an echogenic rim (i.e., the **gestational sac**). The gestational sac grows at a rate of 1.0–1.3 mm/day and normally lies toward the fundus of the uterus. It contains the **chorionic cavity** (i.e., the **extraembryonic coelom),** which lies between the amniotic and chorionic membranes.
   - the embryo, known at this stage as a **bilaminar embryonic disc,** is in the **amniotic cavity.**
   - **chorionic villi** cover the outer walls of the blastocyst and project into the decidua. The villi closest to the decidua are called the **chorion frondosum,** which becomes the fetal contribution to the **placenta.**

   - the embryonic disc with three germ cell layers becomes an **embryo.**
3. At **5 weeks**
   - the gestational sac measures approximately 1 cm. It may be identified by endovaginal sonography when the blood HCG levels are approximately 1000 mlu (milliunits) 2nd IS (second international standard) and by transabdominal sonography when the blood HCG levels are approximately 1800 mlu 2nd IS.
   - a yolk sac may be identified by endovaginal sonography.

II. YOLK SAC

A. The yolk sac is located in the chorionic cavity between the amniotic and chorionic membranes.

B. Only the **secondary yolk sac** is visualized by sonography.

C. The yolk sac dominates the small chorionic

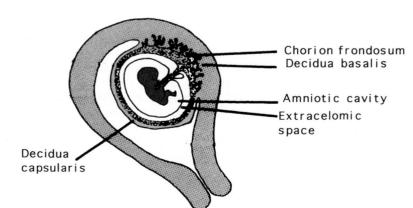

FIGURE 14-2 Gestational sac showing the embryo and the trophoblastic reaction.

cavity until it is possible to discern a clear crown-rump length adjacent to it, at around 6 weeks' gestation.

III. EMBRYO (NORMAL PHYSIOLOGIC DEVELOPMENT AND SONOGRAPHIC APPEARANCE)

A. At **5 weeks**
+ heart motion is detected in 4-mm embryos when scanning with the endovaginal probe.

B. At **6 weeks**
- the embryo measures approximately 5 mm.
- there is closure of the neural tube and the ventral surface.
- there is initial formation of the digestive system and mesonephros.
- limb buds appear.

C. At **7 weeks**
- the gestational sac measures approximately 2.4 cm and the embryo measures approximately 1.0 cm by crown-rump length.
- the developing fourth ventricle and posterior fossa are seen as a cystic area and together are called the **rhombencephalon.**

D. At **9 weeks**
- there are recognizable human features, the face is formed, the choroid plexus and palate are developing, and the naso-oral communication is closed.
- swallowing is initiated.
- there are patent urinary pathways, the nephrons start to produce urine, the bladder communicates with the urachus, and the primitive cloaca is formed.
- the lower limbs are well developed.

E. At **10 weeks**
- **embryogenesis** ends and the embryo is a **fetus.**
- the head is large compared to the fetal body.
- the **choroid plexus** is dominant within the fetal brain.

F. At **12 weeks**
- the brain structures are well developed, the heart has four chambers, and the amnion lies close to the chorion.
- fetal biometry includes measurement of the **biparietal diameter, head circumference,** and **femur length.**
- the placenta is clearly demonstrated.

IV. OVARIES (CORPUS LUTEUM)

A. The corpus luteum develops in the ovary, producing progesterone to support the pregnancy.

B. The corpus luteum cysts can become quite large, sometimes more than 10 cm; they generally regress near the end of the first trimester.

V. CUL-DE-SAC

A. The cul-de-sac lies posterior to the uterus.

B. It is a frequent site for blood collections related to ectopic pregnancy or ruptured corpus luteum cysts.

VI. PREGNANCY FAILURE

A. **Embryo** or **fetal demise** occurs frequently in the first trimester. If 100 ova are exposed to fertilization, 84 will become zygotes, 69 will implant, 27 will abort immediately, and 42 will be clinically recognized as a pregnancy.

B. **Anembryonic pregnancy** (previously called **blighted ovum**) is seen sonographically as a large or small sac with irregular borders and no identifiable embryo or yolk sac.

C. There are several different forms of **abortion.**
1. A **therapeutic abortion** is an elective termination.
2. A **threatened abortion** is bleeding and cramping in the first trimester with a fetus that is still viable.
3. An **inevitable abortion** (i.e., pending abortion) is identified by cervical dilation, gestational sac movement toward the cervix, and rupture of membranes with no chance of pregnancy survival.
4. A **missed abortion** is retention of a dead embryo.
5. **Habitual abortions** are repeated spontaneous abortions.
6. A **complete abortion,** or **spontaneous abortion,** is a spontaneous loss of the pregnancy in the first trimester.

VII. ECTOPIC PREGNANCY

- occurs when the blastocyst implants anywhere other than the endometrial lining at the fundus of the uterus.
- occurs in 1.4% of pregnancies in the United States.
- typically presents between 5 and 6 weeks.

A. **Ectopic sites** (Figure 14–3) include the
- **ampullary (widest) portion of the fallopian tube,** which is the most frequent site.
- **isthmus.**
- **fimbria.**
- **cornual area** (i.e., the interstitial area in the wall of the uterus), which is a dangerous site because of the potential for massive hemorrhage. Ectopic pregnancies in the cornual area present later than most

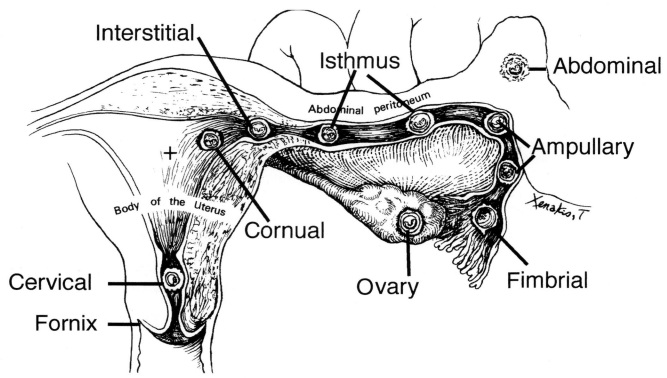

FIGURE 14-3 Possible sites for ectopic pregnancy. Note that the type of ectopic pregnancy is named after its site. The fornix is the structure in which the vaginal probe is normally placed. The fornices are very distendible, so the end of the vaginal probe can be at miduterine level. (Reprinted with permission from Sanders RC: *Clinical Sonography,* 3rd ed. Philadelphia, Lippincott, 1998, p 86.)

ectopic pregnancies (i.e., at approximately 8 weeks).
- **cervix** (i.e., cervical pregnancy), which is a dangerous site because of the potential for massive hemorrhage. Cervical pregnancies present later than most ectopic pregnancies.
- **ovary,** which is a very rare site.
- **abdominal cavity** (i.e., abdominal pregnancy), which presents much later because it is not confined by a tube or the uterus. The placenta implants on peritoneum and cannot be removed without massive bleeding. Diagnosis is difficult because the uterus will be seen between the bladder and the pregnancy; the myometrium is not seen around the fetus as is usual.

B. Risk factors for ectopic pregnancy include
- pelvic inflammatory disease.
- intrauterine contraceptive devices.
- history of fallopian tube surgery.
- assisted reproductive technologies.
- multiparity.
- advanced maternal age.

C. Clinical features of ectopic pregnancy include
- lower abdominal pain.
- abnormal vaginal bleeding.
- an adnexal mass (i.e., on gynecologic examination).
- amenorrhea.
- cervical tenderness.

D. Laboratory values—biochemical markers
1. β-HCG levels double every 2 days in a normal pregnancy but usually plateau, decrease slowly, or increase slowly in an ectopic pregnancy.
2. If a β-HCG level greater than 1000–1500 IS units is found with no intrauterine pregnancy on endovaginal examination, an ectopic pregnancy is probably present.

E. Sonographic findings
1. Most cases referred as possible ectopic pregnancies are actually intrauterine pregnancies. An enlarged uterus with a thick endometrial cavity and no evidence of intrauterine pregnancy is typical of ectopic pregnancy. Additional findings that indicate ectopic pregnancy include
   - a mass in the adnexa that is usually composed of blood.
   - the **adnexal ring sign,** which is a gestational sac–like appearance in the adnexa.
   - an **extrauterine embryo with heart motion.**
   - **fluid in the posterior cul-de-sac** with

internal echoes, which indicates rupture or leakage of blood and usually requires urgent surgery.
- **fluid in Morison's pouch or in paracolic gutters,** which is also a sign of rupture.
- low-resistance flow on pulsed wave Doppler that is similar to the low-resistance flow seen with a corpus luteum.

2. If no viable fetal pole or yolk sac is visible, distinction of a gestational sac from a decidual cast is necessary.

    a. A true **gestational sac** has a double decidual outline consisting of
- an inner ring (decidua capsularis and chorion laeve).
- an outer ring (decidua vera).
- a fluid-filled chorionic cavity in the center.

    b. A **decidual cast** resulting from ectopic pregnancy has a single decidual outline and often contains echogenic blood.

3. **Chronic ectopic pregnancies** are seen as complex masses in the adnexa and result from numerous leaks of blood into a walled-off area. No viable fetus is present.

VIII. SONOGRAPHIC EXAMINATION IN THE FIRST TRIMESTER (based on guidelines from the American College of Radiology, American Institute of Ultrasound in Medicine, and American College of Obstetricians and Gynecologists)

- Scanning may be done transabdominally, provided all of the following information is obtained; it may be necessary to do an endovaginal scan when possible.

    A. Location of the gestational sac

    B. Presence of embryo and crown-rump length
- If no embryo is seen, gestational sac measurements can be used to determine age.
- Late in the first trimester, it may be possible to use biparietal diameter and femur measurements.

    C. Presence or absence of fetal life
- Real-time ultrasonography is imperative; if the embryo is not yet seen, follow up may be required.

    D. Fetal number

    E. Evaluation of uterus (including cervix) and adnexal structures
- The location and size of any myomas or adnexal masses should be recorded.

CHAPTER 15

SECOND AND THIRD TRIMESTERS (NORMAL ANATOMY) (8%-12%)

I. BASIC GUIDELINES FOR OBSTETRIC SONOGRAMS (based on criteria from the American College of Radiology, American Institute of Ultrasound in Medicine, and American College of Obstetricians and Gynecologists)

    A. Obstetric sonograms can be used to evaluate
- the number of embryos and fetuses.
- fetal position.
- embryonic and fetal cardiac activity.
- amniotic fluid volume.
- placental position and appearance.
- fetal cord insertion and number of vessels in the cord.
- measurements, including biparietal diameter, head circumference, femur length, and abdominal circumference.
- the ovaries and adnexa.

    B. A **basic survey of fetal anatomy** should include (but is not necessarily limited to) evaluation of the
- kidneys.
- bladder.
- stomach.
- heart (four-chamber view).
- cerebral ventricles.
- cerebellum and cisterna magna.
- spine (transverse and sagittal views).
- diaphragm (not currently included in the criteria of the American Institute of Ultrasound in Medicine).

    C. A **targeted fetal anatomy survey** is performed if an abnormality is suspected. Based on the suspected abnormality, additional structures examined may include the
- orbits.
- profile.
- nostrils.
- lips and palate.
- outflow tracts of the heart.
- liver.
- clavicles.
- genitalia.
- limb bones (including measurement).
- feet and hands.
- nuchal region.
- cord insertion into the placenta.
- cervix.

    D. Scanning is usually performed with a fully distended maternal bladder, although this is not essential after approximately 20 weeks.

II. EVALUATION OF ANATOMY

    A. Cranium
- Important structures to visualize include all of the following:
  1. Cerebellum
  2. Cisterna magna
  3. Lateral and third ventricles
  4. Cavum septi pellucidi
  5. Cerebral peduncles
  6. Thalamus
  7. Choroid plexus

    B. Spine
  1. The entire spine is demonstrated; however, the spinal cord normally ends at L2. L5-S1 is located at the superior margin of the iliac crest, where the spine angles posteriorly.
  2. The spine is examined in a coronal, sagittal, and transverse axis.

3. Images are obtained of the cervical, thoracic, and lumbosacral areas.

C. Heart (Figure 15–1)

1. A normal four-chamber view of the heart excludes the majority of cardiac abnormalities.
2. The addition of the **left ventricular and right ventricular outflow tracts** may exclude anomalies such as transposition of the great vessels.
3. The apex of the heart should point to the fetal left side at a 45° angle. The right and left sides of the heart should be about equal in size; however, the right side is often slightly larger than the left side.
4. A normal heart rate and rhythm (i.e., 100–180 bpm) should be documented using M-mode.
5. It is common to see fetal heart slowing if the fetal thorax is compressed by the transducer.

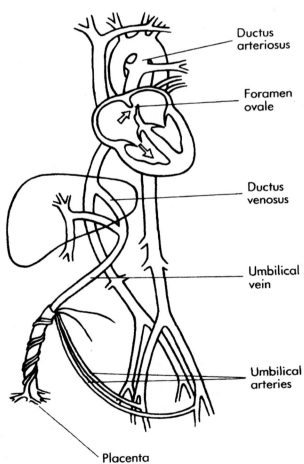

FIGURE 15-1 Diagram of fetal circulation. Blood from the umbilical vein is shunted through the ductus venosus to the right atrium and then across the foramen ovale to the left atrium. Blood returns to the placenta via the two umbilical arteries. (Reprinted with permission from Rumack CM, Wilson SR, Charboneau JW: *Diagnostic Ultrasound,* vol 2. St. Louis, Mosby, 1998, p 1127.)

6. Fetal circulation differs from the circulation after birth. Because the lungs in the fetus do not exchange oxygen, they do not need the large oxygenated blood supply that is required after birth.

a. Fetal oxygen is supplied by blood perfusion from the placenta through the umbilical vein and left portal vein, which connects to the right atrium through the ductus venosus and inferior vena cava.
b. Most of the oxygenated blood flows from the right atrium, through the foramen ovale (i.e., a hole in the atrial septum), and into the left atrium. Subsequently, it enters the left ventricle and is passed to the aorta and fetal brain.
c. Poorly oxygenated blood from the inferior vena cava and superior vena cava also enters the right atrium, and is preferentially sent to the right ventricle and pulmonary artery.
d. Most of the poorly oxygenated blood shunts through the ductus arteriosus, which connects the pulmonary artery and aorta. The blood is conveyed via the descending aorta to the umbilical arteries, which arise from the iliac arteries. The blood then returns to the placenta by way of the cord.
e. The ductus arteriosus, ductus venosus, and foramen ovale close when the cord is clamped after birth.

D. Thorax

1. The diaphragm is seen as a curved, echogenic line that separates the liver and lungs.
2. The lungs are usually more echogenic than the liver.

E. Abdomen

1. **Gastrointestinal**

a. The **liver**
   – is a right-sided organ that contains the umbilical vein, which becomes the left portal vein.
   – is relatively larger in a fetus than in a child.
b. The **spleen**
   – is located posteriorly, lateral to the stomach.
   – is seen sonographically at approximately 18 weeks.
c. The **gallbladder**
   – forms at 7 weeks.
   – is seen sonographically by 20 weeks.
   – lies to the right of the portal (umbilical) vein.
d. The **stomach**
   – is a fluid-filled structure that varies in size and shape. The fetus swallows

amniotic fluid, which fills the stomach.
- can be seen starting at approximately 12 weeks.
- must be demonstrated on every scan.

2. Genitourinary

a. The **kidneys**
- develop in the pelvis and migrate up to their retroperitoneal location.
- excrete urine into the fetal bladder, then into the amniotic fluid. Diminished urine production results in oligohydramnios after 15–18 weeks.
- can be seen starting at approximately 14 weeks.
- Fetal kidneys have less sinus fat than they will later in life.
- A mild degree of pelvic dilation (i.e., 43 mm or less) is accepted as a normal variant.

b. The **bladder**
- appears as a fluid-filled structure in the pelvis.
- fills and empties approximately every 30–60 minutes.
- can be seen starting at approximately 12–14 weeks.

- is bordered by the two umbilical arteries.
- must be demonstrated on every scan.

c. The **genitalia**
- can be seen reliably starting at approximately 16 weeks.
- The testicles descend into the scrotum at 28 weeks.

F. Extremities

1. The limbs, hands, and feet can be measured beginning at 12–13 weeks.

2. The limbs are formed by 10 weeks.

G. Fetal position

1. The head-first position is normal.

   a. If the back of the head is first, it is a **vertex (or cephalic) presentation.**

   b. If the front of the head is first, it is a **face presentation.**

2. If the fetal rump is the presenting part, it is a **breech presentation.**

   a. If the legs are extended, it is an **extended breech presentation.**

   b. If the legs are flexed, it is a **flexed breech presentation.**

3. If the shoulder is the presenting part, it is a **shoulder presentation.** This is a dangerous presentation that results in dystocia.

CHAPTER 16

PLACENTA (1%–5%)

I. DEVELOPMENT

– The placenta begins to develop early in the first trimester and contains two components.

  A. The larger portion, the **chorion frondosum,** is derived from the **blastocyst** (i.e., the fetal portion).

  B. The portion adjacent to the endometrium evolves from the **decidua basalis** (i.e., the maternal portion).

II. POSITION

  A. The placenta may be located in many normal variant positions, including
– anterior.
– posterior.
– right.
– left.
– fundal.
– any combination of the previous positions.

  B. If the placenta overlies the internal os of the cervix, it is called a **placenta previa** (see VII A).

III. ANATOMY

  A. The placenta is organized into lobules called **cotyledons** (Figure 16–1).

  B. A normal placenta weighs between 450 and 550 g.

  C. The placenta has a diameter of 16–20 cm. Normally, the anteroposterior thickness is less than 4 cm.

  D. There are several normal anatomical variants.
    1. Venous lakes are hypoechoic areas with slow vascular flow. Apart from a questionable relationship to increased α-fetoprotein, they are of no clinical significance.
    2. Subchorionic fibrin deposits appear sonographically as cystic areas just be-

neath the chorionic plate. They are of no clinical importance.
    3. Transient myometrial contractions may be confused with retroplacental problems [e.g., myomas (fibroids), hematomas] or with placenta previa. If one rescans after approximately 20 minutes, a myometrial contraction will show a change in shape, size, or location.

IV. MEMBRANES

  A. The **amnion** and **chorion** may be normally separated by fluid in the extracelomic space until approximately 15–16 weeks.

  B. Apparent membranes in the amnion may include elevated amnion, amniotic bands, amniotic sheets, remnants of a resorbed twin, and marginal bleeds.
    1. An **elevated amnion** (i.e., **chorioamniotic separation**) results in a collection of blood or amniotic fluid between the chorion and amnion.
    – It can be the result of an amniocentesis.
    – Although an elevated amnion is usually of no consequence, it can be associated with prematurity.
    2. Amniotic bands are seen in 1 in approximately 1300 live births and are thought to represent a disruption of the amnion at approximately 5 weeks.
    – Fetal contact with the chorion or entrapment of the limbs, trunk, or head by amniotic bands may result in **limb amputation, encephalocele,** or **limb/body wall complex.**
    3. Amniotic sheets result from preexisting synechiae; amnion and chorion surround the synechiae, creating open-ended cavities.
    – These membranous sheets do not in-

Uterine wall

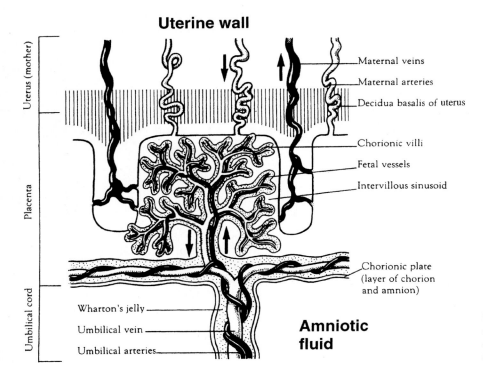

Maternal veins
Maternal arteries
Decidua basalis of uterus
Chorionic villi
Fetal vessels
Intervillous sinusoid
Chorionic plate
(layer of chorion
and amnion)

Wharton's jelly
Umbilical vein
Umbilical arteries

**Amniotic
fluid**

Uterus (mother)
Placenta
Umbilical cord

FIGURE 16-1 Diagram showing the composition of a cotyledon and the exchange process across the placental barrier.

volve the fetus because the amnion stays intact.

4. **Remnants of a resorbed twin** appear as a small sac that remains adjacent to the normal sac. The sac may contain a dead fetus.
5. **Marginal bleeds** occur adjacent to the placenta.
   – A membrane parallel to the uterine wall and adjacent to the placenta may represent a marginal bleed from large maternal vessels at the edge of the placenta.
   – Because it contains blood, there are more echoes in the walled-off area than in true amniotic fluid. These echoes may not be appreciated unless the gain is raised; therefore, the border of the bleed may be confused with an amniotic membrane at standard gain settings.

V. UMBILICAL CORD

A. A normal umbilical cord contains two arteries and one vein. Approximately 1% of patients have a two-vessel cord with only one umbilical artery. This finding may be isolated and of no clinical importance, or it may be associated with chromosomal or fetal abnormalities.

B. The vessels within the cord are surrounded by Wharton's jelly.

C. The cord insertion into the placenta should be central. If it inserts at one edge and into the membranes (i.e., a **velamentous inser-**

tion), growth may be poor, and a c-section indicated.

D. Allantoic cysts occur where the cord enters the fetal abdomen. Cysts at other sites in the cord are associated with chromosomal anomalies.

VI. ABRUPTION

– is a bleed between the placenta and the myometrium or on the amniotic surface of the placenta.
– is an obstetric emergency because severe maternal hemorrhage may occasionally result in fetal or maternal death.
– Marginal bleeds (see IV B 5) are more common, but have less clinical importance.

A. Risk factors for placental abruption include
   – high blood pressure.
   – cocaine use.
   – cigarette smoking.
   – previous history of abruption.
   – trauma.
   – a leiomyoma.
   – placenta previa.

B. Clinical features include
   – severe pain.
   – vaginal bleeding.

C. Sonographic findings
1. Cystic, complex, or hypoechoic areas may be seen between the placental substance and the uterine wall.

2. The hematoma may be isoechoic with the myometrium or placental tissue.

VII. PREVIA

A. Placenta previa
 – occurs when the placenta implants on the internal os of the cervix.
 1. Types of placenta previa (Figure 16–2)
  a. Marginal previa: placenta is adjacent to the internal os
  b. Partial previa: placenta covers a portion of the internal os
   – Partial previa is indistinguishable from marginal previa in practice.
  c. Total or central previa: placenta completely covers the internal os
  d. Low-lying placenta: placenta is close to the os, but does not cover any of it.
   – This is not a placenta previa because it does not prevent vaginal delivery.
 2. Clinical features
  a. Painless vaginal bleeding in the second and third trimesters is the classic symptom.
  b. Placenta previa is often asymptomatic.
 3. Sonographic findings
  a. The examination should be done with an **empty bladder** because the cervix appears spuriously lengthened by a full bladder and a false placenta previa may be created.
  b. The cervix often cannot be seen adequately with an empty bladder from a transabdominal approach.
  c. The cervix can be adequately visualized using a **translabial,** a **transperineal,** or, preferably, an **endovaginal** approach.
  d. A placenta previa seen in the second trimester usually **"migrates"** away from the internal os on follow-up scans. This apparent change in position is principally the result of the differential growth of the uterus, which mostly takes place in the lower uterus and cervix.

B. Vasa previa with **velamentous cord insertion**
 – occurs when the fetal vessels from the placenta cross between the internal cervical os and the presenting fetal part.
 – Color flow Doppler is helpful in diagnosing this rare and dangerous condition.

VIII. MASSES AND LESIONS

A. Chorioangioma
 – is a benign, vascular tumor seen in 1% of placentas.
 1. Sonographic findings
  a. Chorioangiomas vary from homogeneous and solid to hypoechoic and cystic.
  b. They are highly vascular, containing many arterial vessels.
 2. Complications of large chorioangiomas include
  – polyhydramnios.
  – fetal hydrops, which is a rare complication that occurs when increased blood supply to the tumor results in decreased

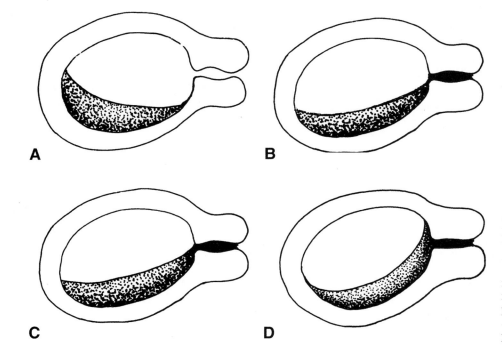

A **B** **C** **D**

FIGURE 16–2 The types of placenta previa. (*A*) Low-lying—abutting on the internal os but not covering it. (*B*) Partial—extending to the internal os. (*C*) Marginal—just covering the internal os. (*D*) Total—completely covering the internal os. (Reprinted with permission from Sanders RC: *Clinical Sonography*, 3rd ed. Philadelphia, Lippincott, 1998, p 110.)

blood supply to the fetus, leading to fetal anemia.

B. A **succenturiate lobe**
- is an accessory lobe of placental tissue connected to the primary placenta by blood vessels.
- is an important diagnosis because postpartum hemorrhage and infection can occur if the succenturiate lobe is left in the uterus.
- can cover the internal cervical os and form a placenta previa.
- If the vessels connecting the main placenta and the accessory lobe cross the internal os, vessel rupture during delivery can occur.

IX. MATURITY AND GRADING

A. **Placental calcification**
1. Approximately 10% of placentas develop intraplacental calcification.
2. Extensive calcification seen before 36 weeks may indicate **intrauterine growth restriction.**
3. Significant placental calcification is probably an indication that the fetal lungs are mature.

B. **Placental grading**
- is a well-known system that has minimal clinical significance.
1. Grade 0: no calcifications
2. Grade 1: scattered calcifications
3. Grade 2: basal calcifications
4. Grade 3: basal and interlobar septal calcifications

X. DOPPLER

A. Doppler measurement of the **umbilical artery,** taken in the cord, is a way of assessing fetal well-being. Normally, there is considerable diastolic flow.

B. The ratio of systolic to diastolic flow (i.e., the **S/D ratio**) can be obtained. Absence of diastolic flow is associated with fetal sickness.

C. **Middle cerebral artery** flow can also be analyzed with Doppler in at-risk fetuses.
1. Normally, there is high-resistance flow with little diastolic flow.
2. Fetal sickness is associated with increased diastolic flow.

XI. PHYSIOLOGY

A. The fetus is supplied with oxygen and nutrients through the umbilical vein by a complex exchange system between the maternal and fetal circulations across the placental barrier.

B. The maternal and fetal circulations surround each other, and the exchange takes place across the chorionic villi (see Figure 16–1). There is no intermixing of fetal and maternal blood.

C. Deoxygenated blood and waste products exit the fetus via the two umbilical arteries.

XII. ACCRETA

- Placenta **accreta, increta,** and **percreta** represent varying degrees of growth of placental villi into the myometrium, usually at the site of a previous cesarean section incision.

A. **Sonographic findings**
1. There is local thinning of the myometrium at the cesarean section site.
2. Perpendicularly aligned intraplacental vessels can be seen adjacent to the involved area. These are better demonstrated on color flow.
3. Vessels may extend into the bladder wall with placenta percreta, the most severe variety.

B. The major complication of all three conditions is **retained placental tissue with massive bleeding at delivery,** often necessitating hysterectomy.

CHAPTER 17

ASSESSMENT OF GESTATIONAL AGE (2%-6%)

I. GESTATIONAL SAC

A. To determine the mean sac diameter, add length by width by height and divide by 3.

B. Gestational sac measurements are relatively inaccurate (i.e., +/− 2 weeks).

II. EMBRYONIC SIZE/CROWN-RUMP LENGTH (CRL)

– is used between approximately 5 and 12 weeks; fetal position is too variable to use after 12–13 weeks.

A. Measure the embryo from head to rump.

B. CRL is the preferred technique in the first trimester because its accuracy is +/− 5 days.

III. BIPARIETAL DIAMETER (BPD)

– is obtainable starting at approximately 12 weeks.

A. Obtain the measurement from an axial plane.

B. Measure from the outer soft tissue surface near the transducer to the inner margin of the opposite side of the skull (i.e., leading edge to leading edge). Landmarks that should be included are the
  – falx (midline structure).
  – thalamus.
  – third ventricle.
  – cavum septi pellucidi.

C. The BPD is inaccurate if
  – the measurement is taken in an oblique plane.
  – the scanning plane is too high or too low in the fetal head.
  – the fetal head is dolichocephalic or brachycephalic.

IV. FEMUR LENGTH (FL)

– is usable starting at approximately 12 weeks.

A. Measure from the neck of the femur to the distal end of the femoral condyle, excluding the epiphysis.

B. FL is less affected by intrauterine growth restriction than other measurements.

V. ABDOMINAL CIRCUMFERENCE (AC)

– is useful from about 15 weeks gestational age on; it is used in conjunction with the BPD and the FL to obtain fetal weight estimates.

A. To obtain the AC, measure the circumference of the abdomen, or average the lateral and anteroposterior diameters and multiply by 1.57.

B. The AC measurements are obtained at a level that includes the
  – fetal stomach.
  – spine.
  – umbilical portion of the left portal vein.
  – aorta.
  – adrenal glands (but not the kidneys).
  – symmetrical ribs.

C. Always remember the following pitfalls when determining the AC.
  1. An oblique view will give an inaccurate measurement.
  2. A flattened appearance may be the result of excessive transducer pressure.
  3. If the measurement is taken at an incor-

rect level (e.g., including the kidneys), the result will be suboptimal.

D. A combination of the AC, BPD, and FL is compared to a scale to allow the estimation of weight, which is expressed as a percentile. The 90th and 10th percentiles are the upper and lower limits of normal.

VI. HEAD CIRCUMFERENCE (HC)

– This measurement is used in addition to the BPD because it is not dependent on the shape for accuracy. It will give a usable measurement even if the head is long and thin (dolichocephaly) or short and broad (brachycephaly).

A. Use the same image that was used to determine the BPD.

B. Measure the circumference of the head, or add the BPD and occipital frontal diameter (OFD) and multiply by 1.57.

C. Measurements are taken from the outer edges of the cranial interface.

VII. TRANSCEREBELLAR MEASUREMENTS

– Transcerebellar measurements are an additional method of dating the pregnancy in the second trimester.

A. Measure the transverse diameter of the cerebellum at the level of the cerebellar hemispheres in an axial plane.

B. Until approximately 20 weeks, the transcerebellar measurement (in mm) is approximately equivalent to gestational age.

C. Transcerebellar measurement is useful when the BPD is distorted (e.g., by an intracranial cyst).

VIII. OCULAR MEASUREMENTS

– Measurements related to the eyes are used when there is a possible facial anomaly.

A. Binocular measurements are measured in an axial plane that is inferior to the BPD.

B. **Binocular distance** is from the outer margin of one orbit to the outer margin of the other orbit.

C. **Interocular distance** between the orbits is measured from the inner orbit to the other inner orbit. This is the measurement most helpful in the diagnosis of hyper- or hypotelorism (i.e., a large or small distance between the eyes).

IX. CEPHALIC INDEX (CI)

– is used to confirm an impression that the head shape is long and thin or short and wide.

A. CI is used to correct for a **brachycephalic** (too wide and short) or **dolichocephalic** (too long and narrow) head.

B. CI is calculated by dividing the BPD by the OFD and multiplying by 100.

C. A normal CI is between 70% and 85%.

X. FETAL LUNG MATURITY

– cannot be established with ultrasound.

A. Fetal lung maturity can be assumed to be present if the fetus is 38 weeks or greater.

B. If the fetus is less than 38 weeks and delivery is contemplated, lung maturity can be established by performing an amniocentesis and analyzing the lecithin/sphingomyelin (L/S) ratio.

XI. OTHER

A. **Lateral ventricular width**
  1. Obtain a view of the lateral ventricles on an axial view, superior to the BPD.
  2. Measure atrium diameter near the posterior portion of the fetal head, at the posterior end of the choroid plexus.
  3. A lateral ventricular width **less than 11 mm** is normal.

B. **Cisterna magna**
  1. The cisterna magna is measured on the same inferiorly angled axial view that shows the cerebellum.
  2. The cisterna magna distance, from cerebellum to skull, is normally **less than 10 mm but greater than 2 mm.**

C. **Nuchal fold**
  – measurement is useful at approximately 15–21 weeks to determine if the fetus is at risk for **Down syndrome** and other anomalies.
  1. The nuchal fold is measured on the same plane as the view of the cerebellum.
  2. Measure from the outer skull to the outer skin surface. **Less than 6 mm** is normal.
  3. Between 11 and 13 weeks, nuchal translucency is measured on a sagittal view at the back of the neck. A measurement of **3 mm or more** is abnormal.

CHAPTER 18

COMPLICATIONS (6%-10%)

I. INTRAUTERINE GROWTH RESTRICTION (IUGR)

- The diagnosis of IUGR is made when a fetus **weighs below the 10th percentile or is less than 2500 g at 36 weeks' gestation.**
- Small for gestational age (SGA) is a term used for small neonates who are not premature.

A. Causes

1. **Maternal characteristics** associated with growth-restricted fetuses include
   - poor nutrition.
   - substance abuse, particularly smoking.
   - heart conditions.
   - diabetes.
   - history of an SGA fetus.
   - chronic renal disease.
   - age (i.e., younger than 17 years of age or older than 35 years of age).
   - high altitude.
   - irradiation.
2. **Placental reasons** for IUGR include
   - placental ischemia and infarcts.
   - abruption.
3. **Fetal causes** of IUGR include
   - intrauterine infections (**TORCH: t**oxoplasmosis, **r**ubella, **c**ytomegalic inclusion disease, **h**erpes simplex).
   - chromosomal anomalies.
   - multiple gestation.
   - other congenital anomalies.

B. Sonographic findings

1. In IUGR, abdominal circumference is smaller than the 10th percentile for known dates.
   - The liver is the first structure to decrease in size if intrauterine nutrition is inadequate.
2. If no earlier scan or reliable dating is available, growth between sonograms will establish the diagnosis (i.e., the fetus will grow less than expected during the known interval).
3. If the liver size and abdominal circumference are the only measurements that are small, **asymmetrical IUGR** is diagnosed. If all measurements are small, the IUGR is considered **symmetrical.**
   - There is a weak association between symmetrical IUGR and chronic causes (e.g., maternal cardiac failure).
   - Abrupt-onset causes (e.g., placental infarction) are more often associated with asymmetrical IUGR.
4. **Oligohydramnios** is normally seen in IUGR.
5. A **grade 3 placenta** seen before 36 weeks may be an indicator of IUGR.
6. Look hard for additional findings because there are many causes of IUGR.

C. Biophysical profile

- Fetuses with IUGR are followed with biophysical profile tests to assess well-being.
1. **Indications** for biophysical profile testing in IUGR include
   - maternal diabetes.
   - umbilical cord abnormalities.
   - fetal anomalies.
   - history of previous fetal demise.
   - maternal hypertension.
2. **Scoring system**
   a. The patient should be scanned approximately 1 hour after eating, if feasible. Scanning is performed for 30 minutes.
   b. **Five variables** are observed. Each variable is assigned a score of 2 points if present and 0 points if absent.

– **Fetal breathing** is given a score of 2 if breathing is seen for 30 seconds during a 30-minute examination.
– **Fetal motion** is given a score of 2 if there are at least three gross movements (trunk and limbs) in 30 minutes.
– **Fetal tone** is given a score of 2 if there is at least one episode of opening and closing of the hand or rolling movement of the trunk in 30 minutes.
– **Amniotic fluid volume** is given a score of 2 if there is a space larger than 2 cm in vertical diameter.
– **Heart rate,** determined by a **nonstress test (NST),** is given a score of 2 if there are at least two accelerations of 15 bpm, each lasting at least 15 seconds, during a 20-minute examination. Each acceleration must be accompanied by fetal movement.

3. **Score interpretation**
   a. A score of 8 (10 with NST) is considered normal.
   b. A score of 4–6 (6–8 with NST) is an indication to repeat the test in 24 hours.
   c. A score of 0–2 (2–4 with NST) is very suspicious for possible chronic asphyxia.

D. **Doppler flow studies**
1. The **umbilical cord** has three vessels, **one vein** to transport oxygen and nutrients to the fetus and **two smaller arteries** to return blood to the placenta.
2. **Umbilical artery pulsed Doppler** gives information about placental resistance. It is performed in at-risk fetuses in the third trimester, particularly if the biophysical profile score is low.
   a. Normally, there is considerable diastolic flow in the umbilical artery.
   b. As placental resistance increases, less diastolic flow is seen and flow reversal in diastole may occur.
   c. Absence of diastolic flow in the umbilical artery is considered ominous.
3. Sampling of the **middle cerebral artery** is performed when diastolic flow is decreased or absent in the umbilical artery.
   a. Normally, little diastolic flow is seen in the middle cerebral artery.
   b. Increased diastolic flow in the middle cerebral artery is an ominous finding.
4. If too much transducer pressure is placed on the fetal head there may be decreased flow in diastole.

E. **Chromosomal analysis** may be indicated if IUGR
– is very severe.

– occurs at an early gestational age.
– is associated with polyhydramnios.

F. **Postpartum complications** of IUGR include
– hypoglycemia.
– acidosis.
– asphyxia.
– meconium aspiration.
– hyperthermia.

II. MULTIPLE GESTATION

A. **Epidemiology**
1. Multiple pregnancy is increasing in frequency because of the impact of assisted reproductive technology.
2. If unaltered by infertility therapy
   – twins occur in 1 in 85 normal births.
   – triplets occur in 1 in 7500 normal births.
   – quadruplets occur in 1 in 670,000 normal births.
   – quintuplets occur in 1 in 41,600,000 normal births.
3. In the United States, twins are seen most frequently in African Americans and least frequently in Asians.

B. **Forms of multiple pregnancy** (Table 18–1)
1. **Dizygotic dichorionic diamniotic twins**
   – comprise 65%–70% of multiple births.
   – are fraternal, nonidentical twins.
   – are the result of fertilization of two separate ova by two different sperm.
   – have an inherited predisposition to fraternal twins.
   – **Sonographic findings**
   a. There is a thick membrane with four components: two amnions and two chorions.
   b. The finding of different genders confirms the diagnosis.
   c. Placental tissue can be seen entering the base of the intersac membranes (twin peak sign).
   d. Two placentas may be seen, but they may lie adjacent to each other and appear as one.
   e. If twins are seen in the first trimester and one later dies, the sac disappears (**vanishing twin**).
   f. After the demise of a twin in the second trimester, the dead twin may persist as a **fetus papyraceous.**
2. **Monozygotic monochorionic diamniotic twins**
   – result from the fertilization of one ovum that divides into two zygotes.
   – are always the same gender because they are identical twins.
   – There is one chorion and two amnions. Therefore, a thin intervening septum

TABLE 18–1	Types of Twins			
Type	**Day of Division**	**Placental Number**	**Amniotic Membrane Number in Septum**	**Complications**
Dizygotic diamniotic dichorionic (70%)	1	2	4	IUGR
Monozygotic diamniotic dichorionic (6%)	3	2	4	IUGR
Monozygotic monochorionic diamniotic (23%)	4–8	1	2	Stuck twin syndrome, twin-to-twin transfusion syndrome
Monozygotic monochorionic monoamniotic (2%)	8–13	1	0	Twisted cords, locking twins, twin-to-twin transfusion syndrome
Acardiac parabiotic (TRAP)	8–13	1	2	"Pump" twin, hydrops
Conjoined	8–13	1	0	

IUGR = intrauterine growth retardation; TRAP = twin-reversed arterial perfusion sequence.

with two membranous components (one on either side) can be seen.

  – The placenta is shared if the division occurs between 4 and 8 days postconception. If the division is within the first 3 days of conception, there may be two chorions (a rare event).

3. Monochorionic monoamniotic twins
  – result from a late division at 7–13 days.
  – are rare (i.e., less than 1% of twins).
  – There is a shared amniotic and chorionic sac with a single cavity for both twins.

C. Complications of multiple pregnancy
  – All forms of twins have a higher incidence of IUGR.
  1. Syndromes related to monochorionic diamniotic or monoamniotic twins
    a. Twin-to-twin transfusion syndrome (also called **placental steal** syndrome)
      – Large arteriovenous anastomoses connect the twins' circulations in a shared placenta.
      – The recipient twin becomes large and may develop hydrops.
      – The donor twin is small and anemic and usually has features of IUGR.
      – If one twin dies, emboli can cross into the other twin's circulation and cause infarcts.
    b. Stuck twin syndrome
      – occurs in monochorionic diamniotic twins. Although it can occur in dichorionic diamniotic twins, in which one twin has an anomaly causing oligohydramnios (e.g., renal anomaly), it is much less frequent.
      – is usually the result of severe twin-to-twin transfusion syndrome.
      – Amniotic fluid around the growth-restricted fetus disappears and the fetus appears "shrink-wrapped" by the sac membrane. This fetus is stuck in

one site, even when the mother's position changes.
      – Severe polyhydramnios develops around the larger twin.
      – The syndrome is usually treated with serial, large-volume amniocenteses. Without treatment it is usually fatal.
    c. Acardiac parabiotic twins [also called twin-reversed arterial perfusion sequence (TRAP) and acardiac acephalic twins]
      – There is a normal "pump" fetus and an acardiac fetus (without a heart).
      – The head and upper extremities of the acardiac twin are malformed or absent. Despite the absence of a heart, leg movement is seen. Grossly thickened skin, often with cystic hygromas, is present in half of the trunk. There is a reversed circulation in which the arteries of the "pump" twin supply oxygenated blood to the acardiac fetus.
      – The "pump" twin may become edematous and hydropic.
  2. Syndromes specific to monochorionic monoamniotic twins
    a. Cord entanglement
      – With no intervening membrane, cord twisting is common, resulting in abrupt fetal death in approximately 50% of cases.
    b. Increased risk of malposition (i.e., **locking twins**)
      – The limbs of the twins become intertwined so the fetuses have to be delivered together.
    c. Conjoined twins
      – are the result of a late division (i.e., 13 days or more postconception).
      – Thoracopagus (i.e., twins joined in the thoracic region) is most common.
      – This syndrome is very rare and is usually lethal.

III. MATERNAL ILLNESS

A. **Diabetes mellitus**
   – is a familial disease.
   – Insulin deficiency causes excess sugar in the urine and blood.
   1. **Grading of diabetes**
      – is based on its severity.
      a. **Gestational diabetes mellitus (type A)** is acquired during pregnancy. It affects 2%–3% of pregnancies and usually leads to **macrosomnia.** It is detected with a **glucose tolerance test** in the second half of the pregnancy.
      b. **Insulin-dependent diabetes (type B, C, D, F, R, or H, depending on complications)** is a more severe, preexisting problem that requires treatment with injected insulin. It is often associated with **IUGR** and is more likely to be associated with congenital malformations.
      c. **Non–insulin-dependent diabetes** is the most common form of diabetes mellitus. It is most common in Native Americans and can be controlled by diet alone.
   2. **Sonographic findings**
      a. **Macrosomia** with polyhydramnios is defined as a fetal weight above the 90th percentile (or 4000 g at term). Macrosomic fetuses are more difficult to deliver and suffer more postdelivery complications, such as Erb palsy (a paralyzed arm). Sonographically, macrosomia is associated with
         – skin thickening.
         – mild polyhydramnios.
         – an enlarged placenta.
      b. **IUGR** is more common in juvenile-onset diabetes.
      c. **Congenital anomalies** are more common in diabetics. The VACTERAL syndrome (**v**ertebral anomalies, **a**norectal abnormalities, **c**ardiac anomalies, **tr**acheal anomalies, **e**sophageal atresia, **r**enal abnormalities, **a**nal atresia, and **l**imb deformities) occurs in approximately 2% of the fetuses of diabetic mothers. A single umbilical artery may also be present.
   3. **Maternal diabetic complications in pregnancy** include
      – frequent urinary tract infections.
      – increased frequency of pregnancy-induced hypertension with toxemia.

B. **Pregnancy-induced hypertension**
   1. Hypertension during pregnancy is often associated with **IUGR.**
   2. **Preeclampsia** is a syndrome related to hypertension with the following components:
      – pregnancy.
      – maternal edema.
      – proteinuria.
   3. **Eclampsia** is the end stage of preeclampsia. It can be detected and treated in the preeclamptic stage. Eclampsia includes
      – very high blood pressure.
      – seizures and coma, if left untreated.
      – possible maternal and fetal demise.
      a. **Risk factors** for eclampsia include
         – an older primigravida.
         – multiple gestation.
         – chronic maternal vascular disease.
         – trophoblastic disease.
      b. **Clinical features** of eclampsia include
         – hypertension.
         – rapid onset of weight gain.
         – edema in maternal extremities.
         – proteinuria.
      c. **Sonographic findings** of eclampsia include
         – IUGR.
         – oligohydramnios.
         – placental abruptio (rare).

IV. ANTEPARTUM

A. Preterm labor, cervical incompetence, and premature rupture of fetal membranes (PROM) change the appearance of the cervix and can cause prematurity.
   1. Preterm labor
      a. The early onset of uterine contractions causes **shortening of the cervix** and **funneling** (i.e., fluid in the internal os and proximal cervical canal). Watching the cervix will show contractions enlarging the funneling intermittently.
      b. An early delivery may be induced, even if drugs such as terbutaline, a tocolytic that decreases contractions, are given.
   2. **Cervical incompetence**
      a. Spontaneous weakening and **shortening of the cervix in the absence of contractions** results in cervical incompetence. It is usually treated with a cervical suture.
      b. The cervix is examined sonographically using a translabial or endovaginal approach.
      c. Normal cervical length is approximately **3.5 cm.** Cervical incompetence reduces the length and causes funneling.
   3. **PROM**
      a. If the cervix opens sufficiently, the membranes rupture and amniotic fluid is released through the vagina.
      b. PROM is one of the causes of **anhy-**

dramnios. Therefore, unexpected severe oligohydramnios or anhydramnios is an indication to examine the cervix.

B. Rh isoimmunization

1. When the maternal blood group is Rh negative and the paternal blood group is Rh positive, the fetus may have the father's blood group. Maternal antibodies to the fetal blood develop and the fetal red blood cells are destroyed.

2. The consequent anemia occurs in the second pregnancy, and is worse in successive pregnancies. RhoGAM is normally given to prevent this problem.

3. **Sonographic findings** of Rh isoimmunization consist of the findings of
   – hydrops.
   – pleural effusion.
   – pericardial effusion.
   – ascites.
   – skin thickening.
   – an enlarged placenta.
   – polyhydramnios.

4. Treatment is by **exchange transfusion.**
   a. Under sonographic guidance, a needle is placed in the umbilical artery [i.e., cordocentesis or percutaneous umbilical blood sampling (PUBS)] are performed to determine antibody titers.
   b. If a transfusion is required, blood is injected under ultrasound guidance into the umbilical vein near its insertion into the placenta or within the liver. Sampling of the umbilical artery is a possible alternative but is associated with bradycardia and more postprocedure bleeding. If the umbilical vessels are technically inaccessible, blood can be placed in the fetal peritoneum, where it is slowly and unpredictably absorbed.
   c. There is an associated risk of fetal blood loss and fetal death with exchange transfusion.

V. FETAL THERAPY—INTRAUTERINE TRANSFUSION

– is used to correct fetal anemia.

A. Indications include
   – erythroblastosis fetalis (i.e., Rh incompatibility).
   – a fetus with an elevated bilirubin level in the amniotic fluid.
   – anemia caused by parvovirus.

B. Procedure

1. Under ultrasound guidance, a 22-gauge needle is inserted into the umbilical vein in the cord.

2. Blood of the same group as the fetus is placed in the vessel. The quantity varies with the size of the fetus.

C. Complications include
   – hemorrhage from the cord.
   – fetal death.

VI. POSTPARTUM

– The uterus, greatly enlarged by pregnancy, slowly contracts over the 6 weeks following delivery.

A. Retained products of conception
   – After delivery, echogenic material is left in the uterus.

1. If there are bony structures, echogenic material with shadowing is present.

2. More often there is placental material, which is evenly echogenic.

3. Blood is difficult to distinguish from placental, noncalcified fetal material. Color flow Doppler will show vascularity if the placenta is still attached to the myometrium.

B. Cesarean section

1. Cesarean section is usually performed by a low transverse abdominal approach with a transverse uterine incision posterior to the bladder, about 2 cm above the cervix. A classic incision is a vertical incision made in the uterine wall.

2. Complications related to the procedure may occur.
   a. Hematomas and infection can develop
      – at the uterine incision site.
      – in the broad ligament.
      – beneath the abdominal wall fascia (subfascial).
      – in the abdominal wall.
      – in the cul-de-sac or the adnexa.
      – in a flap surgically created in the bladder.
   b. A defect in the myometrium may persist at the incision site just above the cervix.

C. Infections
   – may develop in any hematoma.
   – may occur in the **endometrium** after **vaginal delivery or elective termination.**

1. Endometrial infection (endometritis) results in fluid-filled, thickened endometrium on ultrasound.

2. Clinical features of endometritis are the traditional signs associated with infection anywhere, including
   – fever.
   – leukocytosis.
   – local tenderness.

CHAPTER 19

AMNIOTIC FLUID (1%-5%)

I. CHARACTERISTICS

A. Amniotic fluid consists of 98% water and 2% solids (i.e., proteins, enzymes, urea, fetal cells, and vernix).

B. There is a 22-L exchange of fluids every 24 hours by way of the placental membranes.

C. The fetus swallows approximately 500 mL of amniotic fluid in a 24-hour period and at term is urinating up to 600 mL/day.

II. FUNCTIONS

– Protects the fetus
– Equalizes pressure
– Maintains temperature
– Allows fetal movement
– Allows symmetrical growth
– Prevents membrane adherence
– Aids lung maturity

III. ASSESSMENT

– The amount of amniotic fluid is estimated by calculating the **amniotic fluid index (AFI).**

A. The uterus is divided into four quadrants. The depth of the deepest pocket of amniotic fluid without umbilical cord or fetal parts in each quadrant is measured.

B. The four measurements are added. Normal amounts range from 5–20 cm, depending on gestational age.

C. The AFI is not an ideal technique because it does not take into account the width of the fluid pocket. Measuring the dimensions of the largest pocket is an alternative approach.

IV. POLYHYDRAMNIOS

– is an excess amount of amniotic fluid.
– results in premature labor, premature rupture of membranes, premature separation of the placenta, and a prolapsed cord.

A. Causes include
– skeletal dysplasias.
– sacrococcygeal teratoma.
– fetal central nervous system anomalies that depress swallowing (e.g., anencephaly).
– fetal gastrointestinal anomalies with obstruction.
– maternal diabetes mellitus and macrosomia.
– hydrops.
– complications of multiple gestation.
– chest masses.
– abdominal masses.
– chorioangioma.
– cardiac anomalies.
– Rh incompatibility.
– unknown (over 60%).

B. Clinical features include
– large for dates.
– maternal discomfort.
– maternal shortness of breath.

C. Sonographic findings
– Polyhydramnios is diagnosed when the **AFI measures more than 20 cm** or when the largest single fluid pocket is more than 8 cm in two diameters.

V. OLIGOHYDRAMNIOS

– is an insufficient amount of amniotic fluid.
– is seen in approximately 4% of the pregnant population.
– The amount of amniotic fluid normally diminishes in the third trimester.

A. Causes include (**DRIPPC**)
– **d**emise.
– **r**enal anomalies.
– **i**ntrauterine growth restriction.
– **p**remature rupture of membranes.

– **p**ostdates.
– **c**hromosomal anomalies.

B. Sonographic findings
1. An **AFI of less than approximately 5–10 cm,** depending on gestational age, is the threshold for oligohydramnios.
2. Severe oligohydramnios is present when there is an AFI of less than 2 cm or the largest fluid-filled space is smaller than 2 cm.

C. Complications
1. Absence of amniotic fluid (**anhydramnios**) leads to hypoplastic lungs.
2. Severe oligohydramnios may lead to fetal deformities (e.g., clubfoot, flattened facies, pulmonary hypoplasia).

CHAPTER 20

GENETIC STUDIES (1%–3%)

I. MATERNAL SERUM TESTING

A. Maternal serum α-fetoprotein (MSAFP)
  – is produced by the maternal liver and fetal tissues.
  1. Normal levels are above 0.5 and below 2.0 multiples of the median (MoM).
  2. Levels are **decreased in Down syndrome.**
  3. Levels are **increased** in a number of conditions, including
     – neural crest anomalies.
     – spina bifida (95% of cases are discovered with a threshold of approximately 2.1 MoM).
     – anencephaly.
     – encephalocele.
     – iniencephaly.
     – abdominal wall defects.
     – gastroschisis.
     – omphalocele.
     – triploidy.
     – placental masses and thickening.
     – multiple pregnancy.
     – fetal death.

B. "Triple screen"
  1. The combination of decreased **MSAFP,** decreased **estriol,** and increased **human chorionic gonadotropin** levels can be used in combination with maternal age and size to screen for trisomy 21 (Down syndrome).
  2. Sixty percent of trisomy 21 cases can be discovered with the triple screen.

II. AMNIOTIC FLUID TESTING

A. Chromosomal analysis (karyotyping)
  1. The fetal cells found in amniotic fluid can be grown in an incubator over a period of 6–21 days (usually 10 days).
  2. When examined with a microscope, an abnormal number or configuration of the chromosomes can be used to identify chromosomal anomalies.

B. Maternal amniotic fluid α-fetoprotein (MAAFP)
  – is usually more accurate in detection of anomalies than MSAFP because only fetal causes are assessed.

C. Acetylcholinesterase
  – is a protein that is elevated in the amniotic fluid in the presence of **neural crest anomalies.**
  – is mildly elevated in abdominal wall defects.

III. AMNIOCENTESIS

A. Indications include
  – an abnormal sonogram that suggests a chromosomal anomaly.
  – a woman older than 35 years of age to exclude a chromosomal anomaly.
  – follow up of abnormal triple screen results to exclude chromosomal anomaly.
  – suspected spina bifida to obtain the acetylcholinesterase level.
  – determination of the lecithin/sphingomyelin ratio in a third-trimester pregnancy to see if the fetus can be delivered with mature lungs.

B. Technique
  1. A 20- or 22-gauge needle is placed into the amniotic fluid alongside the fetus.
  2. The location, angle, and depth are guided by ultrasound.
  3. Approximately 20 cc of amniotic fluid is withdrawn and the fetus is rescanned briefly to document fetal heart activity.

C. Complications include
  – contractions, resulting in delivery.
  – intra-amniotic infection.
  – amniotic fluid leakage through the puncture site.

IV. CHORIONIC VILLI SAMPLING (CVS)

– is used in the first trimester, at approximately 10 weeks, to determine chromosomal abnormalities (e.g., trisomy 21).

A. Technique
1. Under ultrasound guidance, a small catheter is inserted into the cervix.
2. The catheter is guided into the chorion and a small sample of chorionic villi is removed.

B. Complications include
– spontaneous abortion.
– infection.
– possible limb defects.

V. DOMINANT AND RECESSIVE RISK OCCURRENCE

A. The embryo contains genes derived from both parents; these inherited characteristics are transmitted by way of the chromosomes.

B. **Chromosomes** are composed of genes.
1. There are 46 chromosomes (23 pairs) located in the nucleus of a cell.
2. The pair of sex chromosomes is normally XX (female) or XY (male).

C. **Mutations** are changes in genetic makeup.
1. Mutations are responsible for some fetal anomalies (e.g., **chromosomal abnormalities**).
2. If a mutation is compatible with life, it may be passed on to succeeding generations.
    a. **Dominant genes** have an inheritance pattern whereby 50% of children are affected if **one** parent carries the gene.
    b. **Recessive genes** have a hereditary pattern whereby 25% of children are affected if **both** parents carry the gene.
3. While most mutations are spontaneous, some are caused by radiation and environmental factors.

D. **Chromosomal abnormalities** are seen in 1 in 200 live births, and many more are found in spontaneous abortions. Five common chromosomal anomalies survive long enough to be seen on a routine obstetric ultrasound examination, and include
– Down syndrome (**trisomy 21**).
– Edwards' syndrome (**trisomy 18**).
– Patau's syndrome (**trisomy 13**).
– **Turner's syndrome** (monosomy X); a second sex chromosome is not present.
– **triploidy** (all chromosomes are triplicated).

VI. TERATOGENS

A. Teratogens are processes external to the uterus or mother that result in fetal malformations and intrauterine growth restriction.

B. Teratogens act at the time of **organogenesis,** between 4 and 10 weeks' gestation, when major structures are being formed.

C. Teratogens include
– radiation.
– heavy metals.
– drugs (e.g., antiepileptics, alcohol, nicotine).
– chemicals.

CHAPTER 21

FETAL DEMISE (0%–3%)

I. MISSED ABORTION

– is fetal death before 20 weeks' gestation with a retained fetus.

II. FETAL DEATH

– is the term used when the fetus dies after 20 weeks' gestation.

  A. Clinical features include
    – no audible fetal heart tones with a fetal stethoscope.

  B. Sonographic findings
    1. Fetal death is indicated by
      – no fetal heart motion on ultrasound examination.
      – no fetal movement on ultrasound examination.

2. Signs that appear after the fetus has been dead several days include
  – overlapping of skull bones (i.e., Spaulding's sign).
  – gas in the fetal vascular system.
  – massive skin thickening caused by edema.
  – maceration of trunk contents with loss of organ structure.
  – crunched up or extended fetal position.
  – echogenic material in the amniotic fluid.
  – Long term, a shrunken, deformed group of bones known as a fetus papyraceous may remain.
3. A fetal anomaly responsible for the fetal death may be seen.

CHAPTER 22

FETAL ABNORMALITIES (10%–15%)

I. CRANIAL ABNORMALITIES

A. Anencephaly
- is the most common open neural defect, occurring in 1 in 1000 births.
- is absence of the brain above the level of the brainstem. It is a lethal condition.
- results in a markedly increased level of maternal serum α-fetoprotein (MSAFP) because the brain is exposed.
- **Sonographic findings**
  1. The skull and scalp are absent with a mound at the top of the remaining tissue comprised of blood vessels.
  2. The orbits are prominent because the skull is absent.
  3. It is often associated with spina bifida.
  4. Polyhydramnios may be present because of the absence of fetal swallowing.

B. Ventriculomegaly
- is enlargement of the cerebral ventricles. **Hydrocephalus** is a more specific term that implies obstruction and increased pressure. Hydrocephalus would be correct when an obstruction is identified.
- The lateral ventricle is considered dilated if it is 11 mm or more in width. The third ventricle is considered dilated if it is 3 mm or more in width.
  1. **Aqueduct stenosis**
     - is enlargement of the third and lateral ventricles caused by obstruction of the aqueduct of Sylvius.
     - may develop late.
     - has a poor prognosis.
  2. **Dandy-Walker syndrome**
     - is a condition in which the fourth ventricle is obstructed and dilated. Secondary dilation of the third and lateral ventricles may occur.
     - has a poor prognosis.
     - A hypoplastic cerebellar vermis is present.
  3. **Arnold-Chiari II malformation**
     - is almost always associated with spina bifida *in utero*.
     - results in a **banana-shaped** cerebellum, which is displaced posteriorly, and a **lemon-shaped** cranium.
     - results in an absent cisterna magna because the cerebellum is pulled posteriorly and may be in the upper cervical spinal canal.
     - may cause secondary dilation of the third and lateral ventricles.
     - has a good intellectual prognosis if there are no shunt complications and the hydrocephalus is not very severe.
  4. **Cerebral atrophy**
     - results in enlarged ventricles, yet the cranial size is normal or small. There may be asymmetry of ventricular size.
     - is accompanied by inevitable mental deficiency.
     - **Microcephaly** is a form of cerebral atrophy that may or may not be associated with ventriculomegaly. If no ventriculomegaly is present, the head size needs to be at least **three standard deviations below the mean** to diagnose microcephaly.
  5. **Hydranencephaly**
     - is brain infarction with subsequent destruction of parenchyma in the frontal and parietotemporal regions.
     - is a lethal anomaly.
     - There may be complete absence of the brain above the level of the brainstem, but the skull is present.

6. Holoprosencephaly
 - is the result of failure of the prosencephalon to divide and form right and left hemispheres. Consequently, the lateral ventricles are partially or completely fused, the thalamus is fused, the third ventricle is absent, and the fused common ventricle expands into a dorsal cyst.
 - is strongly associated with midline facial malformations (e.g., cleft lip, cleft palate, hypotelorism, proboscis) and **trisomy 13** (a chromosomal anomaly).
 - There are three forms of holoprosencephaly.
 a. Alobar holoprosencephaly is the most severe form, with a large, **horseshoe-shaped** ventricle.
 b. Lobar and **semilobar** holoprosencephaly are more subtle forms, with partial separation of the ventricles.

C. Other cranial processes
 1. Arachnoid cysts
 - are intracranial cysts attached to the meninges that surround the brain.
 - have a good prognosis unless very large.
 - A retrocerebellar arachnoid cyst may be mistaken for a Dandy-Walker cyst; however, it will not separate the cerebellar lobes, just displace them as a unit.
 2. Choroid plexus cysts
 - are cysts in the choroid plexus that are seen on approximately 1 in 100 sonograms.
 - are usually an incidental finding. There is a 0.04% association with **trisomy 18.**
 - always resolve by 25 weeks' gestation.
 3. Cephaloceles and encephaloceles
 - are neural crest anomalies seen in 1 in 4000 births.
 - are associated with Meckel-Gruber syndrome (see VII C).
 - The meninges protrude through a bony defect in the skull, sometimes containing brain substance in addition to the cerebrospinal fluid within the sac.
 - The defect is usually in the occipital region, but may be in the frontal or parietal regions.
 - There is often secondary hydrocephalus.

II. FACIAL ABNORMALITIES

A. Ocular problems
 1. Hypotelorism
 - is a decrease in the interorbital distance.
 - is associated with holoprosencephaly.
 - **Cyclopia** is an extreme form in which there is one midline orbit.
 2. Hypertelorism
 - is an increase in the interorbital distance.

 - may be caused by a frontal encephalocele.

B. Cleft lip and palate
 - occur when the lip and palate fail to fuse.
 - There are three forms: **bilateral, unilateral,** and **central.**
 1. Central defects are strongly associated with trisomy 13 and holoprosencephaly.
 2. Unilateral and bilateral defects are associated with chromosomal anomalies and amniotic bands.
 - A high palatal defect cannot be diagnosed with ultrasound.

C. Micrognathia
 - is a small jaw.
 - is associated with chromosomal anomalies (e.g., trisomies 13 and 18).

D. Proboscis is associated with holoprosencephaly
 - is a condition in which the nose is absent.
 - A flap of tissue superior to the orbits (i.e., a proboscis) may develop.

III. NECK ABNORMALITIES

A. Cystic hygromas
 - are lymph collections related to obstruction of the lymphatic system.
 - occur when the normal communication between the cisterna chyli and the jugular vein fails to develop.
 - develop on either side of the neck in a posterolateral location. Eventually, the collections become so large that they lie adjacent to each other.
 - are associated with Turner's syndrome (70% association) and trisomies 21, 18, and 13 (lesser associations).
 - Skin thickening, pleural effusion, ascites, and other findings of hydrops often appear as the lymphatic blockage worsens.
 - If hydrops is present, cystic hygromas are lethal; however, without hydrops, they may regress and disappear.

B. Thyroid enlargement
 - may be congenital or a result of maternal thyroid disease.
 - results in polyhydramnios when the thyroid compresses the esophagus.

IV. SPINAL ABNORMALITIES—SPINA BIFIDA
 - is a **congenital** midline vertebral defect whereby the contents of the neural canal are exposed. The spinal cord is tethered and split at the defect.
 - is most common at the lumbosacral junction.
 - is almost always accompanied by **Arnold-Chiari II malformation** (see I B 3).
 - often results in secondary hydrocephalus.

– **Clubfoot** may develop in severe cases. Leg movement cannot be definitely predicted from *in utero* appearances unless movement is absent.

A. **Open spina bifida** (i.e., **spina bifida cystica**) comprises 85% of spina bifida cases. The neural tube is exposed or covered by a thin membrane.

1. In open spina bifida related to a **meningocele,** the meninges that surround the cord protrude through the defect and form a sac that surrounds cerebrospinal fluid.

2. In open spina bifida related to a **myelomeningocele,** neural elements and cerebrospinal fluid protrude into a sac enclosed by meninges.

3. Open spina bifida is almost always associated with elevated AFP levels.

B. **Closed spina bifida** is a tethered, split cord with a bony deformity covered by skin or a thick membrane.

– Closed spina bifida is not associated with elevated AFP.

C. **Spina bifida occulta** is a small bony defect that is completely covered by skin. It is a common, unrelated, asymptomatic condition not seen *in utero*.

D. **Diastematomyelia** is a related defect in which a bony spur splits and tethers the cord.

V. **ABDOMINAL WALL ABNORMALITIES**

A. **Omphalocele**

– is a protrusion of bowel and/or liver through the abdominal wall at the umbilical cord insertion site. A membrane covers the protruding organs, which may contain ascites.

– Omphaloceles that contain bowel have an **80%** association with **chromosomal anomalies.** Liver-containing omphaloceles have a **20%** association with chromosomal anomalies.

– There is a **50% association with anomalies** elsewhere, especially cardiac anomalies.

– MSAFP levels are typically increased.

B. **Gastroschisis**

– is a defect in the abdominal wall, typically to the right of the umbilical cord insertion site, through which small and large bowel (sometimes stomach and bladder also) protrude.

– No membrane covers the mass.

– **Gut obstruction** of the extra- or intra-abdominal bowel may occur if the defect is small, resulting in dilation of the bowel.

– There is **almost no association** with other anomalies or with an abnormal karyotype.

– **MSAFP** levels are typically increased.

C. **Pentalogy of Cantrell**

– is a rare defect in which an omphalocele and the heart are located outside of the chest.

– is accompanied by other defects, such as an absent sternum and interrupted diaphragm.

D. **Bladder extrophy**

– occurs when the bladder has no anterior wall and lies on the surface of the abdominal wall.

– The bladder often forms a mound below the umbilical cord insertion site.

E. **Limb/body wall syndrome**

– is a lethal defect in which there may be absent limbs and most of the abdominal contents are not covered by the abdominal wall.

– is thought to be caused by **amniotic sac disruption.**

– is often accompanied by a **myelomeningocele.**

VI. **THORACIC ABNORMALITIES**

– A small amount of fluid normally moves in and out of the fetal lungs.

A. **Cystic adenomatoid malformation (CAM)**

– is a condition in which numerous small or large cysts replace one or more lobes of the lung.

– often resolves spontaneously.

– Large CAMs may inhibit venous return and result in fetal ascites and other features of hydrops.

– Surgical removal of the affected lobe *in utero* has been successful in preventing hydrops and lung hypoplasia.

– **Sonographic findings**

1. A multicystic or solid-looking mass can be seen in the thorax, often displacing the heart.

2. However, specific sonographic findings are determined by the type of CAM.

a. In **type 1** CAMs, the cysts are large and appear as large, anechoic areas.

b. In **type 2** CAMs, there are numerous small to medium-sized cysts.

c. In **type 3** CAMs, multiple tiny cysts form a solid, echogenic mass (individual cysts are too small to be appreciated).

B. **Sequestration** of the lung

– occurs when a segment of the lung has a **separate blood supply** and is not connected to the trachea.

– The sonographic appearance is indistinguishable from a type 3 CAM, except that a prominent supplying vessel from the aorta may be seen.

C. **Diaphragmatic hernia**

- is herniation of the abdominal contents into the chest.
- can occur on the left side or the right side; however, a diaphragmatic hernia is eight times more likely to occur on the left side.
- is strongly associated with **chromosomal anomalies and cardiac problems.**
- has a relatively poor prognosis that depends on the size of the defect, whether the liver is in the chest, and the presence of pulmonary hypoplasia.
- Sonographic findings depend on the location of the hernia.

1. **Sonographic findings of left-sided hernias** include
   - cardiac displacement to the right (i.e., dextroposition).
   - absent diaphragm on the left.
   - a fluid-filled stomach seen in the chest.
   - small bowel seen in the chest that may not be distinguishable from the lung.
   - possible polyhydramnios.
   - a distorted portal vein if the liver is in the chest.
   - stomach not seen in the abdomen.

2. **Sonographic findings of right-sided hernias,** a difficult diagnosis to make, include
   - stomach displaced to the right.
   - liver seen in the chest.

D. Pleural effusions
- are a component of hydrops.
- usually regress with time when isolated.
- are associated with **chromosomal anomalies.**
- can be bilateral.
- Fluid in the pleural space outlines the lung.
- Very large effusions push the diaphragm inferiorly and cause hydrops.
- If large and persistent, fluid drainage into the amniotic fluid via a catheter *in utero* may be helpful.

VII. GENITOURINARY ABNORMALITIES

- Fetal contribution to the production of amniotic fluid starts at 12 weeks' gestation but does not become the only factor until approximately 18 weeks' gestation.
- The fetus swallows and urinates approximately 500 mL of urine in every 24-hour period.
- **Oligohydramnios** is a condition in which there is an insufficient amount of amniotic fluid.
- **Anhydramnios** is a condition in which there is no amniotic fluid and will occur when the fetus cannot urinate due to obstruction or nonfunctioning kidneys (e.g., urethral atresia, renal agenesis).

A. Renal agenesis
- is commonly unilateral, and rarely bilateral.

- is fatal if bilateral. Death is secondary to anhydramnios. Because no kidneys are present, no urine is produced from 15–18 weeks' gestation on, and pulmonary hypoplasia develops.
- The fetal bladder and kidneys cannot be visualized on ultrasound.
- The **adrenals** move laterally and become linear in shape. They can be mistaken for small kidneys.

B. Autosomal recessive (infantile) polycystic kidney disease
- can occur *in utero,* and usually results in stillbirth.
- is an inherited autosomal recessive condition with a **25% chance of recurrence** in successive offspring.
- results in oligohydramnios or anhydramnios.
- The kidneys are both enlarged and highly echogenic. The cysts are too small to be seen sonographically.
- The bladder is consistently small or nonvisualized.

C. Meckel-Gruber syndrome
- is a condition in which small, visible cysts (dysplasia) are present in both kidneys.
- is a lethal, autosomal recessive disorder.
- results in severe oligohydramnios.
- Additional features include occipital encephalocele, polydactyly, and, less often, cardiac anomalies and cleft palate.

D. Multicystic dysplastic kidney disease
- is the most common cystic renal abnormality in neonates.
- is not usually a genetic syndrome. Rather, it is thought to be a consequence of early *in utero* obstruction.
- can be unilateral, bilateral, or, rarely, may affect only a portion of one kidney. If bilateral, it is fatal.
- The affected kidney is large with multiple noncommunicating, cystic structures interspersed with echogenic tissue.

E. Hydronephrosis
- is seen in more than 75% of fetal renal abnormalities.
- is an obstruction of the fetal urinary tract.
- can be unilateral or bilateral. Severe bilateral hydronephrosis, in which fetal urination is diminished, results in oligohydramnios.
- leads to dilation of the pelvicalyceal system.

1. Renal pelvic dilation less than 10 mm is often a normal variant, but needs follow up.
2. Fetuses with Down syndrome show a greater than usual (25% versus 2.8%) incidence of mildly dilated renal pelves (greater than 3 mm).

F. Ureteropelvic junction obstruction
  – is common.
  – is a stenosis at the junction of the ureter and pelvis.
  – results in a dilated renal pelvis and calyces. The pelvis is at least 10 mm in width; smaller widths may be physiologic.
  – is often bilateral, although the two sides may be dilated to different degrees.
  – The renal parenchyma may be narrowed, indicating poor function.

G. Posterior urethral valve obstruction
  – is a developmental anomaly of male fetuses with a malformation of valves in the posterior urethra.
  – results in a dilated, thick-walled bladder with a dilated posterior urethra (i.e., the **keyhole sign**).
  – causes bilateral hydronephrosis and hydroureter.
  – If the renal parenchyma is very echogenic and cortical cysts are present, bilateral renal **dysplasia** is present and the prognosis for long-term renal function is poor.
  – Fetal ascites may develop if the bladder ruptures.
  – **Oligohydramnios** is often present and is followed to assess how much useful renal function persists.
  – **Catheter insertion** to drain the obstructed bladder is occasionally performed *in utero* if obstruction is severe and amniotic fluid levels are falling.

H. Vesicoureteral reflux
  – is common *in utero*.
  – is ten times more common in **males** than females *in utero*. Females, however, get postnatal renal infections because of their short urethras.
  – results in a mildly dilated renal pelvis and calyces, which vary in size over the course of the examination.
  – Ureteral dilation and peristalsis may be seen.
  – The bladder may be distended with a thin wall. As it empties, the renal pelvis may distend.

I. Mesoblastic nephroma
  – is a benign, unilateral neoplasm.
  – is seen in the third trimester.
  – appears as a solid renal mass.
  – always results in severe polyhydramnios.

J. Fetal hydroceles
  – are a normal variant when seen *in utero*.
  – The processus vaginalis, a connection between the peritoneal sac and the scrotum, exists *in utero*, and peritoneal fluid may pool in the scrotum.

K. Fetal ovarian cysts
  – are intraperitoneal cysts that develop in the middle of the second trimester.
  – only seen in females.
  – are a response to maternal hormones and disappear spontaneously after birth, unless they have twisted and hemorrhaged.
  – A crescent-shaped group of internal echoes develops if the cyst has bled.
  – Ovarian cysts may be seen anywhere between the bladder and the liver.

VIII. GASTROINTESTINAL ABNORMALITIES

  – **Gut obstruction** can occur at any level from the mouth to the anus.
  – When the obstruction is located above the large bowel it is associated with polyhydramnios.
  – Most gut obstructions carry a low-grade association with karyotypic abnormalities.

A. Tracheoesophageal abnormalities
  – are associated with other cardiac, musculoskeletal, and gastrointestinal abnormalities.
  – There are four variants, but only the variant in which there is no connection between the stomach, esophagus, and trachea can be recognized with ultrasound.
  – Sonographic findings may include absence of a fluid-filled stomach or a very small stomach, a small abdominal circumference, and severe polyhydramnios.

B. Duodenal atresia
  – occurs when the duodenum is obstructed just beyond the antrum.
  – has a 30%–50% association with **Down syndrome.**
  – is associated with an increased risk of intrauterine growth restriction (IUGR).
  – may be associated with congenital heart disease.
  – results in severe polyhydramnios.
  – A distended stomach and proximal duodenum (the **double bubble sign**) may be seen.
  – No other bowel loops contain fluid.

C. Jejunoileal atresia
  – is a condition in which multiple loops of small bowel are dilated.
  – results in polyhydramnios.

D. Meconium cysts and meconium peritonitis
  – result from leakage of gut contents at the site of perforation.
  – have a slight association with cystic fibrosis.
  – may be associated with dilated loops of bowel.
  – appear as pseudocysts with echogenic and possibly calcified walls.
  – There may be some free intra-abdominal fluid.

E. Isolated ascites
- is usually associated with hydrops.
- may be caused by renal obstruction with rupture of the bladder or a calyx or lymphatic problems.

IX. SKELETAL ABNORMALITIES

- **Rhizomelia** is a short proximal limb.
- **Mesomelia** is a short middle segment of a limb.
- **Micromelia** is shortening of the entire limb.
- **Acromelia** is short distal segments (e.g., hands, feet).

A. Achondrogenesis
- is a rare, lethal, short-limb dysplasia seen in 1 in 40,000 live births.
- results in polyhydramnios.
- results in short ribs, very short limbs (micromelia), and a bell-shaped abdomen.
- may include features such as lack of vertebral ossification, cystic hygromas, and a large head with normal to decreased ossification of the cranium.

B. Thanatophoric dysplasia
- is the most common **lethal** form of dwarfism (i.e., 1 in 5000 births).
- results in polyhydramnios, as do all lethal forms of dwarfism.
- is characterized by very short bones (micromelia), bowed femurs shaped like telephone receivers, and flattened vertebrae (platyspondylia).
- There is a protruding, bell-shaped abdomen with a small thorax.
- Macrocephaly with a **cloverleaf skull** may occur in some cases.
- A "trident" hand with short, stubby fingers that are widely separated may also be present.

C. Achondroplasia
- is a common (i.e., 1 in 1000 births) autosomal dominant, heterozygous condition.
- is lethal in the homozygous form (i.e., both parents have achondroplasia).
- is similar to thanatophoric dwarfism, only milder.
- The fetus appears normal until approximately 24 weeks' gestation.
- After about 24 weeks' gestation, features such as short limbs, a bell-shaped trunk, a large head, a flat nose, and a prominent forehead may be seen.

D. Osteogenesis imperfecta
- exists in three forms: very severe, severe, and mild. Patients with the severe and mild forms usually survive birth; however, patients with the severe form are wheelchair-bound for life.
- results in bowed, irregular, fragile bones with fractures.

- Limb lengths are variable.
- Hypomineralization of the entire skeleton is most obvious in the skull, which can be flattened with transducer pressure in the severe form. Only a single bone may be abnormal in the mild form.

E. Clubfoot
- occurs in 1 in 1000 live births.
- may be familial.
- is associated with many entities, particularly oligohydramnios or anhydramnios, neurologic disorders, spina bifida, caudal regression syndrome, and chromosomal disorders.
- Of all cases, **95% are equinovarus** (i.e., inverted foot) with medial deviation and plantar flexion.
- There is an abnormal angle between the lower leg and the foot.
- Both the tibia and fibula can usually be seen on the same view as the foot.

F. Polydactyly
- is a condition in which there are too many digits.
- is common, especially in African Americans.
- is associated with **trisomy 13.**

X. CARDIAC ABNORMALITIES

A. Heart rate abnormalities
1. **Bradycardia** is a heart rate under 100 bpm.
2. **Tachycardia** is a heart rate over 180 bpm.

B. Pericardial effusion
- is too much fluid in the pericardium that surrounds the heart.
- is often a component of hydrops. If not a component of hydrops, it is usually associated with cardiac anomalies.
- A "fat pad" that surrounds the heart can be easily mistaken for a small pericardial effusion on ultrasound.

C. Ectopia cordis
- is a condition in which the heart lies partially or completely outside of the thorax.
- is associated with omphalocele.
- The combination of ectopia cordis and omphalocele with a fusion defect of the anterior thoracic wall, diaphragm, and sternum is known as **pentalogy of Cantrell** (see V C).
- Fetal survival is almost unknown; there are usually other cardiac anomalies.

D. Ventriculoseptal defect
- is the **most common form** of cardiac defect.
- is a condition in which there is a hole in the muscular wall between the two ventricles.
- The septum is normally thinner just below the aortic root, making this area especially

prone to false-positive defects on ultrasound; color flow Doppler is helpful in making the diagnosis.

XI. SYNDROMES

– A syndrome is a grouping of abnormalities in different parts of the body, perhaps on a familial basis.
– A chromosomal abnormality may be present when there are a number of defects.

  A. Beckwith-Wiedemann syndrome
   – is an autosomal dominant syndrome characterized by **enlargement of all organs.**
   – is associated with an increased risk of omphalocele.
   – is associated with cardiac anomalies.
   – results in macroglossia (i.e., an enlarged tongue), hepatosplenomegaly, and enlarged kidneys.

  B. Down syndrome (trisomy 21)
   – is a chromosomal anomaly seen in 1 in 850 fetuses.
   – is more common in women older than 35 years of age.
   – is associated with duodenal atresia, endocardial cushion defects, and posterior urethral valve abnormalities.
   – can only be diagnosed definitively by amniocentesis with karyotyping.
   – Estriol, AFP, and human chorionic gonadotropin levels in maternal blood can be used to assign an increased risk in approximately 60% of cases.
   – **Sonographic findings** include:
    1. Cardiac defects (50% of cases)
    2. Duodenal atresia
    3. Nuchal thickening or translucency
    4. Mild renal pelviectasis
    5. A short femur and humerus
    6. Echogenic bowel
    7. Clinodactyly
    8. Nuchal translucency (between 11 and 13 weeks) or a thickened nuchal fold of more than 6 mm (up to 22 weeks)
    9. Mild lateral ventricular dilation
    10. A sandal gap between the big toes and remaining toes
    11. Small ears

  C. Trisomy 18 (Edwards' syndrome)
   – is a chromosomal anomaly that occurs in approximately 1 in 5000 births.
   – is more common in older women.
   – **Sonographic findings** include:
    1. Diaphragmatic hernia
    2. Congenital heart defects
    3. Clubfeet and clubhands
    4. Choroid plexus cyst
    5. Omphalocele
    6. IUGR
    7. Renal dilation
    8. Two-vessel cord
    9. Hydrocephalus
    10. Micrognathia

  D. Trisomy 13 (Patau's syndrome)
   – occurs in approximately 1 in 50,000 births.
   – is more common in older women.
   – **Sonographic findings** include:
    1. Holoprosencephaly (strong association)
    2. Facial abnormalities (e.g., hypotelorism, cyclopia, proboscis, central cleft lip and palate)
    3. Congenital heart lesions
    4. Clubfeet
    5. Omphalocele
    6. IUGR
    7. Two-vessel cord

XII. OTHER ABNORMALITIES—MATERNAL INFECTIONS

– Several infections, some of which seem trivial in the mother, have major effects on the fetus. These are known by the acronym **TORCHS** (**t**oxoplasmosis, **r**ubella, **c**ytomegalic inclusion disease, **h**erpes, **s**yphilis).
– Cytomegalic inclusion disease and toxoplasmosis are the most common.
– **Parvovirus and HIV** are modern additions to this list.

  A. Toxoplasmosis is associated with
   – hepatosplenomegaly.
   – intracranial calcifications.
   – IUGR.

  B. Cytomegalic inclusion disease is associated with
   – IUGR.
   – hydrocephalus with periventricular calcification.
   – cardiomegaly, myocarditis, supraventricular tachycardia, and pericardial effusion.
   – intra-abdominal echogenic bowel and calcification.
   – microcephaly.
   – placentomegaly.
   – hydrops.

  C. Parvovirus
   – is associated with cardiomegaly, hypertrophic cardiomyopathy, and pericardial effusion.
   – is treatable with a fetal blood transfusion.
   – Fetal anemia causes hydrops.

  D. HIV
   – can cross the placenta.
   – infects one third of fetuses of infected mothers.
   – HIV-exposed pregnancies are at risk for IUGR and cytomegalovirus.

CHAPTER 23

COEXISTING DISORDERS (0%-3%)

I. LEIOMYOMAS (FIBROIDS)

– are commonly found in pregnancy, particularly in older women.

A. Clinical complications
1. If the fibroids are located in the cervix, they can prevent vaginal delivery.
2. Hemorrhage may occur into a fibroid (i.e., "red degeneration"), which is very painful.
3. Large fibroids can compress the fetus and prevent it from moving freely.
4. Clinical misdating occurs if the fibroid makes the gestational age by fundal palpation seem more advanced.

B. Sonographic findings
1. A mass with an organized internal texture is seen arising from the uterine wall. Although it can be mistaken for a myometrial contraction (see V), it tends to bulge outward rather than inward and persists if the examination is repeated half an hour later.
2. Fibroids tend to move toward the fundus with time; therefore, a cervical fibroid may move superiorly as the pregnancy proceeds.
3. In "red degeneration," a cystic area may develop at the center of the fibroid.

II. CYSTIC DISORDERS

A. Corpus luteum cysts
– are present in the first trimester in a minority of pregnancies.
– disappear spontaneously by 16–18 weeks.
– can be echo-free or complex in appearance.

B. Dermoids
– are very common in pregnancy.
– appear in the adnexa in a variety of patterns.

– have to be followed to make sure they are not growing because they can be mistaken for malignancy.

III. GESTATIONAL TROPHOBLASTIC DISEASE

– is a complication of pregnancy or conception. No fetus coexists with these forms.

A. There are three forms: hydatidiform moles, invasive moles, and choriocarcinoma.
1. **Hydatidiform moles**
   – are benign, but have an approximately 10% risk of becoming invasive moles.
   – develop from the placenta of missed abortions.
   – Complete hydatidiform moles have a normal diploid karyotype of paternal origin.
2. **Invasive moles**
   – persist and locally invade the myometrium after a dilation and curettage to remove a hydatidiform mole has been performed.
   – are treated with hysterectomy and chemotherapy.
3. **Choriocarcinoma**
   – is an epithelial tumor that rarely occurs in pregnancy.
   – can develop at any time during or after pregnancy, and can follow an anembryonic pregnancy or abortion.
   – is malignant and metastasizes early.
   – responds well to chemotherapy.

B. Incidence
1. Hydatidiform and invasive moles occur in approximately 1 in 1500 to 1 in 2000 pregnancies in the United States.
2. Hydatidiform and invasive moles are much more common in Southeast Asia; for exam-

ple, the incidence in Taiwan is 1 in 82 pregnancies.

3. Molar pregnancies are more common in women older than 40 or younger than 20 years of age.

C. Clinical features

1. **Hydatidiform and invasive moles** are characterized by
   - hyperemesis.
   - abnormal vaginal bleeding.
   - an enlarged uterus for gestational age.
   - very high β-human chorionic gonadotropin (β-HCG) levels.

2. **Choriocarcinoma** is characterized by
   - elevated HCG levels.
   - metastases to the liver, brain, and lungs.

D. Sonographic findings

1. **Hydatidiform and invasive moles**
   a. Moles can appear similar to an incomplete or missed abortion; however, no fetus is present.
   b. Moles are described as having a grape-like, heterogeneous appearance.
   c. Color flow shows increased vascularity.
   d. **Theca-lutein cysts,** the result of high HCG levels, are seen in up to 50% of cases. Multiple large cysts, actually enlarged follicles, occupy both ovaries.
   e. Residual molar tissue with invasive moles is vascular and can be seen with color flow. On the initial sonogram, the two look similar.

2. **Choriocarcinoma**
   a. An echogenic uterine mass with cystic areas is seen.
   b. The mass is vascular on color flow.
   c. Choriocarcinoma can resemble a distorted blighted ovum.
   d. Liver metastases should be sought; they are hypoechoic and vascular.
   e. Choriocarcinoma does not resemble hydatidiform moles sonographically, but may look similar to an invasive mole after a dilation and curettage.

IV. PARTIAL MOLES

   - are usually related to **triploidy,** a chromosomal anomaly in which all chromosomes are triplicated. Either two paternal and one maternal or two maternal and one paternal set of chromosomes are present.
   - usually result in early fetal demise.
   - There is amniotic fluid, and a fetus present.
   - The placenta is enlarged and filled with sonolucent areas. It looks like a hydatidiform mole within a formed placenta.
   - Severe intrauterine growth restriction and fetal anomalies (e.g., spina bifida) are often present.

V. MYOMETRIAL CONTRACTIONS

   - are common in the first and second trimesters.
   - A portion of the myometrium painlessly contracts and thickens over a period of 20–30 minutes and then spontaneously disappears or moves along the uterine wall.
   - The thickened area of myometrium has the same features as the myometrium elsewhere.

SECTION B • GYNECOLOGY

CHAPTER 24

NORMAL PELVIC ANATOMY (10%-15%)

I. UTERUS (Figure 24–1)

A. The uterus is retroperitoneal. It is housed between the urinary bladder and rectum, and is attached to the broad ligaments.

B. The uterus has four components, including the
- fundus.
- corpus (body).
- isthmus.
- cervix.

C. The uterus is comprised of three layers.
  1. The **parametrium** is the outer layer, and is lined by a **serous** coat.
  2. The **myometrium** is the middle, **muscular** layer.
  3. The **endometrium** is the inner layer.

D. The uterus is a pear-shaped, muscular organ. Uterine shape is maintained in postmenopausal females; however, the uterus is a tubular shape in infants.

E. The size of the uterus varies with age and parity.
  1. The uterus is approximately $9 \times 3 \times 4$ cm in nulliparous females. It is larger in multiparous females and smaller in prepubertal and postmenopausal females.
  2. The size difference between the cervix and the uterus varies with age. The cervix: uterus ratio is 2:1 in infants and 1:2 in menstruating and postmenopausal females.

F. Various uterine positions are possible (Figure 24–2).
  1. An **anteverted** uterus tilts toward the bladder.
  2. In an **anteflexed** uterus, the fundus is folded onto itself anteriorly.
  3. A **retroverted** uterus tilts toward the rectum.
  4. With a **retroflexed** uterus, the fundus folds toward the rectum.

G. Sonographic examination of the endometrial cavity for pathology
  1. Perform an endovaginal sonogram during the **proliferative phase.**
  2. Measure the thickness of the endometrium so that it includes endometrium on both sides of the canal.
  3. If there is questionable intracavity pathology, perform a saline infusion study (i.e., **hysterosonogram**).

II. VAGINA

A. The vagina is an 8- to 10-cm, collapsible, muscular tube.

ANTERIOR

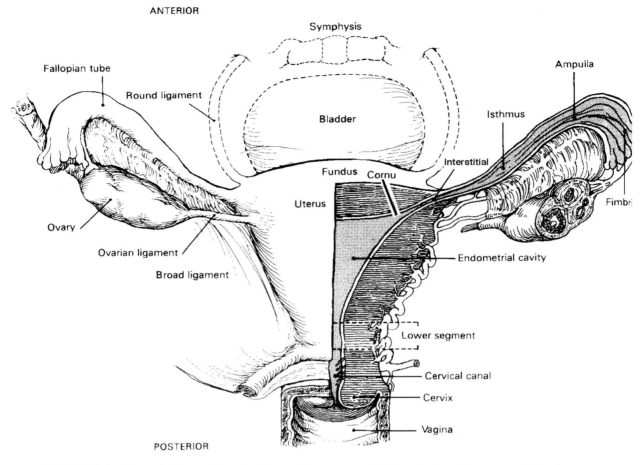

FIGURE 24-1. Normal uterus and ovaries. The ovaries are suspended from the broad ligament and lie adjacent to the ampullary end of the fallopian tube. The fallopian tube arises from the cornu of the uterus. The lumen is rarely visible. (Reprinted with permission from Sanders RC: *Clinical Sonography: A Practical Guide,* 3rd ed. Philadelphia, Lippincott, 1998, p 40.)

B. The vagina extends from the external os to the external genitalia.

III. OVARIES (see Figure 24–1)

A. The ovaries are almond-shaped, paired endocrine glands that are not covered by peritoneum.

B. The ovaries are suspended by **ovarian ligaments** and supplied by the **ovarian artery** and **uterine artery.**

C. The size of the ovaries varies with age.
  1. In prepubertal females, the ovaries are approximately $1 \times 1 \times 1$ cm; however, they may contain cysts.
  2. In menstruating females, the ovaries are approximately $3 \times 2 \times 2$ cm or larger.
  3. In postmenopausal females, the ovaries are $2 \times 2 \times 1$ cm or smaller.

D. The ovaries have an outer **cortex** and an inner **medulla.**

1. The cortex consists of follicles and connective tissue.
2. The medulla consists of blood vessels, connective tissue, and primitive oocytes.

IV. FALLOPIAN TUBES

A. The fallopian tubes (also called the **oviducts** or **salpinges**) are paired tubular structures that arise from the cornu of the uterus and extend into the peritoneal cavity.

B. There are six named portions of each fallopian tube.
  1. The **cornual** portion is the entrance to the tube from the endometrial cavity.
  2. The **intramural** or **interstitial** portion is the part of the fallopian tube within the uterine wall.
  3. The **isthmic** portion is the tube-shaped area between the uterine wall and close to the fimbria.
  4. The **ampullary** portion is the longest,

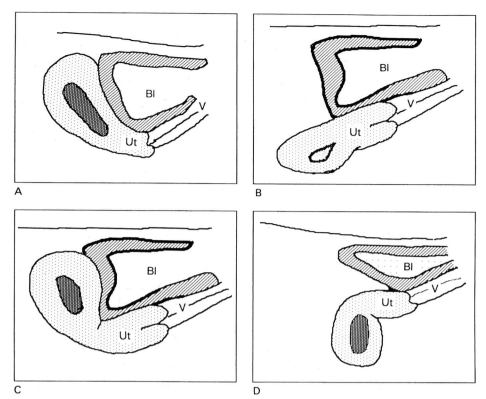

FIGURE 24-2. Various uterine positions. (*A*) Anteverted. (*B*) Retroverted. (*C*) Anteflexed. (*D*) Retroflexed. Note the septum where the uterus folds over on itself. *Bl* = bladder; *Ut* = uterus; *V* = vagina. (Reprinted with permission from Sanders RC: *Clinical Sonography: A Practical Guide*, 3rd ed. Philadelphia, Lippincott, 1998, p 41.)

widest portion close to the peritoneal end.

5. The **infundibular** portion is at the peritoneal end.

6. The **fimbriae** are finger-like extensions from the peritoneal end of the tube.

V. SUPPORTING STRUCTURES (Figure 24–3)

– The pelvis is divided into a **true (lesser)** and **false (greater)** pelvis.

A. The **rectus abdominis** muscle in the anterior abdominal wall extends from the xiphoid to the symphysis pubis.

B. The **iliopsoas** muscles, which are paired cylindrical muscles, are lateral and anterior to the iliac crest.

C. The **obturator internus** muscles are smaller bilateral muscles lining the lateral margin of the true pelvis; they lie lateral to the ovaries.

D. The **piriformis** muscles are paired and transversely aligned posterior to the ovaries, uterus, vagina, and rectum.

E. The **coccygeus, iliococcygeus,** and **pubococcygeus** muscles line the floor of the true pelvis.

F. The **levator ani** muscle is a hammock-like muscle that extends from the body of the pubis and ischial spine to the coccyx. It is the most inferior of the muscles and is too thin to see with ultrasound.

VI. POTENTIAL SITES FOR FLUID ACCUMULATION

– There are several potential spaces for fluid accumulation in the pelvis.

A. The **anterior cul-de-sac** is posterior to the urinary bladder wall and anterior to the uterus.

B. The **posterior cul-de-sac** (i.e., **pouch of Douglas**) is posterior to the uterus and anterior to the wall of the rectum.

C. The **space of Retzius** lies between the symphysis pubis and anterior bladder wall.

D. The **fornices** of the vagina comprise the distal vaginal recesses, which surround the cervix.

VII. VASCULATURE

A. The **uterine artery** arises from the internal iliac artery and supplies blood to the ovaries,

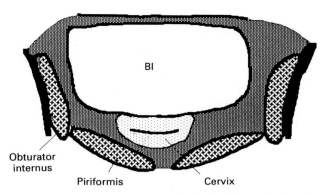

FIGURE 24-3. Transverse view at the level of the cervix showing the muscles that form the side walls of the pelvis. *Bl* = bladder. (Reprinted with permission from Sanders RC: *Clinical Sonography: A Practical Guide,* 3rd ed. Philadelphia, Lippincott, 1998, p 43.)

vagina, cervix, fallopian tubes, and uterus. Branches of the uterine artery include the
 – **radial artery** (perfuses the myometrium).
 – **spiral artery** (perfuses the endometrium).

B. The **ovarian arteries** are branches of the aorta.

C. The **right ovarian vein** drains directly into the inferior vena cava.

D. The **left ovarian vein** drains into the left renal vein.

VIII. DOPPLER

A. Normal flow to the follicle in the proliferative phase is **low resistance.**

B. After ovulation and the development of the corpus luteum, flow changes to **high resistance.**

CHAPTER 25

PHYSIOLOGY (6%–15%)

I. MENSTRUAL CYCLE

– The ovaries and endometrium undergo serial changes under the influence of hormones (Figure 25–1).

  A. The **anterior lobe of the pituitary gland** produces **follicle-stimulating hormone** and **luteinizing hormone.** These hormones determine the amount of **estrogen** and **progesterone** secreted by the ovaries.

  B. The graafian follicles in the ovaries produce **estrogen,** a hormone that
   – regenerates the endometrium after menses.
   – causes the endometrium to thicken.
   – induces salt and water retention.
   – promotes myometrial contractions during normal menses and labor.

  C. During the second half of the cycle and implantation, the **corpus luteum** produces **progesterone,** a hormone that
   – thickens the endometrium in the secretory phase.
   – readies the endometrium for implantation.
   – decreases myometrial contractions.

II. PREGNANCY TEST

  A. To detect pregnancy, the serum level of β-human chorionic gonadotropin is measured using a radioimmune assay. A similar test on urine is not as accurate.

  B. The serum test detects pregnancy approximately 2 weeks after conception.

III. HUMAN CHORIONIC GONADOTROPIN

– is a hormone normally released during the first trimester.

– is produced by placental tissue (i.e., trophoblasts).
– increases in amount with increases in trophoblastic tissue.
– doubles every 48 hours until 8–10 weeks' gestation.
– maintains estrogen and progesterone activity of the corpus luteum.
– is measured by First International Reference or Second International Standard, but typically the latter.

IV. FERTILIZATION

– The formation of an embryo is the result of the union of a sperm and a mature ovum.

  A. The **oocyte** (i.e., mature ovum) is released from a follicle on approximately day 14 of the menstrual cycle.

  B. The oocyte is swept by the fimbriae into the fallopian tube, where union of the sperm and the ovum (i.e., fertilization) takes place. At this point, the sperm and the ovum normally each have 23 chromosomes.

  C. Approximately 24–36 hours after ovulation, the sperm penetrates the zona pellucida of the ovum.

  D. The genetic components of the sperm and ovum unite and form a single fertilized cell called the **zygote,** which is a diploid cell with 46 chromosomes.

  E. The process of mitosis (i.e., cell division) begins 24–36 hours after formation of the zygote. Cleavage occurs and two **blastomeres** are formed.

  F. The cleavage progresses from a 2-part, to an 8-part, to a 16-part, to a 32-part division with

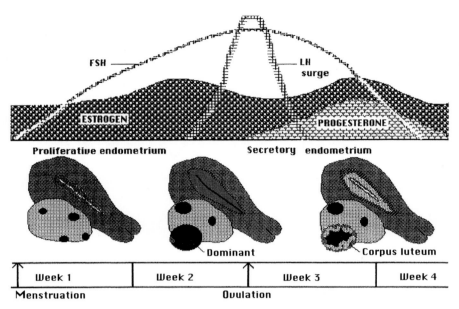

FIGURE 25-1. Graph showing hormone production during the menstrual cycle. Note the high levels of luteinizing hormone and estrogen during ovulation. *FSH* = follicle-stimulating hormone; *LH* = luteinizing hormone. (Reprinted with permission from Sanders RC: *Clinical Sonography: A Practical Guide,* 3rd ed. Philadelphia, Lippincott, 1998, p 39.)

the creation of more blastomeres until a solid ball of 12–15 cells (i.e., the **morula**) is formed.

G. The morula travels through the fallopian tube to the uterus over 3 days until it comes to rest in the uterine cavity.

H. While in the uterine cavity, the morula changes into a hollow ball of cells (i.e., the **blastocyst**) and forms the gestational sac.

CHAPTER 26

PEDIATRIC GYNECOLOGY (1%-5%)

I. NORMAL ANATOMY

    A. The uterus is small and tubular before puberty.

    B. The ovaries are small, but may contain one or more small cysts. Cysts become more frequent as puberty approaches.

II. PRECOCIOUS PUBERTY

    A. Precocious puberty is the development of secondary sexual characteristics (e.g., pubic hair, breasts) and the onset of menstruation before 8 years of age.

    B. Although usually **idiopathic,** precocious puberty may be associated with **intracranial tumors** or, more **rarely, feminizing adrenal tumors.** Therefore, the adrenal glands should be scanned in these patients.

    C. Sonographic findings of precocious puberty include
       – ovaries and uterus enlarged for age.
       – an adult cervix:uterus ratio (i.e., larger fundal than cervical width and length).
       – an echogenic endometrial canal.

III. HEMATOMETRA AND HEMATOCOLPOS

    A. Infantile form
       1. *In utero,* secretions of fluid under the influence of maternal hormones may result in distension of the vagina (**hydrocolpos**) or uterus (**hydrometra**) with fluid.

       2. The fluid may or may not contain echoes.

    B. Pubescent form
       1. If there is an **imperforate hymen** or partial or complete atresia of the vagina by a **transverse vaginal septum,** blood will accumulate in the vagina or uterus at menstruation, leading to
         – **hematocolpos** (vagina only).
         – **hematometra** (uterus only).
         – **hematocolpometra** (vagina and uterus).
       2. The fluid distending the vagina or uterus will be filled with echoes.
       3. Occasionally, blood will extravasate around the ovaries causing a collection of blood called an **endometrioma.**

IV. SEXUAL AMBIGUITY

    A. Female infants may be born with an enlarged clitoris and enlarged labial folds.

    B. Male infants may have a small penis and undescended testicles.

    C. Both female and male genital organs may be present.

    D. Turner's syndrome is the most common form of gonadal dysgenesis. The ovaries are small and flattened. Sonographic findings of the child's pelvis, before hormonal therapy, include
       – small or undetectable ovaries.
       – a uterus with the prepubertal configuration and size, regardless of age.

CHAPTER 27

INFERTILITY AND ENDOCRINOLOGY (2%-6%)

I. CONTRACEPTION—INTRAUTERINE CONTRACEPTIVE DEVICES

– are placed in the uterine cavity to prevent implantation of the fertilized ovum.

A. Types of intrauterine contraceptive devices (IUCDs) [Figure 27–1]

1. **Paragard**
   – is a T-shaped device.
2. **Progestasert**
   – is a T-shaped device.
   – releases progesterone.
3. **Copper 7 and Copper T**
   – are 7- and T-shaped devices.
   – are still seen in the United States, but are no longer being inserted.
   – contain copper.
4. **Lippes loop**
   – is no longer being inserted, but may still be seen in long-term users.
   – has a typical sonographic appearance; the five loops cause a series of five acoustic shadows.
5. **Dalkon shield**
   – is ovoid with many small legs.
   – was removed from the market in the United States because of repeated pelvic infections.

B. Sonographic findings with IUCDs

1. IUCDs appear as a series of reflective areas, known as entrance and exit echoes, with acoustic shadowing.
2. Ultrasound aids in checking the normal position in the cavity at the fundus.

C. Defective sites for IUCDs

1. IUCDs found in the uterine wall are difficult to remove, painful, and ineffective.
2. IUCDs placed near the cervix may fall out.
3. IUCDs that have become displaced outside of the uterus or into a gestational sac are dangerous, leading to infection or spontaneous abortion, and also ineffective at preventing pregnancy.

II. CAUSES OF INFERTILITY

– Infertility is diagnosed when a couple is unable to conceive after **12 months of unprotected intercourse.**
– Infertility is an increasingly common problem, currently involving 18%–20% of married couples.

A. Male factors (approximately 40% of known causes) include

– decreased or abnormal sperm production or motility.
– obstruction or absence of the epididymis, vas deferens, or ejaculatory ducts.
– ejaculation malfunction.
– large varicocele.
– idiopathic.

B. Female factors (40% of known causes) include

– tubal obstruction (e.g., pelvic inflammatory disease, endometriosis, implants, adhesions).
– ovulation failure.
– abnormalities or absence of the vagina, cervix, or uterus.
– immunologic incompatibility.

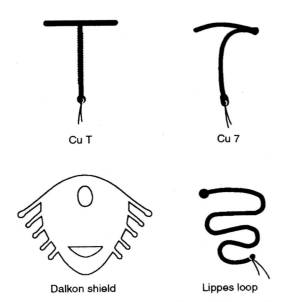

FIGURE 27-1. Diagram of the shape of several intrauterine contraceptive devices. The Paragard device has a similar shape to the copper (Cu) T device.

- nutritional factors.
- metabolic factors.
- ovarian disorders.

C. Of the remaining causes, 5%–10% are unknown, and 5%–10% are related to both partners.

III. SONOGRAPHIC INVESTIGATION OF INFERTILITY

A. Preliminary sonograms can show some of the causes of **female infertility,** including
- a congenital abnormality of the uterus or vagina.
- an endometrioma.
- adnexal adhesions.
- unruptured follicles.

B. Uterine causes of female infertility that can be seen sonographically include
- an intracavitary mass in the endometrium.
- a submucosal fibroid.
- uterine adhesions.
1. **Synechiae** form after curettage and spontaneous abortion, and appear as bright linear echoes in the cavity.
2. In **Asherman's syndrome,** there are so many adhesions that the cavity is completely closed.

C. Hysterosonosalpingograms can show additional problems. By injecting saline or ultrasonic contrast into the uterus and observing for the presence or absence of peritoneal spill, it is possible to assess for
- tubal patency.
- hydrosalpinx.

IV. MEDICATIONS AND TREATMENT

A. Hormones are used to assist infertile patients.
1. **Clomid (clomiphene citrate)**
   - stimulates the pituitary gland to secrete increased follicle-stimulating hormone (FSH).
   - can be followed by the administration of human chorionic gonadotropin (HCG) at the time of ovulation to help release the ovum.
2. **Pergonal (human menopausal gonadotropin)**
   - is a natural hormone derived from the urine of postmenopausal women.
   - is comprised of FSH and luteinizing hormone.
   - is used if Clomid does not work.

B. Ovulation induction (follicle monitoring)
   - Monitoring the development of follicles under ultrasound is performed so that the ideal time for **follicle aspiration, timed intercourse,** or **HCG administration** is known.
1. **Dominant follicles** are identified when they reach a size of approximately **1.6 cm.**
2. The **luteinized unruptured follicles syndrome** is present if follicles reach a size of 3 cm or more.

C. Assisted reproductive technology is the broad term used to describe the numerous methods used in assisting a woman to achieve a pregnancy. Some of these methods use the assistance of ultrasound.
1. **In vitro fertilization (IVF), embryo transfer, follicular aspiration, gamete intrafallopian transfer (GIFT), and zygote intrafallopian transfer (ZIFT)**
   a. Fertilization of the ovum by the sperm takes place in the laboratory.
   b. The follicles are aspirated through a needle placed with endovaginal ultrasound guidance.
   c. The fertilized ovum is then placed in the fallopian tube (GIFT or ZIFT) or endometrium.
2. **Artificial insemination**
   a. The sperm is derived from a donor. The fertilized ovum is then placed in the endometrial cavity.
   b. Ideal placement in the endometrial cavity may be monitored with ultrasound.
3. **Complications of assisted reproductive technology**
   a. Ovarian hyperstimulation syndrome
   - is caused by high levels of HCG.
   (1) **Clinical features** include
   - hypotension.
   - polycythemia.

(2) Sonographic findings include
- huge multiple cysts on the ovaries (i.e., theca-lutein cysts).
- pleural effusion.
- ascites.

b. Multiple gestation
- is more common after *in vitro* fertilization because of increased hormonal stimulus.
- results in increased fetal and neonatal morbidity.
- Triplets, quadruplets, or quintuplets are often reduced in number by **selective reduction,** which is performed under ultrasound control.

c. Ectopic pregnancy
- is more common in patients undergoing infertility treatment.

CHAPTER 28

POSTMENOPAUSAL GYNECOLOGY (6%-10%)

I. ANATOMY AND PHYSIOLOGY

– There are normal changes in appearance and function at menopause.

A. Uterus
1. Menstruation ceases.
2. The uterus gradually shrinks, but retains the adult shape (i.e., pear shaped).
3. The fundus is larger than the cervix.
4. The endometrium is normally less than 8 mm in width.

B. Ovaries
1. Ovulation ceases, although simple intraovarian cysts, which change little, may be found.
2. The ovaries shrink in size.

II. HORMONE REPLACEMENT THERAPY

A. Estrogen, with or without progesterone, is often administered. Benefits of estrogen replacement therapy include
– decreased risk of osteoporosis.
– decreased risk of heart disease.

B. Progesterone is added to counteract the side effects of estrogen in the second half of the cycle.
1. The combination of estrogen and progesterone induces a false period and endometrial thickening.
2. An endometrial thickness of greater than **8 mm** is normally investigated.

C. Sequential estrogen and progesterone administration can cause the endometrium to measure up to 15 mm in the estrogen phase. Endometrial thickness decreases with the addition of progesterone.

D. Continuous combined estrogen and progesterone is associated with a thin endometrium.

III. PATHOLOGY

A. Clinical manifestations of pathology
1. **Vaginal bleeding** can be caused by
   – poorly controlled hormone replacement therapy.
   – endometrial polyps.
   – submucosal or intracavitary fibroids.
   – endometrial cancer.
   – postmenopausal endometrial atrophy.
   – endometritis.
2. A **thickened endometrial cavity** can be caused by
   – the normal secretory phase.
   – an early intrauterine pregnancy (double sac sign).
   – complications of pregnancy (e.g., ectopic pregnancy).
   – endometritis.
   – blood in the endometrial cavity.
   – benign endometrial hyperplasia.
   – polyps.
   – intracavitary fibroids.
   – hormone replacement therapy.
   – endometrial cancer.

B. Pathologic conditions
1. **Benign endometrial hyperplasia**
   – may present with irregular bleeding.
   – results in a thickened endometrium throughout.
   – Tiny cysts may be seen.
2. **Endometrial polyps**
   – are often asymptomatic, but may cause bleeding.
   – are often multiple.

– are characterized by one or more focal echogenic masses in the endometrium.
– are almost always benign.

3. Endometrial cancer
– is a common gynecologic malignancy in the United States.
– is confined to the uterus at presentation in 75% of cases.

a. Risk factors for endometrial cancer include
– obesity.
– chronic anovulation.
– hormone replacement therapy.
– early menarche.
– late menopause.
– tamoxifen therapy.

b. Sonographic findings associated with endometrial cancer include
– a thickened endometrium with variable echogenicity.
– a polypoid mass.
– low impedance flow with color Doppler.
– absence of a normal hypoechoic halo around the endometrium when there is deep invasion.
– an endometrial halo that remains present in the presence of superficial lesions.

4. Ovarian cancer
a. Ovarian cystadenocarcinoma
– is relatively common.
– is often bilateral.
– is characterized by an irregular outline with papillary material breaking through the capsule.
– **metastasizes** to the liver, para-aortic nodes, and peritoneal cavity.
– **Ascites with peritoneal deposits** of metastases is evidence of spread.

b. Granulosa cell tumors
– are rare tumors with a low malignant potential.

– produce estrogen.
– are mainly seen in postmenopausal patients.
– can appear multilocular, cystic, or solid.

c. Sertoli-Leydig cell tumor (or **arrhenoblastoma**)
– is a masculinizing tumor.
– has a similar appearance to the granulosa cell tumor.

d. Dysgerminoma
– is a rare stromal tumor seen in women 20–30 years of age.
– is similar to the seminoma seen in males.
– grows rapidly and is highly malignant.
– generally appears ovoid, solid, smooth, and homogenous.

e. Krukenberg tumor
– is a pelvic metastasis from stomach cancer that attaches to the ovary.
– is a bilateral, smooth-walled, hypoechoic tumor.
– is often accompanied by ascites and fixed bowel.

5. Other pathology
a. Atrophy
(1) In postmenopausal patients, the endometrium may atrophy and bleed when it is very thin.
(2) Atrophy is diagnosed if the endometrium is **4 mm or less** in width and of the same thickness throughout.

b. Submucosal and intracavitary fibroids
(1) Fibroids may cause bleeding if they abut on the endometrial cavity, even after menopause.
(2) Moderately echogenic masses with a smooth echogenic border are seen when fibroids are located in the endometrial cavity.

CHAPTER 29

PELVIC PATHOLOGY (6%-10%)

I. CONGENITAL UTERINE MALFORMATIONS

– are seen in 1% of the population.

– are associated with genitourinary anomalies because the reproductive organs and kidneys develop at approximately the same time.

– often result in infertility or miscarriage.

A. Congenital vaginal malformations

1. The vagina may be partially or completely absent or obstructed by a membrane. **Vaginal atresia** or **imperforate hymen** can result in **hematocolpos** (blood-filled vagina), **hematometra** (blood-filled uterus), or **hematocolpometra** (blood-filled vagina and uterus) at puberty.

2. At birth or *in utero*, fluid may fill the vagina or uterus, a condition called **hydrocolpometra**.

B. Congenital uterine malformations (Figure 29–1)

1. **Unicornuate uterus**
   a. Incomplete development of one side of the uterus leads to a unicornuate uterus (i.e., a uterus with one tube).
   b. The uterus will appear small and more lateral in position on the sonogram.
   c. A rudimentary horn may be visible.

2. **Uterus didelphus**
   a. Double vaginas, cervices, and uteri function separately.
   b. The two uteri are at approximately a 45° angle to one another.

3. **Bicornuate uterus**
   a. Improper fusion leads to two partially or completely separate bicornuate uterine cavities.
   b. The uterus is heart shaped.

4. **Arcuate uterus**
   – The uterus is normally shaped but there is an indentation on the superior aspect of the endometrial cavity.

5. **Septate uterus**
   a. Two partially or completely separate endometrium form.
   b. The uterus is normally shaped.

C. Diethylstilbestrol (DES) exposure malformations

1. DES was prescribed from the 1940s to the 1960s to prevent spontaneous abortion and premature labor.

2. Female offspring of DES-exposed mothers can be affected. A T-shaped uterus occurs (i.e., a small uterus without the normal bulbous fundus and with a short cervix).

D. Agenesis

1. Agenesis is the congenital absence of the uterus (uterine aplasia) or the cervix.

2. Agenesis is a rare condition.

II. UTERINE MASSES

A. Clinical features that indicate the need for an ultrasound study include

– heavy periods (**menorrhagia**).

– frequent periods (**metrorrhagia**).

– heavy and frequent periods with bleeding in between (**menometrorrhagia**).

– painful periods (**dysmenorrhea**).

B. Fibroids (or leiomyomas)

– are common, benign muscle masses.

– are estrogen sensitive and, therefore, may regress after menopause.

1. **Types of fibroids**
   a. **Subserosal** fibroids occur on the surface of the uterus.
   b. **Pedunculated** fibroids extend away

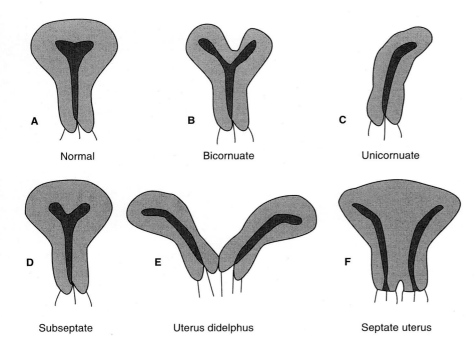

A Normal

B Bicornuate

C Unicornuate

D Subseptate

E Uterus didelphus

F Septate uterus

FIGURE 29-1. Congenital uterine anomalies. (*A*) Normal uterus. (*B*) Bicornuate uterus. Note the V-shaped indentation in the fundus of the endometrial cavity. (*C*) Unicornuate uterus that has only one horn. No fallopian tube leads to the left ovary. (*D*) Uterus subseptate. There is no deformity of the uterine outline, but the two horns of the uterus are split. (*E*) Uterus didelphus. There are two uteri that are separate, two cervices, and two vaginas. (*F*) Septate uterus. Two completely separate uterine cavities are enclosed within a single uterine outline. (Reprinted with permission from Sanders RC: *Clinical Sonography: A Practical Guide,* 3rd ed. Philadelphia, Lippincott, 1998, p 47.)

from the uterus and are attached by a stalk.

  c. Intramural fibroids occur in the wall of the uterus.

  d. Submucosal fibroids abut on the endometrial cavity.

  e. Intracavitary fibroids occur in the endometrial cavity.

  f. Cervical fibroids extend into or arise from the cervix.

2. Clinical features of fibroids include

  – menometrorrhagia.

  – dysmenorrhea.

  – local pain.

  – pressure on the bladder or rectum.

  – infertility.

  – spontaneous abortion.

  – obstruction of a normal vaginal delivery.

3. Sonographic findings

  a. Fibroids have smooth borders with hypoechoic, whorl-like patterns within.

  b. Fibroids may contain hypoechoic areas of **degeneration** or **calcification.**

    (1) Degeneration in fibroids is common. Degenerative changes occur in 60% of fibroids.

    (2) Smooth muscle may be replaced with fibrous tissue (hyaline degeneration), and cystic changes may occur.

    (3) In "red degeneration," there is bleeding into the center of the fibroid. "Red degeneration" is painful and occurs most often in pregnancy.

    (4) Calcification is common, and usually occurs around the edge of the fibroid.

C. Adenomyosis

  – is a condition in which there are deposits of endometrial tissue in the myometrium that bleed at menstruation.

  1. Clinical features include

    – pain.

    – painful, lengthy, heavy menstruation.

    – a clinically enlarged uterus.

  2. Sonographic findings include

    – an enlarged or normal-sized uterus.

    – multiple cystic or ill-defined hypoechoic areas in the myometrium, close to the endometrium.

D. Nabothian cysts

  – are small (less than 3 cm) cysts in the cervix.

  – may be multiple.

  – are asymptomatic.

  – contain mucous secretions.

  – are a common, normal variant finding.

E. Cervical cancer

  – is common.

  – is almost never diagnosed with ultrasound unless large. A bulky cervix is seen.

III. OVARIAN MASSES

  A. Physiologic masses

    1. Follicles

    – are echo-free cysts that grow to a size of approximately 2.6 cm by day 14 of the cycle.

a. A dominant follicle usually develops in one ovary in one cycle and in the other the next cycle.

b. With clomiphene citrate (Clomid) or human menopausal gonadotropin (Pergonal) stimulation, more than one dominant follicle is seen.

2. Follicular cysts
- are echo-free cysts.
- are follicles that failed to ovulate.
- may grow to be as large as 10 cm.
- eventually regress spontaneously.

3. Corpus luteum
- develops once ovulation has taken place.
- can vary in appearance from echo-free to complex, depending on presence and degree of hemorrhage; the corpus luteum is also called a hemorrhagic cyst.
- can vary in size up to about 7 cm.
- regresses spontaneously over the next few weeks following ovulation.

4. Theca-lutein cysts
- are multiple large cysts that appear in both ovaries and are derived from follicles.
- can persist for several weeks.
- appear in the presence of **multiple pregnancies** (and occasionally in singletons), **hyperstimulation syndrome** (from fertility drug administration), and **trophoblastic disease.**

B. Benign ovarian masses
1. Benign cystic teratomas
- represent 25% of all ovarian masses.
- can occur at any age, but are most common in women 20–30 years of age.
- may be asymptomatic or painful.

a. **Dermoids**
- are always benign.
- contain only ectodermal tissue.
- are bilateral in 10%–25% of cases.

b. **Benign cystic teratomas**
- contain tissue from all three germ layers.
- rarely become malignant.

c. **Sonographic findings** of dermoids and benign cystic teratomas vary and may include
- an echogenic focus with shadowing in a cyst.
- an echogenic anterior portion of the mass with shadowing posteriorly (**"tip of the iceberg" sign**).
- a densely echogenic area, making it difficult to separate the mass from mesenteric fat.
- fluid-fluid levels, with the superior area more echogenic.

- a cyst containing a floating, shadowing hairball.
- an entirely cystic mass.
- a cystic mass with multiple septa and papillary masses.

d. The diagnosis can be confirmed by performing a CT scan or plain x-ray, which will show fat or teeth in the mass.

2. Cystadenomas of the ovary (serous and mucinous)
- are common.
- can become large, and yet remain benign.

a. **Serous cystadenomas**
- are more common.
- contain thin, serous fluid; therefore, they are echo-free.
- may contain septa or papillary projections.
- are often bilateral.

b. **Mucinous cystadenomas**
- are usually unilateral, but can be bilateral.
- contain thick gel or mucin.
- may contain papillary projections, but they are less common than in serous cystadenomas.

3. Stromal tumors
a. **Fibromas**
- are benign, solid tumors.
- have a peak incidence between 50 and 60 years of age.
- often present as **Meigs' syndrome** (75% of fibromas), which consists of ovarian fibromas, abdominal ascites, and right pleural effusion.

b. **Thecomas**
- are benign, solid masses.

IV. ENDOMETRIOSIS

- **Endometrial cysts** (i.e., **endometriomas, chocolate cysts**) are blood collections related to endometriosis deposits.
- Endometrial tissue may implant in the ovaries, on any of the organs in the pelvis, or in surgical scars. However, it may occasionally deposit elsewhere.

A. Clinical features include
- painful, heavy periods.
- pain during intercourse.
- infertility.
- monthly hematuria or gut bleeding.
- bloody stools.

B. Sonographic findings include
- single or multiple masses that lie inside or outside of the ovary.
- an evenly echogenic, cystic, or solid mass.
- a multilocular mass.
- adhesions with fixation of the ovaries, bowel, and uterus.

V. POLYCYSTIC OVARY SYNDROME

– This biochemical disorder is a common cause of infrequent or absent ovulation.

A. Clinical features include
– infertility.
– oligomenorrhea (i.e., infrequent periods).
– obesity and hirsutism (Stein-Leventhal syndrome).

B. Sonographic findings include
– multiple small retention cysts lining the cortical zone at the edge of an enlarged ovary.
– increased central stromal tissue.
– bilateral changes.

VI. PELVIC INFLAMMATORY DISEASE (PID)

– infects up to 1 million people in the United States annually.
– is an infection of the upper genital tract that ascends from the cervix into the uterus, fallopian tubes, and adnexa.
– is most often caused by sexually transmitted diseases (e.g., gonorrhea), but is also caused by bacterial infections, intrauterine contraceptive devices, surgery, tuberculosis, and a ruptured appendix.

A. Acute PID
  1. Clinical features include
  – pain.
  – fever.
  – increased white blood cell count.
  – tenderness to cervical motion.
  – purulent discharge.
  2. Sonographic findings include
  – a thickened endometrium containing fluid due to endometritis.
  – thickened or dilated fallopian tubes containing fluid with internal echoes (i.e., acute salpingitis).
  – abscess formation characterized by bilateral, thick-walled, complex masses in the adnexa that spare the ovaries (**tubo-ovarian abscess**).

B. Chronic PID
  – is a residuum of acute PID.
  1. Clinical features include
  – chronic pain.
  – adhesions.
  – edema.
  2. Sonographic findings include
  – dilated fallopian tubes with thin walls and containing watery fluid (i.e., **hydrosalpinx**). Hydrosalpinx tends to result in dilation at the fimbriated end with a series of distended tubular cystic areas outside of the ovary.
  – **adhesions,** which result in an abnormal location of the ovaries close to the uterus, either far laterally or posterior. The ovaries are tender and immobile when pushed with the endovaginal probe.

VII. DOPPLER FLOW STUDIES

A. Benign adnexal masses have a high-resistance Doppler flow pattern.

B. Malignant ovarian masses tend to have a low-resistance Doppler flow pattern.

C. Corpora lutea and ectopic pregnancies have a low-resistance Doppler flow pattern. A ring of vessels is seen around ectopic pregnancies and corpora lutea with color flow Doppler.

VIII. GYNECOLOGY-RELATED STUDIES

A. Gastrointestinal (GI) studies
  1. Endometrial tissue may implant in the GI tract and bleed monthly. Ovarian cancer also may invade the GI tract.
  2. Possible involvement of the GI tract by gynecologic processes is investigated by barium enema or CT scan.

B. Genitourinary studies
  1. Large pelvic masses may extrinsically compress the ureters and cause hydronephrosis. A renal sonogram is often performed when a large pelvic mass is found.
  2. Invasion of the bladder by pelvic neoplasms occurs and is usually investigated by CT scan.

IX. OTHER PATHOLOGIES

A. Paraovarian cysts
  – grow in the adnexa in the region of the fallopian tube.
  – are usually simple cysts, but intracyst hemorrhage can occur with subsequent septations.

B. Peritoneal inclusion cysts
  – occur in patients who have undergone multiple or complex pelvic surgeries.
  – appear as loculated fluid in the peritoneum walled in by adhesions.
  – have irregular walls and may contain internal echoes.
  –are most commonly located in the cul-de-sac.

C. Gartner's cyst
  – is a congenital cyst that occurs in the anterior wall of the vagina.

CHAPTER 30

EXTRAPELVIC PATHOLOGY ASSOCIATED WITH GYNECOLOGY (1%–3%)

I. ASCITES

– is commonly seen with ovarian lesions, and usually means a malignant ovarian neoplasm.

– may also occur in association with benign fibroma (Meigs' syndrome).

A. Malignant ascites (i.e., ascites related to metastases) is characterized by peritoneal metastatic deposits and adhesions. Bowel is tethered in a fixed location.

B. Benign ascites surrounds bowel in a natural fashion.

C. Infected ascites may contain multiple membranes, forming a cobweb-like pattern.

II. MALIGNANT PELVIC MASSES

– preferentially **metastasize** to the liver and to **para-aortic nodes.**

III. BENIGN OR MALIGNANT UTERINE OR OVARIAN MASSES

– can compress the ureters and cause secondary **hydronephrosis** if large enough.

SECTION C • OBSTETRIC AND GYNECOLOGIC PATIENT CARE: PREPARATION AND TECHNIQUE

CHAPTER 31

OBSTETRIC AND GYNECOLOGIC PATIENT CARE: PREPARATION AND TECHNIQUE (1%-5%)

I. REVIEWING CHARTS

– Before performing the sonogram, there are several tasks the sonographer should complete.

  A. Briefly examine the patient's chart, looking for:
- the clinical question being asked.
- the differential diagnosis being entertained.
- relevant laboratory values.
- results of any previous imaging techniques (e.g., mammogram for a breast mass).

  B. Insert the patient's name and number into the ultrasound system.

  C. Make sure the room is clean and the examination table has fresh linen.

II. EXPLAINING EXAMINATIONS

  A. When ready for the patient, the sonographer should greet the patient in a respectful manner, using the patient's second name rather than the patient's first name.

  B. After a careful explanation of the procedure that will be performed (e.g., endovaginal examination), the sonographer should interview the patient. Questions should focus on
- main symptoms.
- age.
- last period date.
- number of pregnancies.
- number of miscarriages.
- number of premature infants.
- number of abortions.

– menstrual characteristics (e.g., heavy, frequent).
– presence and severity of pelvic pain.
– presence and severity of vaginal bleeding.
– history of previous pelvic surgeries.

C. Before performing any procedure (e.g., amniocentesis)
– prepare the equipment required (e.g., amniocentesis tray, sterilizing fluids).
– make sure informed consent has been obtained.
– try to put the patient at ease with conversation.

III. SUPINE HYPOTENSIVE SYNDROME

– is common in the second and third trimesters.
– is thought to be caused by excessive fetal pressure on the inferior vena cava, preventing venous return to the heart when the patient is in the supine position.

A. When attempting to examine a patient with supine hypotensive syndrome in a supine position, the patient may
– feel faint.
– feel lightheaded.
– feel sick.
– become pale and sweaty.

B. Correction techniques when a patient has the supine hypotensive syndrome
– The examination can continue with the patient in a different position.
1. Turn the patient on her left side and the symptoms will generally disappear.
2. If necessary, sit the patient up.

IV. BIOLOGIC EFFECTS

– There are no known biologic effects to the human from the diagnostic ultrasound studies done over the past 35 years.

A. Side effects of ultrasound at dosages above those used for diagnosis include
– tissue heating.
– cavitation.

B. Studies at doses close to those used clinically have suggested low birthweight in laboratory animals.

C. To avoid any possible side effects, practice the ALARA principle (i.e., As Low As Reasonably Achievable).
1. Keep the power output as low as possible and use receiver gain to change the quality of the image.
2. Do not use Doppler in early pregnancies. Doppler puts out high levels of ultrasound, especially when used at one site for a long time.

3. Newer instrumentation is required to give an indication of power output on the display.

V. INFECTIOUS DISEASE CONTROL

A. Infection has been transmitted from patient to patient because of unhygienic sonography.

B. To prevent infection
– use gloves when scanning.
– wash your hands frequently.
– sterilize the vaginal and endorectal probes in glutaraldehyde for at least 10 minutes between patients (see the product requirements).
– always use a sterile condom with endovaginal and transrectal probes.
– use sterile precautions when an invasive procedure is performed.
– wipe down the ultrasound system and surfaces in the examination room every day with a disinfectant solution.

VI. SCANNING TECHNIQUES

A. Preparation
1. The bladder should be full
– for transabdominal gynecologic studies.
– for transabdominal obstetric sonograms during the first trimester and for second trimester obstetric sonograms.
2. The bladder should be empty
– for endovaginal sonograms.
– for views of the cervix.
– to determine if placenta previa is present.
– when assessing the maternal kidneys for hydronephrosis.

B. Position
1. Transabdominal gynecologic and obstetric patients are typically scanned in the supine position.
2. The lithotomy position (patient lying on a gynecologic table with her feet in stirrups) is used for endovaginal scanning.
3. Decubitus views are used if the patient has the supine hypotensive syndrome, has suspected fluid-fluid levels or bladder calculus (which should be demonstrated changing position), or when trying to encourage a change in fetal position.
4. Prone views with the patient in the hand/knee position may be helpful when massive polyhydramnios prevents adequate views of the fetus; the fetus is brought into the field of view.

C. Transducer choice
1. Use the highest transducer frequency with satisfactory penetration.

2. Take into account **endovaginal versus transabdominal considerations.**
   a. The **transabdominal approach**
      - provides a large field of view, so uterine or mass size can be measured and larger fetuses can be examined.
      - A superiorly placed ovary or pelvic mass may only be seen from a transabdominal approach.
   b. The **endovaginal approach** helps
      - to see the details of the ovaries and endometrium.
      - for first trimester obstetric work.
      - when there is a question of placenta previa or cervical incompetence.
      - for detailed views of the fetal head in the second and third trimesters if the fetus is vertex.
      - for views of the fetal sacrum when the fetus is breech, especially if a teratoma or a spina bifida is present.

D. **Transducer techniques** include
   - sliding the endovaginal transducer (e.g., inferiorly to visualize the cervix better or superiorly to show the ovaries).
   - rocking (e.g., moving the endovaginal transducer gently to separate the ovary from the uterus or from a mass).
   - tilting (e.g., moving the transducer under bowel to avoid air).
   - compression, particularly when scanning for appendicitis versus a right lower quadrant mass.

E. **Color flow and pulsed Doppler** are used
   - to look at the number of vessels in the umbilical cord.
   - for umbilical cord assessment of fetal well-being, particularly the umbilical arteries.
   - to assess placental, ovarian, and uterine vascularity.
   - when there is a question of fetal vascular abnormality (e.g., vein of Galen aneurysm).
   - in fetal echocardiography.

VII. ARTIFACTS

   - Artifacts encountered in obstetric and gynecologic scanning are related to the interaction of sound with tissues.

A. **Mirror artifact**
   - With a full bladder, the sound is transmitted from wall to wall and takes a long time to return to the transducer. A spurious cystic mass posterior to the bladder may be created.

B. **Rectus muscle artifact**
   - Sound may be refracted by the rectus muscles, creating a double image of a structure below (e.g., intrauterine contraceptive device, gestational sac).

C. **Grating artifact**
   - Caused by side lobes, this artifact may create curvilinear lines in the image.

D. **Slice thickness artifact**
   - may create low-level echoes in the posterior aspect of a cystic structure due to the sound beam partially striking the wall of the cyst and partially striking the cystic contents.

E. **Reverberation artifact**
   - Caused by the reduplication of main bang echoes, this artifact creates echoes near the anterior abdominal wall.

VIII. PHYSICAL PRINCIPLES

A. Sound is generated by a vibrating source.

B. Humans hear sound at 2–20 kHz. Medical ultrasound is in the range of 1–30 mHz, so it is above the range of human hearing.

C. Ultrasound waves are mechanical, longitudinal waves that travel slowly through air and quickly through dense material (e.g., bone).

D. Gel is used to eliminate air and to create a coupling between the transducer and the skin so that the speed of sound in the body is similar to the speed in the coupling medium between the transducer and the body, allowing sound to be conducted into the body.

E. A crystal that is electrically pulsed creates ultrasound. As it changes shape and vibrates, a sound beam is produced that propagates through the tissue.

F. Important machine controls that control the production of ultrasound include
   - **power,** which controls the amount of sound produced by the transducer.
   - **gain,** which varies the overall amplification of the echoes.
   - **time gain compensation, depth gain compensation, or swept gain,** which compensates for the attenuation of the returning echoes as sound travels through time and depth (i.e., controls returning signal).
   - **calipers,** which are used to measure structures.
   - **pre- and postprocessing,** which can be used to alter the gray scale amplitude levels of an image by computerized manipulation (e.g., emphasizing the low-level echoes may allow a diagnosis).
   - **dynamic range,** which can be used to vary the range of the highest to lowest sound decibels that can be displayed.
   - **persistence,** which controls the length of time that an echo is present in the display.

PART III

Comprehensive Examinations

ABDOMEN REVIEW TEST

Each numbered statement or question is followed by a minimum of four options. Select the ONE that is BEST.

1. A transducer with small rectangular elements lined up side by side and firing in a straight line is a
   A. curved linear (curved array) transducer
   B. phased array transducer
   C. mechanical sector transducer
   D. intracavitary transducer
   E. linear array transducer

2. A 30-year-old hemophiliac with a decrease in hematocrit presents for an abdominal sonogram. Where is the sonographer **MOST** likely to find an explanation for the abnormal hematocrit value?
   A. Psoas muscle
   B. Spleen
   C. Beneath the diaphragm
   D. Liver
   E. Posterior cul-de-sac

3. A 24-year-old man was referred for a CT scan after experiencing penetrating trauma to his abdomen. The CT scan showed a hematoma in the right psoas muscle. Two weeks later he was referred to ultrasound for an abdominal sonogram to follow up the initial CT scan. Which of the following techniques would afford the **BEST** view of the area of the bleed?
   A. Supine, scanning intercostally
   B. Prone oblique decubitus, using the kidney as an acoustic window
   C. Supine, scanning through the distended bladder
   D. Supine, after administering a water enema
   E. None; this area cannot be imaged sonographically

4. All of the following are indications for ultrasound evaluation of the retroperitoneum **EXCEPT**
   A. to rule out a splenic abscess
   B. to follow up a hematoma in the quadratus lumborum muscles
   C. an unexplained decrease in hematocrit
   D. to rule out a hematoma in Gerota's fascia
   E. following a renal transplant

5. All of the following findings are consistent with Crohn's disease **EXCEPT**
   A. an increased white blood cell count
   B. bloody stools
   C. lack of color flow Doppler signals in the bowel wall
   D. a thickened bowel wall
   E. lack of peristalsis

6. All of the following may be features of benign prostatic hypertrophy **EXCEPT**
   A. renal failure
   B. unexplained fever
   C. frequent urination
   D. poor urinary stream
   E. abnormal serum creatinine levels

7. Which of the following is **NOT** a transrectal ultrasound diagnosis?
   A. Infertility
   B. A seminal vesicle cyst
   C. Prostatic calculi
   D. Congenital vas deferens absence
   E. Peyronie's disease

8. All of the following are indications for ultrasound evaluation of the neck **EXCEPT**
   A. a cold nodule on a nuclear medicine study
   B. difficulty swallowing
   C. a palpable neck mass
   D. abnormally low serum calcium levels
   E. a history of tongue carcinoma

9. Which of the following is **NOT** true concerning the parathyroid glands?
   A. They may be located posterior to the thyroid gland
   B. They may be located in the thyroid gland
   C. A normal parathyroid gland is 1 cm
   D. A parathyroid mass is often not palpable
   E. A typical patient has four parathyroid glands

10. When performing an ultrasound evaluation of the thyroid, color flow Doppler may be helpful when
    A. determining whether a mass is malignant or benign
    B. looking for calcifications in the lesion
    C. proving that a mass is real and not an artifact
    D. a mass is echogenic
    E. a mass is in the near field

11. A round, echo-free mass seen high in the midline of the neck, above the thyroid, is **MOST** likely
    A. a thyroglossal duct cyst
    B. a branchial cleft cyst
    C. a lymph node
    D. a normal parathyroid gland
    E. an adenoma

12. A 42-year-old man is found to have a 14-mm parathyroid gland on ultrasound evaluation. Based on this finding, the sonographer should look
    A. at the abdomen for a primary neoplasm
    B. at the jugular vein for tumor invasion
    C. at the esophagus to rule out obstruction
    D. along the major vessels for adenopathy
    E. at the kidneys for calcifications

13. Which of the following is the **BEST** transducer to use when imaging the thyroid gland?
    A. 3.5 MHz sector
    B. 5.0 MHz curved linear array
    C. 7.5 MHz electronically focused
    D. 7.5 MHz mechanical sector
    E. 10 MHz sector

14. A 35-year-old woman with a palpable neck mass presents for a thyroid sonogram. Two solid, echogenic masses, each surrounded by a halo of hypoechoic tissue, are seen in the thyroid gland. The **MOST** likely diagnosis is
    A. thyroid adenomas
    B. Graves' disease
    C. thyroid cancer
    D. Hashimoto's disease
    E. thyroid cysts

15. Which of the following correctly describes the placement of structures in the neck from medial to lateral?
    A. Left lobe of the thyroid, internal jugular vein, common carotid artery
    B. Right lobe of the thyroid, internal carotid artery, internal jugular vein
    C. Internal carotid artery, right lobe of the thyroid, internal jugular vein
    D. Left lobe of the thyroid, common carotid artery, internal jugular vein
    E. Right lobe of the thyroid, internal carotid artery, external carotid artery

16. A patient is sent to ultrasound to follow up a CT scan that showed an ill-defined mass in the isthmus of the thyroid. The sonographer is unable to visualize the mass on the initial sonogram. All of the following may be helpful in demonstrating the pathology **EXCEPT**
    A. a standoff pad
    B. a higher frequency transducer
    C. a slight increase in pressure
    D. color flow Doppler
    E. more acoustic gel

17. A 6-year-old patient with a history of a recent streptococcus throat infection treated with a 10-day course of antibiotics is referred for a neck sonogram to evaluate a large, tender, palpable mass. Which of the following is the sonographer **MOST** likely to find?
    A. A hypoechoic, homogeneous mass with an echogenic center lateral to the internal jugular vein
    B. A solid, echogenic mass in the thyroid gland surrounded by an echopenic halo
    C. A diffusely enlarged thyroid gland
    D. An echogenic mass lateral to the carotid artery
    E. A well-circumscribed, echo-free structure adjacent to the thyroid gland

18. Which of the following laboratory values will **MOST** likely be abnormal in a patient with a multinodular goiter?
    A. Serum calcium
    B. Potassium
    C. Triiodothyronine (T_3) and thyroxine (T_4)
    D. White blood cells
    E. Thyroid-stimulating hormone

19. The artery(ies) that carries(y) 15%–30% of the total cardiac output is(are) the
    A. left gastric artery
    B. left common carotid artery
    C. superior mesenteric artery
    D. renal arteries
    E. common iliac arteries

20. Which of the following structures is **NOT** retroperitoneal?
    A. Aorta
    B. Inferior vena cava
    C. Kidneys
    D. Spleen
    E. Adrenal glands

21. The liver is an intraperitoneal organ surrounded by peritoneum. Which portion, if any, is **NOT** covered by peritoneum?
    A. Right lobe
    B. Caudate lobe
    C. Bare area
    D. Left lobe
    E. It is all covered

22. A remnant of the fetal ductus venosus that divides the caudate lobe of the liver from the left lobe of the liver is the
    A. main lobar fissure
    B. ligamentum venosum
    C. falciform ligament
    D. ligamentum teres
    E. hepatoduodenal ligament

23. The vessel that is responsible for supplying the liver with the most nutrients is the
    A. main portal vein
    B. hepatic artery
    C. common bile duct
    D. celiac artery
    E. hepatic vein

24. Which of the following vessels is associated with waveforms that do **NOT** vary with respiration in a normal patient?
    A. Hepatic vein
    B. Portal vein
    C. Jugular vein
    D. Femoral vein
    E. Inferior vena cava

25. The cells of the intestinal mucosa secrete a hormone that causes the gallbladder to contract and release bile. This hormone is
    A. lecithin
    B. cholecystokinin
    C. cholesterol
    D. bilirubin
    E. renin

26. Serum glutamic pyruvic transaminase (SGPT) is also referred to as
    A. bilirubin
    B. alanine aminotransferase (ALT)
    C. serum protein
    D. alkaline phosphatase
    E. α-fetoprotein (AFP)

27. All of the following increase in hepatocellular disease **EXCEPT**
    A. alanine aminotransferase (ALT)
    B. aspartate aminotransferase (AST)
    C. prothrombin time (PT)
    D. bilirubin
    E. acid phosphatase

28. Which of the following decreases in hepatocellular disease?
    A. Vitamin K
    B. Alkaline phosphatase
    C. Alanine aminotransferase (ALT)
    D. Aspartate aminotransferase (AST)
    E. Indirect bilirubin

29. Fatty infiltration of the liver is associated with all of the following **EXCEPT**
    A. diabetes mellitus
    B. ethanol abuse
    C. obesity
    D. intravenous antibiotics
    E. oral contraceptives

30. After a cholecystectomy, the common bile duct measures 8 mm in a patient experiencing right upper quadrant and back pain. Which of the following may **NOT** be true?
    A. The "duct" is actually a large hepatic artery
    B. There is a stone lodged in the common bile duct or ampulla of Vater
    C. This may be a normal finding in an elderly patient
    D. This may be a normal finding in a postcholecystectomy patient
    E. This is a normal response to food in a 25-year-old patient

31. In a fasting state, the superior mesenteric artery has
    A. a low-resistance waveform
    B. a high-resistance waveform
    C. reversed diastolic flow
    D. no resistance
    E. a high dicrotic notch

32. Which of the following is **NOT** an indication for renal artery Doppler imaging?
    A. Possible renal artery stenosis
    B. Hypertension
    C. Abdominal bruit
    D. Unilateral small kidney
    E. Renal calculi

33. Five patients from a renal transplant ward are sent to ultrasound for postoperative sonograms. The following is a list of the indications for their postoperative examinations. Based on these indications, which patient was **NOT** sent to a machine equipped with Doppler?
    A. Renal artery stenosis
    B. Renal vein thrombosis
    C. Rejection
    D. Urinoma formation
    E. Acute tubular necrosis

34. In certain geographical areas, a widespread disease caused by an infection from parasites that involves the bladder is
    A. schistosomiasis
    B. glycogen storage disease
    C. malaria
    D. hydatid disease
    E. ascaris infection

35. A complex cystic area is seen in the liver. Which of the following patients, whose occupations are listed, is **MOST** at risk to contract this condition?
    A. Asbestos worker
    B. Coal miner
    C. Shepherd
    D. Glass blower
    E. Carpenter

36. Which of the following is a rare malignant tumor, most commonly found in infants and children, that causes abdominal distention and hepatomegaly?
    A. Hepatoblastoma
    B. Hepatocellular carcinoma
    C. Focal nodular hyperplasia
    D. Hematoma
    E. Rhabdomyosarcoma

37. Complete blockage of the cystic duct can result in
    A. a dilated distal common bile duct
    B. hydrops of the gallbladder
    C. Mirizzi syndrome
    D. gallbladder polyps
    E. jaundice

38. A bile duct neoplasm that carries a poor prognosis and is located at the hepatic duct bifurcation is **MOST** likely to be
    A. Budd-Chiari syndrome
    B. Arnold-Chiari malformation
    C. a Klatskin tumor
    D. cystadenocarcinoma
    E. intraductal metastasis

39. Which of the following cells are responsible for the endocrine function of the pancreas?
    A. Islet cells
    B. T cells
    C. Islets of Langerhans
    D. Acinar cells
    E. Red blood cells

40. A patient presents with severe abdominal pain, nausea, vomiting, abdominal distention, increased lipase levels, and decreased hematocrit. What should the sonographer suspect?
    A. Hepatitis
    B. Duodenitis
    C. Cholecystitis
    D. Hemorrhagic pancreatitis
    E. Cholelithiasis

41. A fatal tumor that involves the exocrine portion of the pancreas and predominately occurs in elderly male smokers is
    A. an islet cell tumor
    B. adenocarcinoma
    C. cystadenocarcinoma
    D. a pseudocyst
    E. phlegmon

42. The most sensitive laboratory test for determining renal dysfunction is
    A. serum creatinine
    B. blood urea nitrogen
    C. 24-hour urine collection
    D. specific gravity
    E. urinalysis

43. Which of the following is a true cyst?
    A. Parenchymal renal cyst
    B. Biloma
    C. Parapelvic cyst
    D. Pancreatic pseudocyst
    E. Seroma

44. A hypoechoic mass is seen in the renal pelvis of the kidney. Which of the following is the **MOST** likely diagnosis?
    A. Transitional cell carcinoma
    B. Angiomyolipoma
    C. Adenoma
    D. Hypernephroma
    E. Renal lymphoma

45. A 75-year-old man presents with abdominal pain, hematuria, and a palpable upper abdominal mass. The sonographer performs an abdominal scan. When scanning the kidney, a solid mass with calcifications is noted. Further investigation reveals tumor involvement in the inferior vena cava. Which of the following is the **MOST** likely diagnosis?
    A. Wilms' tumor
    B. Transitional cell carcinoma
    C. Renal cell carcinoma
    D. Multicystic dysplastic kidney disease
    E. Hemangioma

46. What renal disease is associated with berry aneurysms?
    A. Renal cell carcinoma
    B. Autosomal recessive polycystic kidney disease
    C. Autosomal dominant polycystic kidney disease
    D. Multicystic dysplastic kidney disease
    E. Transitional cell carcinoma

47. Extrinsic causes of hydronephrosis include all of the following **EXCEPT**
    A. a calculus
    B. uterine fibroids
    C. trauma
    D. pregnancy
    E. ovarian neoplasms

48. To exclude a false-positive diagnosis of hydronephrosis, the sonographer should
    A. change to a lower frequency transducer
    B. perform prevoid and postvoid images of the kidneys
    C. defer to CT scan
    D. repeat the scan in 24–48 hours
    E. defer to MRI

49. A 39-year-old renal transplant patient arrives in the ultrasound department. The patient is referred for all of the following **EXCEPT**
    A. to rule out hydronephrosis
    B. to rule out fluid collections around the kidney
    C. Doppler imaging of the arcuate artery to rule out rejection
    D. Doppler imaging of the renal vein to rule out a kinked vein
    E. to rule out cyclosporine toxicity

50. Two days after a renal transplant, the most common cause of acute renal failure is
    A. cyclosporine toxicity
    B. acute tubular necrosis
    C. renal obstruction
    D. acute pyelonephritis
    E. acute rejection

51. All of the following are sonographic indications of rejection in a transplanted kidney **EXCEPT**
    A. increased parenchymal echogenicity
    B. bladder distension
    C. high-resistance Doppler pattern
    D. abnormal decrease in renal size
    E. presence of hydronephrosis

52. A 25-year-old man with a myelomeningocele has a sonogram of the urinary bladder. All of the following conditions might be found **EXCEPT**
    A. renal calculi
    B. a dilated ureter
    C. a large bladder with trabeculation
    D. benign prostatic hypertrophy
    E. a dilated renal pelvis

53. A 17-year-old boy presents in the emergency room with scrotal pain. The sonogram reveals an enlarged testicle, decreased echogenicity, thickening of the scrotal wall, a hydrocele, and no arterial flow. These findings are consistent with
    A. cryptorchidism
    B. torsion
    C. acute orchitis
    D. epididymitis
    E. a spermatocele

54. In a patient with cryptorchidism, which of the following is **MOST** likely to occur?
    A. A seminoma
    B. Torsion
    C. Epididymitis
    D. A hydrocele
    E. A spermatocele

55. Infarction of the spleen is associated with all of the following **EXCEPT**
    A. splenic artery thrombosis
    B. bacterial endocarditis
    C. sickle cell anemia
    D. a splenic cyst

56. An elderly man falls on a wooden chair and strikes his left side. He catches the fall with both hands, but has to struggle to get back to a standing position. Although in pain, he does not report his injury. One day later he falls again and is unable to sit up. Paramedics arrive to find the patient pale and clammy with a blood pressure of 60/40. At the hospital, a sonogram is ordered. The sonographer should be careful to search for
    A. splenic rupture
    B. prostate obstruction
    C. gallbladder rupture
    D. an abscess
    E. a renal artery aneurysm

57. A 36-year-old woman is referred for a breast sonogram after a mass is seen on a mammogram. This mass appears small and homogeneous with smooth borders and contains low-level internal echoes. The **MOST** likely diagnosis is
    A. a cyst
    B. a fibroadenoma
    C. cystosarcoma phyllodes
    D. ductal carcinoma
    E. a galactocele

58. The most common malignant breast tumor in the United States is
    A. medullary carcinoma
    B. fibroadenoma
    C. lobular carcinoma
    D. infiltrating ductal carcinoma
    E. Paget's disease

59. Arteriovenous fistulas may be caused by all of the following **EXCEPT**
    A. surgery
    B. trauma
    C. aneurysm
    D. atherosclerosis
    E. congenital factors

60. Extrahepatic collections of extravasated bile from abdominal trauma, biliary surgery, or gallbladder disease are known as
    A. hematomas
    B. choledochal cysts
    C. lymphoceles
    D. urinomas
    E. bilomas

61. The C-loop of the duodenum is bordered by all of the following **EXCEPT**
    A. the main lobar fissure
    B. the sphincter of Oddi
    C. the gallbladder
    D. the pancreatic head
    E. the renal artery

62. A young male patient with rebound tenderness, an elevated white blood cell count, a fever, and periumbilical and right lower quadrant pain **MOST** likely has
    A. gallstones
    B. appendicitis
    C. pancreatitis
    D. renal colic
    E. ulcerative colitis

63. When scanning the appendix for appendicitis, the differential diagnosis typically includes all of the following **EXCEPT**
    A. a tubo-ovarian abscess
    B. a torsed ovarian cyst
    C. a ruptured ectopic pregnancy
    D. rectal polyps
    E. Crohn's disease

64. Chronic inflammatory disease of the thyroid is known as
    A. multinodular goiter
    B. endemic goiter
    C. Hashimoto's disease
    D. follicular adenoma
    E. follicular adenocarcinoma

65. An aneurysm caused by a bacterial infection is called a
    A. pseudoaneurysm
    B. mycotic aneurysm
    C. berry aneurysm
    D. saccular aneurysm
    E. fusiform aneurysm

66. The vessel(s) in the liver that is(are) important in defining lobar anatomy for hepatic resection is(are) the
    A. inferior vena cava
    B. hepatic veins
    C. portal artery
    D. hepatic arteries
    E. umbilical vein

67. Choppy, triphasic flow patterns are seen in the
    A. hepatic veins
    B. portal veins
    C. hepatic arteries
    D. superior mesenteric artery
    E. iliac veins

68. Which of the following techniques is the **MOST** satisfactory for recording and maintaining an accurate representation of the image seen on the ultrasound screen?
    A. Thermal paper
    B. Radiographic film
    C. Polaroid film
    D. Picture-archiving systems (PACs)
    E. VHS videotape

69. A gallbladder contains gallstones and one wall shows localized, severe thickening. Which of the following is the **MOST** likely diagnosis?
    A. Empyema
    B. Cholecystitis
    C. Adenomyomatosis
    D. Hemobilia
    E. Gallbladder cancer

70. When measuring gallbladder wall thickness in suspected acute cholecystitis, the wall should be measured
    A. on the posterior surface
    B. on the lateral surface
    C. on the anterior surface
    D. on any surface
    E. at the fundus

71. An echo-free gallbladder that is 12 cm in length is
    A. a biloma
    B. a papilloma
    C. hydropic
    D. megacystic
    E. consistent with acalculous cholecystitis

72. Renal sinus lipomatosis
    A. is another term for a renal cyst
    B. causes an increase in echogenicity and size of the renal sinus
    C. is a term for anechoic areas secondary to obesity
    D. results in increased cortical echoes
    E. is a form of angiomyolipoma

73. The muscle groups of the anterior abdominal wall include all of the following **EXCEPT**
    A. the internal oblique
    B. the diaphragm
    C. the external oblique
    D. the transversus abdominus
    E. the rectus abdominus

74. A common site for fluid collections in the pelvis is
    A. Morison's pouch
    B. Hartmann's pouch
    C. the pouch of Douglas
    D. the sacral pouch
    E. the Chiari pouch

75. The typical position for scanning the spleen is
    A. reverse Trendelenburg
    B. prone
    C. erect
    D. left lateral decubitus
    E. right lateral decubitus

76. A health care worker contracted hepatitis B from an accidental needle stick. Which of the following is **NOT** likely to be seen on her abdominal sonogram?
    A. Prominent portal vessels
    B. A thickened gallbladder wall
    C. Splenomegaly
    D. A lobular outline to the liver
    E. A hypoechoic liver

77. Dilation of the inferior vena cava may be seen in
    A. portal hypertension
    B. congestive heart failure
    C. uremia
    D. hypertension
    E. mitral valve prolapse

78. All of the following vessels arise from the aortic arch **EXCEPT**
    A. the left common carotid artery
    B. the right innominate artery
    C. the left subclavian artery
    D. the right common carotid artery
    E. the brachiocephalic artery

79. Sonographic depiction of acute renal vein thrombosis includes all of the following **EXCEPT**
    A. renal vein dilation distal to the occlusion
    B. an enlarged, hypoechoic kidney
    C. low-level echoes in the renal vein
    D. absent or reversed diastolic flow in the intrarenal arteries
    E. decreased or no flow on Doppler study

80. A 1-week-old patient presents with left flank pain associated with a mass in the same area. Laboratory tests indicate hematuria and proteinuria. The patient is afebrile. Sonography depicts an enlarged kidney. Which of the following is the **MOST** likely diagnosis?
    A. Renal cyst
    B. Multicystic kidney
    C. Left renal vein thrombosis
    D. Pyonephrosis
    E. Neuroblastoma

81. Cirrhosis of the liver can be caused by all of the following **EXCEPT**
    A. alcohol abuse
    B. obstruction by cholelithiasis
    C. hepatitis B
    D. chemical toxicity
    E. diabetes mellitus

82. All of the following are typical of long-standing cirrhosis **EXCEPT**
    A. a small liver
    B. an enlarged liver
    C. a nodular outline to the liver
    D. increased echogenicity
    E. hepatofugal flow of the portal veins

83. Which of the following is a liver function test related to a blood clotting mechanism?
    A. Bilirubin level
    B. Aspartate aminotransferase (AST) level
    C. Alanine aminotransferase (ALT) level
    D. Prothrombin time
    E. Lactic acid dehydrogenase level

84. A subcapsular hematoma may appear
    A. hypoechoic and curvilinear
    B. anechoic and circular
    C. echogenic and square
    D. hypoechoic and rectangular
    E. echogenic and straight

85. The gallbladder is divided into all of the following regions **EXCEPT**
    A. the neck
    B. the body
    C. the fundus
    D. the isthmus
    E. Hartmann's pouch

86. The typical symptoms of gallbladder disease include all of the following **EXCEPT**
    A. nausea and vomiting
    B. melena
    C. right shoulder pain
    D. right upper quadrant pain
    E. chest pain

87. Most gallstones are composed of
    A. sludge
    B. xanthine
    C. cholesterol
    D. uric acid
    E. cysteine

88. All of the following can be surgically removed without need of replacement **EXCEPT**
    A. the gallbladder
    B. the appendix
    C. the uterus
    D. the pancreas
    E. the spleen

89. Common conditions in which the gallbladder wall is thickened include all of the following **EXCEPT**
    A. fatty infiltration of the liver
    B. acute cholecystitis
    C. AIDS
    D. ascites
    E. hypoalbuminemia

90. The principal functions of the urinary system include all of the following **EXCEPT**
    A. excretion of waste products
    B. formation of urine
    C. regulation of body temperature
    D. regulation of blood pressure
    E. control of fluid balance

91. Which of the following is **NOT** normally found in renal metabolic waste material?
    A. Water
    B. Red blood cells
    C. Carbon dioxide
    D. Nitrogenous waste
    E. Protein

92. Fusion anomalies of the kidneys include all of the following **EXCEPT**
    A. ectopic kidneys
    B. pancake kidneys
    C. crossed renal ectopia
    D. horseshoe kidneys
    E. duplicated kidneys

93. Absence or failure of formation of the kidney is
    A. renal noesis
    B. renal dysgenesis
    C. renal dysamyomenosis
    D. arenaluria
    E. renal agenesis

94. A known drug user presents with a high fever and right flank pain. The sonogram reveals a complex mass with low-level echoes, debris, and bright echoes with ring down artifacts. These findings **MOST** likely represent
    A. hypernephroma
    B. an abscess
    C. a complex cyst
    D. a hematoma
    E. transitional cell carcinoma

95. The presence of pus in a dilated collecting system is referred to as
    A. acute pyelonephritis
    B. a renal abscess
    C. pyonephrosis
    D. focal pyelonephritis
    E. lobar nephronia

96. What structure surrounds the kidney?
    A. Tunica albuginea
    B. Perirenal fat
    C. Glisson's capsule
    D. Renal capsule
    E. Renal cortex

97. **MOST** prostate cancers occur in the
    A. peripheral zone
    B. central zone
    C. transitional zone
    D. seminal vesicles
    E. ejaculatory ducts

98. The **MOST** sensitive indicator of the presence of prostate cancer is
    A. an abnormal digital rectal examination
    B. increased prostate-specific antigen (PSA)
    C. a hypoechoic nodule on a sonogram
    D. decreased PSA
    E. a hyperechoic nodule on a sonogram

99. A 25-year-old man with scrotal swelling is referred for a scrotal sonogram. A large cystic space is found surrounding the normal testicle. All of the following could be appropriate descriptors for the finding **EXCEPT**
    A. congenital
    B. acquired
    C. traumatic
    D. malignant
    E. infective

100. Which of the following increases the blood urea nitrogen level?
    A. Decreased protein intake
    B. Pregnancy
    C. Liver failure
    D. Dehydration
    E. Excessive fluid intake

101. Which of the following conditions causes leukocytosis?
    A. Benign prostatic hypertrophy
    B. AIDS
    C. Anemia
    D. Goiter
    E. Pyelonephritis

102. Multiple, sizeable areas of splenic tissue in the splenic fossa are referred to as
    A. accessory spleens
    B. polysplenia
    C. ectopic spleen
    D. agenesis of the spleen
    E. wandering spleen

103. All of the following cause splenomegaly **EXCEPT**
    A. infectious mononucleosis
    B. thalassemia
    C. portal vein thrombosis
    D. splenic infarct
    E. cirrhosis

104. A congenital disease of the aorta is
    A. Marfan's syndrome
    B. Morison's pouch
    C. atherosclerosis
    D. dissecting aortic aneurysm
    E. aortic thrombosis

105. A highly vascular, benign tumor in the liver is referred to as a
    A. hepatoma
    B. hemangioma
    C. lymphoma
    D. hepatic adenoma
    E. focal nodular hyperplasia

106. Small outpouchings of the mucosa of the gallbladder that extend into the underlying gallbladder wall are called
    A. Morison's pouch
    B. Rokitansky-Aschoff sinuses
    C. Maxillary sinuses
    D. the pouch of Douglas
    E. Hartmann's pouch

107. All of the following are possible causes of hyperbilirubinemia **EXCEPT**
    A. increased red blood cell destruction
    B. congenital disease
    C. common duct stone
    D. presbyductia
    E. severe cirrhosis

108. Chronic inflammation of the bile ducts resulting in scarring and destruction is known as
    A. sclerosing cholangitis
    B. pneumobilia
    C. Mirizzi syndrome
    D. choledocholithiasis
    E. Klatskin tumor

109. The majority of intratesticular masses are
    A. benign
    B. malignant
    C. echogenic
    D. cystic
    E. complex

110. The majority of extratesticular masses are
    A. benign
    B. malignant
    C. echogenic
    D. solid
    E. complex

111. Which of the following is a rare, highly malignant testicular tumor in which levels of circulating human chorionic gonadotropin are high?
    A. Teratoma
    B. Seminoma
    C. Choriocarcinoma
    D. Adenoma of the tunica albuginea
    E. Fibroadenoma

112. Which of the following is the **MOST** common germ cell tumor of the testicles?
    A. Testicular metastases
    B. Teratoma
    C. Dermoid
    D. Seminoma
    E. Embryonal cell carcinoma

113. Which of the following is a common cause of infertility in men?
    A. Spermatoceles
    B. Varicoceles
    C. Epididymal cysts
    D. Hydroceles
    E. Hematoceles

114. A scrotal hernia occurs when bowel protrudes through the inguinal canal into the scrotal sac. The presence of which of the following confirms the diagnosis?
    A. Fluid-filled mass
    B. Solid mass
    C. Peristalsis
    D. Cystic mass
    E. Hydrocele

115. Enlarged lymph nodes may do all of the following **EXCEPT**
    A. compress the ureter
    B. compress the aorta
    C. compress the inferior vena cava
    D. displace the superior mesenteric artery
    E. displace bowel

116. Typical locations of lymph nodes include all of the following **EXCEPT**
    A. surrounding or adjacent to the aorta
    B. in the inguinal region
    C. in the renal hilum
    D. surrounding or adjacent to the pancreas
    E. under the diaphragm

117. In the postmenopausal breast
    A. the amount of fatty tissue decreases while the amount of normal breast tissue increases
    B. the amount of fatty tissue increases while the amount of normal breast tissue increases
    C. the amount of fatty tissue increases while the amount of normal breast tissue decreases
    D. the amount of fatty tissue decreases while the amount of normal breast tissue decreases
    E. there are no changes in fatty or normal breast tissue

118. A 50-year-old woman is referred for a breast sonogram. All of the following aspects of her history are important to know **EXCEPT**
    A. pain and tenderness
    B. nipple discharge
    C. family history of breast cancer
    D. localized mass
    E. family history of gynecomastia

119. Which of the following statements is **TRUE?**
    A. Fibroadenomas and medullary cell carcinomas have very different sonographic appearances
    B. Lactating breasts are easy to examine with ultrasound because of milk-filled ducts
    C. A breast hematoma is usually the result of an obstructed duct
    D. A simple cyst demonstrates smooth walls, no internal echoes, and good through transmission
    E. Breast malignancies are always well circumscribed and demonstrate posterior enhancement

120. The first sonographically detectable branch to leave the abdominal aorta is the
    A. common hepatic artery
    B. superior mesenteric artery
    C. celiac axis
    D. portal vein
    E. proper hepatic artery

121. At its distal end, the aorta bifurcates into the
    A. iliac arteries
    B. femoral arteries
    C. right and left renal arteries
    D. superior and inferior mesenteric arteries
    E. iliac veins

122. The superior mesenteric vein and the splenic vein join to form the
    A. inferior vena cava
    B. superior mesenteric artery
    C. right portal vein
    D. main portal vein
    E. hepatic vein

123. On a transverse view of the midabdomen, which of the following can be seen coursing between the aorta and the superior mesenteric artery?
    A. Body of the pancreas
    B. Inferior vena cava
    C. Right renal vein
    D. Left renal vein
    E. Superior mesenteric vein

124. On a longitudinal view, which of the following may be visualized posterior to the inferior vena cava?
    A. Left renal vein
    B. Right renal vein
    C. Right renal artery
    D. Left renal artery
    E. Aorta

125. The portal confluence is composed of the
    A. superior mesenteric vein, splenic vein, and portal vein
    B. right, middle, and left hepatic veins
    C. inferior vena cava, right renal vein, and portal vein
    D. superior mesenteric vein, inferior mesenteric vein, and splenic vein
    E. right portal vein, splenic vein, and inferior mesenteric vein

126. On which of the following views are all three hepatic veins **BEST** seen?
    A. Transverse, midliver
    B. Transverse, close to the diaphragm
    C. Transverse, adjacent to the gallbladder
    D. Longitudinal, midline
    E. Longitudinal, adjacent to the aorta

127. The porta hepatis contains all of the following **EXCEPT**
    A. the sphincter of Oddi
    B. the portal vein
    C. Glisson's capsule
    D. the hepatic artery
    E. the common bile duct

128. Which of the following structures can be seen entering the pancreatic head?
    A. Splenic vein
    B. Common hepatic artery
    C. Gastroduodenal artery
    D. Superior mesenteric vein
    E. Superior mesenteric artery

129. All of the following are characteristics of the hepatic veins **EXCEPT**
    A. they branch away from the diaphragm
    B. they have echogenic walls
    C. they originate close to the diaphragm
    D. they can be traced into the inferior vena cava
    E. all three are best seen on a transverse scan

130. The gastroduodenal artery is a branch of the
    A. common hepatic artery
    B. common bile duct
    C. aorta
    D. splenic artery
    E. gastric artery

131. The vessel that typically runs between the portal vein and the common bile duct is the
    A. porta hepatis
    B. hepatic artery
    C. inferior vena cava
    D. gastroduodenal artery
    E. middle hepatic vein

132. The vessel normally seen lying posterior to the head of the pancreas is the
     A. aorta
     B. pancreatic artery
     C. splenic artery
     D. hepatic artery
     E. inferior vena cava

133. The three layers that compose the aortic wall are
     A. adventitia, visceral, peritoneal
     B. aneurysmal, intima, peritoneal
     C. adventitia, media, intima
     D. ventral, media, intima
     E. pia, arachnoid, dura

134. A patient is sent to ultrasound to rule out Budd-Chiari syndrome. Which of the following vessels require careful interrogation?
     A. Hepatic veins
     B. Portal vein and hepatic artery
     C. Aorta and inferior vena cava
     D. Lower extremity veins
     E. Anterior and middle cerebral arteries

135. All of the following will help to distinguish the hepatic artery from the common bile duct **EXCEPT**
     A. the hepatic artery is pulsatile
     B. the common bile duct is always anterior to the hepatic artery
     C. the hepatic artery can be traced back to the celiac axis
     D. the use of color flow or duplex Doppler imaging will show flow in the hepatic artery
     E. the hepatic artery has more echogenic walls than the common bile duct

136. All of the following will help to distinguish the aorta from the inferior vena cava **EXCEPT**
     A. the aorta lies more midline
     B. color flow or duplex Doppler imaging will show respiratory changes in the inferior vena cava
     C. the inferior vena cava is normally to the left of the aorta
     D. the inferior vena cava is normally compressible while the aorta is not
     E. the aorta has branches arising anteriorly

137. All of the following are features of portal hypertension **EXCEPT**
     A. collaterals
     B. splenomegaly
     C. ascites
     D. hepatic artery thrombosis
     E. recanalization of the paraumbilical veins

138. Hepatofugal flow may be indicative of all of the following **EXCEPT**
     A. common bile duct obstruction
     B. a poor Doppler angle (above 60°)
     C. portal hypertension
     D. a cirrhotic liver
     E. portal vein thrombosis

139. With hepatopetal flow, the blood in the portal vein and the blood in the hepatic artery
     A. flows in the same direction
     B. flows in opposite directions
     C. cannot be detected with Doppler
     D. flows away from the liver
     E. is turbulent

140. The normal Doppler waveform of the portal vein is
     A. triphasic
     B. away from the liver
     C. monophasic
     D. biphasic

141. An inability to detect blood flow in the portal vein may be caused by all of the following **EXCEPT**
     A. a clot in the portal vein
     B. low flow velocity in the portal vein
     C. high flow velocity in the portal vein
     D. a transducer angle perpendicular to the portal vein
     E. an obscuring mass

142. When scanning transversely over the pancreas, which of the following is a tortuous vessel that will be seen coursing superior to the body and tail of the pancreas?
     A. Splenic artery
     B. Pancreatic artery
     C. Splenic vein
     D. Right renal artery
     E. Superior mesenteric vein

143. Which of the following Doppler measurements is **MOST** sensitive in assessing renal artery stenosis?
     A. Resistive index
     B. Acceleration time
     C. Peak-systolic/end-diastolic ratio
     D. Flow velocity
     E. Pulsatility index

144. In the pediatric patient, if a Wilms' tumor is suspected the sonographer should look for related abnormalities in all of the following **EXCEPT**
     A. the opposite kidney
     B. the pancreas
     C. the inferior vena cava
     D. the aorta
     E. the liver

145. When scanning a pediatric patient, a cystic structure is seen in the posterior portion of the bladder and hydronephrosis is present. The structure in the bladder is **MOST** likely
    A. a rhabdomyosarcoma
    B. a bladder diverticulum
    C. a pelvic kidney
    D. a ureterocele
    E. an ovarian cyst

146. In a pediatric patient, the renal pelvis is dilated but the ureter is normal. Which of the following is the **MOST** likely diagnosis?
    A. Multicystic dysplastic kidney
    B. Ureterovesical junction obstruction
    C. Ureteropelvic junction obstruction
    D. Pelvic kidney
    E. Urethral obstruction

147. A heterogeneous malignant tumor found in a newborn in the region of the kidney **MOST** likely represents
    A. a teratoma
    B. an infantile polycystic kidney
    C. adrenal hemorrhage
    D. a neuroblastoma
    E. Wilms' tumor

148. All of the following are typical characteristics of multicystic dysplastic kidney disease **EXCEPT**
    A. bilateral, evenly echogenic kidneys
    B. multiple cysts that do not communicate
    C. little or no renal parenchyma present
    D. fatal if bilateral
    E. cysts of varying size and shape

149. Which of the following is a normal finding when scanning the urinary tract of an infant?
    A. Prominent renal pyramids
    B. Dilation of the proximal portions of the ureters
    C. Decreased echogenicity of the cortices of the kidneys
    D. Increased echogenicity of the sinus echoes
    E. Echoes in the bladder

150. All of the following are characteristics of an infant with prune-belly syndrome **EXCEPT**
    A. hydronephrosis
    B. renal agenesis
    C. an enlarged bladder
    D. a dilated posterior urethra
    E. hydroureter

151. Which of the following conditions affects male children and is characterized by bilateral hydronephrosis, an overly distended bladder, and dilated ureters?
    A. Vesicoureteral reflux
    B. Posterior urethral valves
    C. Cryptorchidism
    D. Ureteropelvic junction obstruction
    E. Multicystic dysplastic kidney disease

152. An obstruction at the junction of the ureter and bladder will **MOST** likely cause
    A. dilation of the bladder only
    B. hydronephrosis only
    C. hydronephrosis and hydroureter
    D. increased echogenicity of the renal cortex

153. Most of the central echogenic area in the normal kidney represents
    A. renal sinus fat
    B. the renal pyramids
    C. the renal cortex
    D. the renal capsule
    E. the medulla

154. Which of the following is the **BEST** approach when scanning the right kidney in a normal patient?
    A. Supine, scanning intercostally
    B. Right lateral decubitus, using the spleen as an acoustic window
    C. Supine, using the liver as an acoustic window
    D. Prone, scanning posteriorly
    E. Supine, using a subxiphoid approach

155. Put the following normal renal structures in order from least to greatest echogenicity.
    A. Pyramids, sinus fat, cortex
    B. Sinus fat, pyramids, cortex
    C. Sinus fat, cortex, pyramids
    D. Cortex, sinus fat, pyramids
    E. Pyramids, cortex, sinus fat

156. All of the following are normal variants in the adult kidney **EXCEPT**
    A. a dromedary hump
    B. multiple renal arteries
    C. an oblique position in the patient
    D. a column of Bertin
    E. greater echogenicity of the renal parenchyma compared to the normal liver

157. Which of the following describes the sonographic features of autosomal recessive (infantile) polycystic kidney disease?
    A. Bilateral, enlarged, echogenic kidneys
    B. Bilateral hydronephrosis
    C. Small, echogenic kidneys
    D. Multiple large, irregular cysts throughout the kidney
    E. Multiple cysts of varying size throughout the kidney

158. All of the following may be present in a patient with autosomal dominant (adult) polycystic kidney disease **EXCEPT**
   A. small, shrunken kidneys
   B. multiple irregularly shaped cysts
   C. renal failure
   D. distortion of the central sinus echoes
   E. liver cysts

159. To assess the degree of echogenicity of the renal cortex, a comparison with the liver would be inaccurate in which of the following instances?
   A. Hydronephrosis
   B. The presence of two liver cysts
   C. A cirrhotic liver
   D. Renal stones
   E. A discrepancy in renal length

160. All of the following are procedures used to relieve apparent or genuine hydronephrosis **EXCEPT**
   A. a nephrostomy tube
   B. having the patient urinate
   C. a renal vein stent
   D. inserting a catheter into the bladder
   E. prostatectomy

161. A benign, highly echogenic, vascular tumor found on a renal sonogram is **MOST** likely
   A. an angiomyolipoma
   B. a Wilms' tumor
   C. a staghorn calculus
   D. a renal lymphoma
   E. an adenoma

162. Which of the following is characteristic of a horseshoe kidney?
   A. Two normal kidneys plus a pelvic kidney
   B. Bilateral, malrotated kidneys
   C. Two kidneys on the same side of the body
   D. A single kidney, in the shape of a horseshoe, with a single collecting system
   E. Bilateral kidneys fused together by an isthmus of tissue

163. Which of the following is a condition in which small stones are present in the renal pyramids?
   A. Staghorn calculus
   B. Cystitis
   C. Pyelonephritis
   D. Nephrocalcinosis
   E. Pyonephrosis

164. Which of the following is necessary to perform a diagnostic transabdominal sonogram of the bladder?
   A. A catheter placed in the bladder
   B. A distended bladder
   C. NPO for 8–12 hours before the examination
   D. Patient in a left lateral decubitus position
   E. The bladder cannot be examined transabdominally

165. Which of the following is **NOT** a cause of gross hematuria?
   A. Bladder calculi
   B. Benign prostatic hypertrophy
   C. Renal stones
   D. A bladder tumor
   E. Renal sinus lipomatosis

166. The presence of hydronephrosis and a renal pelvis filled with low-level echoes may be indicative of
   A. the gain turned down too low
   B. pyonephrosis
   C. staghorn calculus
   D. medullary nephrocalcinosis
   E. peripelvic cysts

167. The extension of the pancreas that lies posterior to the superior mesenteric vein is the
   A. caudate lobe
   B. tail
   C. uncinate process
   D. body
   E. head

168. Wirsung's duct is another name for the
   A. common bile duct
   B. cystic duct
   C. main pancreatic duct
   D. hepatic duct
   E. Donald duct

169. Findings in a patient with acute pancreatitis of recent onset may include all of the following **EXCEPT**
   A. gallstones
   B. a normal sonographic appearance of the pancreas
   C. a pancreatic pseudocyst
   D. low urinary amylase
   E. pain

170. A shrunken, echogenic pancreas is usually indicative of
   A. chronic pancreatitis
   B. acute pancreatitis
   C. cirrhosis
   D. a pancreatic pseudocyst
   E. no pathology; this is a normal finding

171. A normal structure that encircles the pancreatic head and may mimic a pancreatic mass is
   A. the stomach
   B. the duodenum
   C. a pancreatic pseudocyst
   D. the uncinate process
   E. the gastroduodenal artery

172. Having the patient drink water during a pancreatic sonogram may be useful in all of the following ways **EXCEPT**
    A. using the fluid-filled duodenum to image the pancreatic head
    B. distinguishing the stomach from a pancreatic pseudocyst
    C. increasing the gas in the abdomen, thereby pushing the pancreas into a better position for scanning
    D. imaging the pancreatic tail through the fundus of the stomach
    E. distinguishing the duodenum from a pancreatic mass

173. A patient presents with a dilated common bile duct and an ill-defined pancreatic head mass with poor through transmission. Which of the following is the **MOST** likely diagnosis?
    A. Gallstone pancreatitis
    B. Common bile duct calcification
    C. Pancreatic pseudocyst
    D. Pancreatic cancer
    E. Hepatoma

174. Which of the following blood tests is helpful in diagnosing acute pancreatitis?
    A. Bilirubin
    B. Lactate dehydrogenase (LDH)
    C. Alkaline phosphatase
    D. Creatinine
    E. Serum amylase

175. Which of the following is **NOT** an acoustic window to demonstrate the pancreas?
    A. Intercostal approach through the liver, at the lower pole of the right kidney
    B. Left lobe of the liver
    C. Spleen
    D. Fluid-filled stomach
    E. Fluid-filled duodenum

176. Echogenic foci with acoustic shadowing in the pancreas and a dilated pancreatic duct are consistent with which of the following?
    A. Gallstones
    B. Pancreatic pseudocyst
    C. Chronic pancreatitis
    D. Pancreatic cancer
    E. Polycystic disease

177. The distal common bile duct is **BEST** visualized sonographically using which of the following for an acoustic window?
    A. Head of the pancreas
    B. Water-filled second portion of the duodenum
    C. Gallbladder on a decubitus view
    D. Liver on suspended inspiration
    E. Liver on a decubitus view

178. In a normal patient, where are the gallbladder and duodenum located in relation to the pancreatic head?
    A. Superior
    B. To the right
    C. To the left
    D. Posterior
    E. Anterior

179. Which of the following is the **BEST** acoustic window to demonstrate the pancreatic tail?
    A. Right lobe of the liver
    B. Spleen and left kidney
    C. Right kidney
    D. Fluid-filled duodenum
    E. Caudate lobe of the liver

180. An 8-year-old patient presents with midabdominal pain and an elevated serum amylase level after blunt trauma to her abdomen. The abdominal sonogram demonstrates a cystic mass in the lesser sac. The mass **MOST** likely represents
    A. a lymphoma deposit
    B. a pancreatic pseudocyst
    C. an aortic aneurysm
    D. fluid-filled bowel
    E. an ovarian cyst

181. Which of the following is a way to avoid mistaking the duodenum for a pancreatic head mass?
    A. Give the patient cholecystokinin
    B. Look for bile duct dilation
    C. Give the patient fluid by mouth
    D. Apply firm pressure to the midabdominal region
    E. Place the patient in the Trendelenburg position

182. The ampulla of Vater is another name for the
    A. accessory pancreatic duct
    B. entrance of the gastroduodenal artery and the common bile duct into the pancreatic head
    C. junction of the splenic vein, superior mesenteric vein, and portal vein
    D. outlet of the stomach
    E. entrance of the common bile duct and pancreatic duct into the duodenum

183. Common causes for acute pancreatitis include all of the following **EXCEPT**
    A. hypertension
    B. alcoholism
    C. pancreatic duct calculus
    D. blunt midabdominal trauma
    E. gallstones

184. All of the following are common symptoms of pancreatic disease **EXCEPT**
    A. weight loss
    B. chronic severe abdominal pain
    C. an epigastric mass
    D. dysuria
    E. vomiting

185. Which of the following is a condition in neonates in which the ducts of the biliary tree are very small and jaundice is present?
    A. A choledochal cyst
    B. Biliary atresia
    C. Intussusception
    D. Budd-Chiari syndrome
    E. Cirrhosis

186. All of the following are characteristics of pyloric stenosis **EXCEPT**
    A. an abnormally thickened pyloric wall
    B. projectile vomiting
    C. presence of an epigastric mass
    D. a persistently fluid-filled stomach
    E. shortened pyloric length

187. A condition seen mostly in children in which there is telescoping and subsequent obstruction of the bowel is called
    A. intussusception
    B. pyloric stenosis
    C. biliary atresia
    D. Crohn's disease
    E. obstructive bowel disease

Questions 188–191

Refer to the transverse view of the thyroid below:

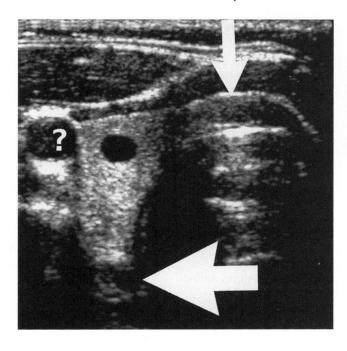

188. The small arrow is pointing to
    A. the esophagus
    B. the strap muscle
    C. reverberation artifact in the trachea
    D. the isthmus
    E. piriform extension of the thyroid

189. The question mark is in
    A. a thyroid cyst
    B. a parathyroid adenoma
    C. the jugular vein
    D. the carotid artery
    E. the strap muscle

190. What does the large arrow represent?
    A. Longus colli muscle
    B. Parathyroid adenoma
    C. Reverberation artifact
    D. Adenoma of the thyroid
    E. Jugular vein

191. What pathology is seen on this image?
    A. Thyroid adenoma
    B. Thyroid cancer
    C. Hürthle cell tumor
    D. Hashimoto's thyroiditis
    E. Thyroid cyst

Questions 192–194

Refer to the transverse view of the prostate below:

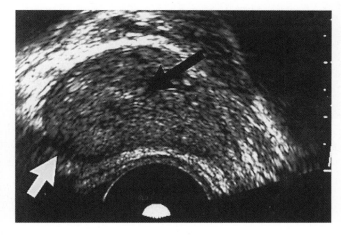

192. Where is the area delineated by the white arrow located?
    A. Peripheral zone
    B. Central zone
    C. Transitional zone
    D. Urethra
    E. Anterior fibromuscular area

193. The black arrow is pointing to
    A. cancer of the prostate
    B. prostatitis
    C. an area of benign prostatic hypertrophy
    D. a prostatic cyst
    E. a prostatic utricle

194. What is the **MOST** likely pathology on this image?
    A. Prostate cancer
    B. Prostatitis
    C. Prostatic hemorrhage
    D. Prostatic cyst
    E. Transurethral resection of the prostate (TURP) defect

Questions 195 and 196

A full-term neonate developed shortness of breath. An x-ray revealed a mass in the left lung, so the patient was referred for a chest sonogram, with the following findings:

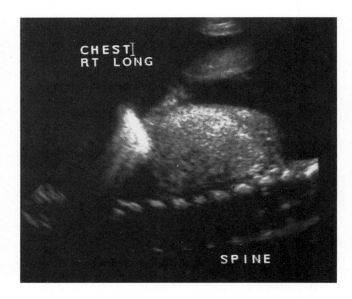

195. Based on the abnormality seen on the image, which of the following is the **MOST** likely diagnosis?
    A. Pleural effusion
    B. Pulmonary sequestration
    C. Left-sided diaphragmatic hernia
    D. Mediastinal teratoma
    E. Bronchogenic cysts

196. What additional modality or technique will clarify the diagnosis?
    A. Lower frequency transducer
    B. Nuclear medicine
    C. Decubitus x-ray
    D. Color flow Doppler
    E. Trendelenburg position

Questions 197 and 198

Refer to the oblique views of the porta hepatis below:

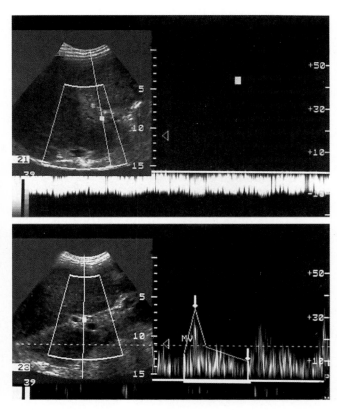

197. Which vessels are being sampled?
    A. Hepatic artery and hepatic vein
    B. Hepatic vein and portal vein
    C. Common bile duct and hepatic artery
    D. Portal vein and hepatic artery
    E. Common bile duct and portal vein

198. These images of the porta hepatis are taken from a patient with cirrhosis. How would you describe the flow pattern in the vessels being examined in the porta hepatis?
    A. Absent diastolic flow
    B. Reversed systolic flow
    C. Absent flow
    D. Hepatofugal flow
    E. Hepatopetal flow

Questions 199–201

A 66-year-old man presents in the emergency department with nausea and vomiting. He has a 30-year history of drug and alcohol abuse. A sagittal view of the left lobe of his liver is shown below:

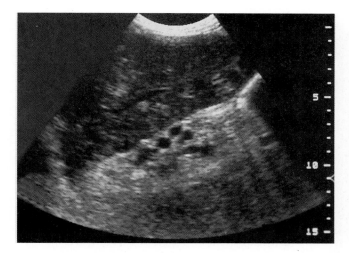

199. Which of the following is the **MOST** likely explanation for the ultrasound findings in this patient?
    A. Budd-Chiari syndrome
    B. Pancreatic pseudocysts
    C. Mesenteric cysts
    D. Varices
    E. Remnants of a multicystic kidney

200. Within which anatomical structure do the "cysts" lie?
    A. Spleen
    B. Kidney
    C. Pancreas
    D. Porta hepatis
    E. Adrenal gland

201. Which of the following would **NOT** be helpful in further investigating the cystic areas?
    A. Perform a Valsalva maneuver to see if the cysts change size
    B. Try to detect flow in the varices using color flow Doppler
    C. Check for an enlarged spleen
    D. Look at the ligamentum teres to see if it is recanalized
    E. Look for reversed flow in the hepatic vein

Questions 202 and 203

A 24-year-old man presented with weight loss, fever, and increased blood urea nitrogen. He underwent a kidney biopsy. Two hours after the procedure, an ultrasound was requested. The sonogram of his bladder is shown below:

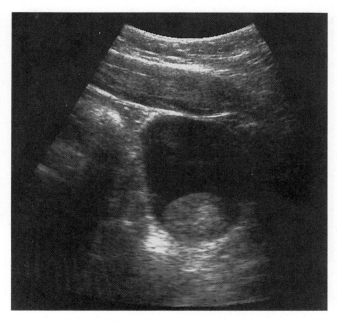

202. Which of the following is the **MOST** likely explanation for the ultrasound findings in this patient?
    A. Fungal balls
    B. Sediment
    C. Blood clot
    D. Bladder tumor
    E. Calculi

203. What ultrasound technique will help to confirm the diagnosis?
    A. Decubitus views
    B. Postvoid imaging
    C. Perineal scan
    D. Change from a 5.0 to a 2.5 MHz transducer

Questions 204 and 205

A 71-year-old woman with abdominal pain and a history of hepatitis C presents with worsening liver function tests. The following image is obtained:

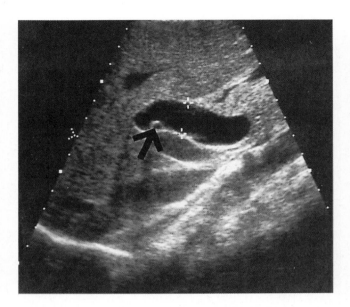

204. Which of the following is the **MOST** likely diagnosis?
    A. Choledochal cyst
    B. Choledocholithiasis
    C. Cholangitis
    D. Cholesterolosis
    E. Common bile duct dilation

205. The arrow is pointing to
    A. a small stone in the common bile duct
    B. the hepatic artery
    C. an intraductal cyst
    D. *Ascaris lumbricoides*
    E. the hepatic vein

Questions 206 and 207

A patient presents with severe right upper quadrant pain, nausea, and vomiting. The patient is referred to ultrasound. A transverse view of the patient's pancreas is shown below:

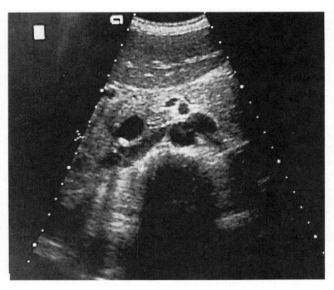

206. What is seen on this image?
    A. Dilated gastroduodenal artery
    B. Dilated pancreatic duct
    C. Duodenal diverticulum containing some air
    D. Choledocholithiasis with a dilated common bile duct
    E. Pseudocyst

207. Which of the following anatomical structures is **NOT** seen on this image?
    A. Superior mesenteric artery
    B. Superior mesenteric vein
    C. Left renal vein
    D. Aorta
    E. Splenic artery

Questions 208 and 209

After total hip replacement, a 76-year-old woman presented with right upper quadrant pain, nausea, and an increased white blood cell count. The following image was obtained:

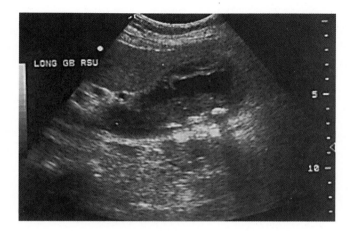

208. Which of the following findings is **NOT** seen on this patient's sonogram?
    A. Gallstones
    B. Gallbladder distension
    C. Gallbladder wall thickening
    D. Pericholecystic fluid
    E. Comet tail artifact

209. Which of the following is the **MOST** likely diagnosis?
    A. Cholesterolosis
    B. Cholangitis
    C. Acute cholecystitis
    D. Chronic cholecystitis
    E. Acalculous cholecystitis

Questions 210 and 211

A 60-year-old bar owner with complaints of abdominal pain was examined. The following image was obtained:

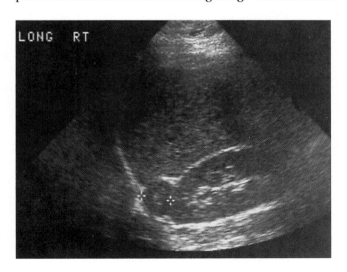

210. What is seen on this patient's sonogram?
    A. Subcapsular mass
    B. Intrahepatic mass
    C. Intraperitoneal mass
    D. Retroperitoneal mass
    E. Renal mass

211. Which of the following is the **MOST** likely explanation for the mass?
    A. Renal metastasis to the adrenal gland
    B. Pheochromocytoma
    C. Metastasis to the adrenal gland from lung cancer
    D. Neuroblastoma
    E. Myelolipoma

Questions 212–214

A 32-year-old woman who is afebrile presents with back pain and an elevated creatinine. The following image is obtained:

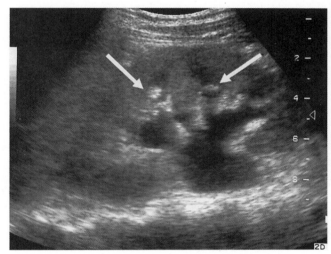

212. The **MOST** likely diagnosis is
    A. pyonephrosis
    B. focal caliectasis
    C. hydronephrosis
    D. hydroureter
    E. duplex collecting system

213. What additional finding is indicated by the arrows?
    A. Hypernephroma
    B. Transitional cell tumor
    C. Calcified arcuate artery
    D. Milk of calcium
    E. Wilms' tumor

214. What technical changes could be made to better demonstrate the pathology indicated by the arrows?
    A. Decrease transducer frequency
    B. Increase transducer frequency
    C. Use color Doppler
    D. Change the patient's position
    E. Fill the patient's bladder

Questions 215 and 216

A 38-year-old man with a history of several attacks of abdominal pain has a renal sonogram done. A left sagittal view is shown below:

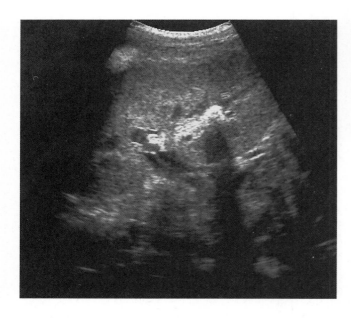

215. What is seen on this patient's sonogram?
    A. Air in the collecting system
    B. Angiomyolipoma
    C. Renal cell carcinoma
    D. Papillary necrosis
    E. Nephrolithiasis

216. In addition to the kidneys and bladder, what other part of this patient's body might be examined with ultrasound?
    A. Parathyroid glands
    B. Pancreas
    C. Para-aortic area
    D. Liver
    E. Breasts

Questions 217–219

A 45-year-old man presents with pain in his testicles. The following image is obtained:

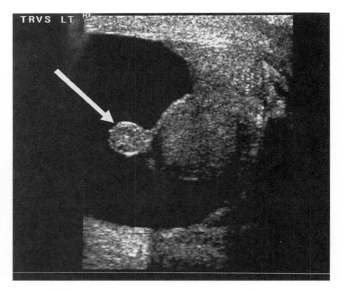

217. The arrow is pointing to
    A. a testicular mass
    B. the appendix epididymis
    C. a blood clot in the scrotum
    D. an epididymal mass
    E. scrotal calculi

218. What else can be seen on the sonogram?
    A. Hydrocele
    B. Spermatocele
    C. Varicocele
    D. Hematocele
    E. Epididymal cyst

219. Where is this collection located?
    A. Deep to the tunica albuginea
    B. Between the tunica albuginea and the tunica vaginalis
    C. Between the two layers of the tunica vaginalis
    D. Between the tunica vaginalis and the scrotal wall
    E. In the scrotal wall

Question 220

A 12-year-old girl presents with fever and back pain. Each of her kidneys is examined with ultrasound. Her left kidney is normal. However, examination of her right kidney reveals the following findings:

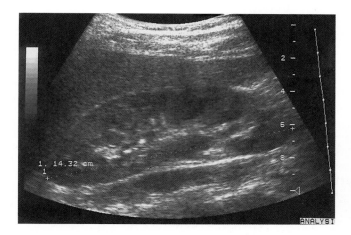

220. Which of the following is the **MOST** likely diagnosis?
    A. Beckwith-Wiedemann syndrome
    B. Hemihypertrophy
    C. Acute pyelonephritis
    D. Chronic glomerulonephritis
    E. Pyonephrosis

Question 221

A 22-year-old man with nephrotic syndrome presents to the emergency department. He is febrile and complaining of sweats and back pain. The following image is obtained:

221. Which of the following is the **MOST** likely diagnosis on this image?
    A. Hepatic cyst
    B. Simple cyst
    C. Renal cell carcinoma
    D. Renal abscess
    E. Parapelvic cysts

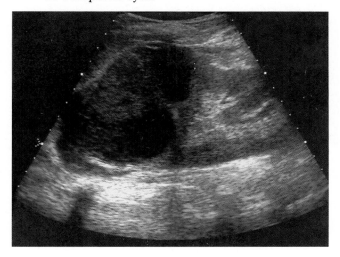

Questions 222 and 223

A 25-year-old drug addict presents with back pain, fever, and painful urination. A sonogram of his bladder is shown below:

222. Which of the following is the **MOST** likely explanation for the ultrasound findings?
    A. Hematoma
    B. Bladder wall tumor
    C. Artifact
    D. Pus
    E. Bladder wall trabeculations

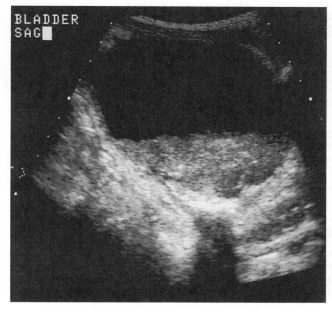

223. What additional pathology can be found on this patient's sonogram?
    A. Hydroureter
    B. Abscess in the psoas muscle
    C. Prostate mass
    D. Seminal vesicle cyst
    E. Bladder calculus

Question 224

Refer to the sagittal view of the liver below:

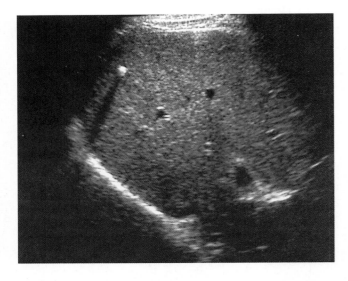

224. Which of the following is **NOT** a possible explanation for the findings on this image?
    A. Calcified granuloma
    B. Calcified hematoma
    C. Air in the biliary system
    D. Tip of a biopsy needle

Questions 225 and 226

A small child with hypertension presented for a renal ultrasound. Both kidneys were examined. It was found that the left kidney was 5 cm long and the right kidney was 10 cm long. A sagittal view of the patient's left kidney is shown below:

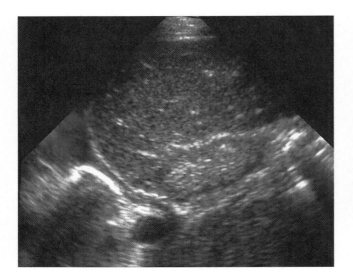

225. Which of the following abnormalities is seen on this sonogram?
    A. Transitional cell tumor of the renal pelvis
    B. Angiomyolipoma of the renal pelvis
    C. Narrowed renal parenchyma
    D. Normal kidney with contralateral renal hypertrophy
    E. Staghorn calculus

226. What additional finding(s) is(are) seen?
    A. Pericardial effusion
    B. Adrenal mass
    C. Splenomegaly
    D. Pleural effusion and splenomegaly
    E. Pleural effusion

Question 227

Refer to the sagittal midline upper abdominal views below:

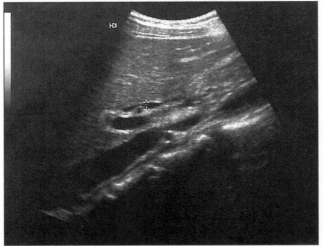

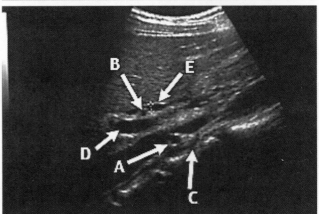

227. Which of the following letters on the image identifies the adrenal gland?
    A.
    B.
    C.
    D.
    E.

Question 228

A 45-year-old woman with a history of alcohol abuse presents with epigastric pain and elevated serum amylase and lipase levels. The following transverse image is obtained:

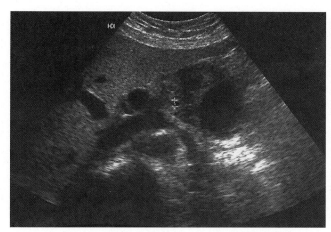

228. Which of the following is the **MOST** likely explanation for the sonographic findings?
    A. Dilated stomach
    B. Pancreatic pseudocyst
    C. Acute pancreatitis
    D. Cystic fibrosis
    E. Mucinous cystadenoma

Questions 229–232

A 40-year-old woman presents for a routine abdominal scan. A transverse left upper quadrant view is shown below:

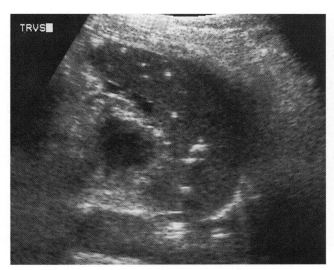

229. Which of the following abnormalities are seen on this abdominal sonogram?
    A. Infarcts
    B. Metastases
    C. Hemangiomas
    D. Granulomas
    E. Hematomas

230. To which of the following diseases has the patient been previously exposed?
    A. Gonorrhea
    B. Typhoid
    C. Hepatitis
    D. Salmonella
    E. Histoplasmosis

231. What does the fluid-filled mass medial to the spleen represent?
    A. Pancreatic pseudocyst
    B. Adrenal cyst
    C. Stomach
    D. Renal cyst
    E. Splenic cyst

232. There is an area of dropout involving the lateral aspect of the spleen that is the result of technical problems. This area would be better defined using all of the following techniques **EXCEPT**
    A. filling the stomach with water
    B. using a transducer with a smaller footprint
    C. scanning the patient in the left-side-up position
    D. standing the patient up and rescanning the area
    E. scanning coronally through the left side with the patient in a supine position

Questions 233 and 234

Refer to the sagittal view of the right upper quadrant below:

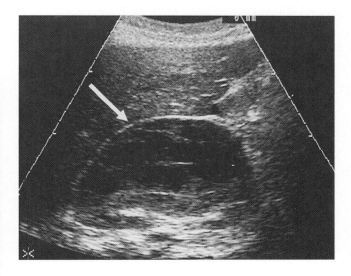

233. The collection indicated by the arrow is in the
    A. subcapsular space
    B. subphrenic space
    C. subdiaphragmatic space
    D. submarine space
    E. perinephric space

234. Which of the following is the **MOST** appropriate history for this case?
    A. Recent kick in the side during a fight
    B. Loss of weight and appetite
    C. High fever for months with abdominal pain
    D. Leg swelling and leg pain
    E. Acute chest pain radiating down one arm the previous night

Question 235

A 30-year-old man presents with endocarditis and fever of unknown origin. A transverse sonogram of his spleen is shown below:

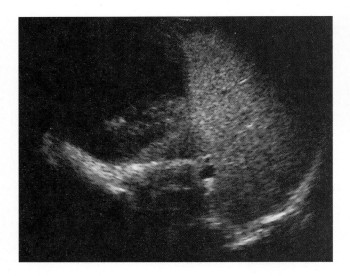

235. The findings on the sonogram **MOST** likely represent a
    A. splenic cyst
    B. pancreatic pseudocyst
    C. splenic abscess
    D. splenic infarct
    E. splenic metastasis

Question 236

After choledochojejunostomy, a 36-year-old man presents with increased bilirubin. The following image is obtained:

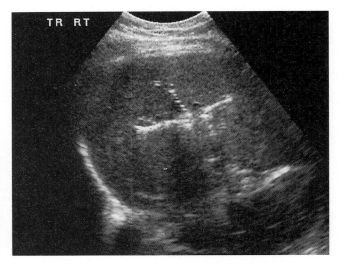

236. The sonographic findings are **MOST** consistent with
    A. biliary obstruction
    B. air in the biliary tree
    C. stones in the biliary tree
    D. Budd-Chiari syndrome
    E. multiple granulomas

Questions 237 and 238

Refer to the longitudianl view of the right kidney below:

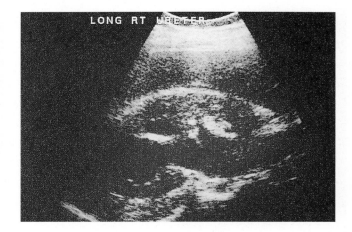

237. Define the level of obstruction in this urinary tract.
    A. Calyceal
    B. Infundibular
    C. Ureteropelvic junction
    D. Glomerular
    E. Ureter

238. In this case, the sonographer should also look at the
    A. prostate, scanning transabdominally with an empty bladder
    B. distal ureter, scanning transabdominally with an empty bladder
    C. distal ureter, scanning transabdominally with a full bladder
    D. appendix, scanning transabdominally
    E. midureter, scanning transvaginally

Question 239

Refer to the sonogram showing Kaposi's sarcoma below:

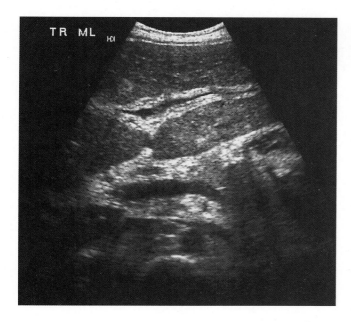

239. The sonogram shows periportal thickening and multiple small, peripheral, hyperechoic nodules. This pathology is **MOST** likely seen in patients suffering from
    A. an infection
    B. allergies
    C. AIDS
    D. trauma
    E. a bleeding disorder

Questions 240 and 241

Refer to the transverse and sagittal views of the gallbladder region below:

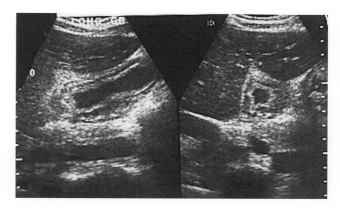

240. Which of the following abnormalities is seen on this image?
    A. *Ascaris lumbricoides* in the gallbladder
    B. Ascites
    C. Gallbladder tumor
    D. Cystic tumor in the liver
    E. Gallbladder wall thickening

241. Which of the following entities would **NOT** cause the findings seen on this sonogram?
    A. Acute cholecystitis
    B. Hepatitis A
    C. Ascites
    D. AIDS
    E. Chronic cholecystitis

Question 242

A 45-year-old HIV-positive man presents with scrotal swelling and pain. A color flow Doppler examination reveals the following findings:

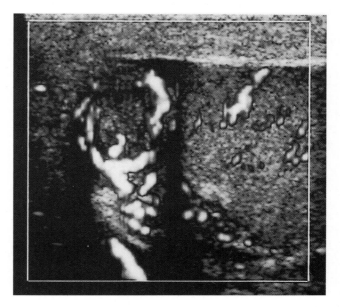

242. Which of the following is the **MOST** likely diagnosis?
    A. Normal testicular sonogram
    B. Acute epididymitis
    C. Seminoma
    D. Torsion
    E. Orchitis

Questions 243–246

A 43-year-old man was struck by a car while crossing the street. The following image was obtained:

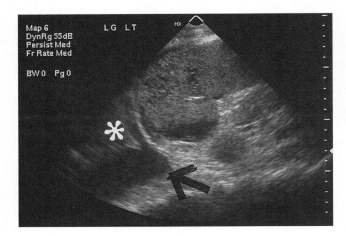

243. What do you see on the sonogram?
    A. Evidence of splenic torsion
    B. Evidence of splenic trauma
    C. Evidence of splenic hemangiomas
    D. Evidence of splenic granulomas
    E. A normal spleen

244. The arrow is pointing to a
    A. pleural effusion
    B. perisplenic hematoma
    C. pericardial effusion
    D. perirenal collection
    E. fluid-filled stomach

245. What does the asterisk indicate?
    A. Heart
    B. Lung mass
    C. Normal or consolidated lung
    D. Rib
    E. Diaphragm

246. The echo-free area posterior to the spleen is
    A. the stomach
    B. an adrenal cyst
    C. a perisplenic hematoma
    D. a renal cyst
    E. the aorta

Question 247

Refer to the transverse view of the left upper quadrant below:

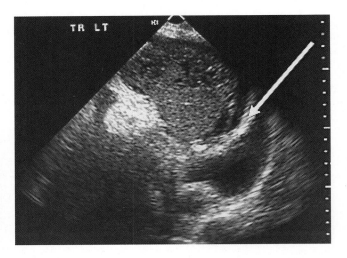

247. The arrow is pointing to
    A. the left hemidiaphragm
    B. a blood clot
    C. the phrenicocolic ligament
    D. the splenic capsule
    E. the stomach wall

Question 248

Refer to the transverse view of the liver below:

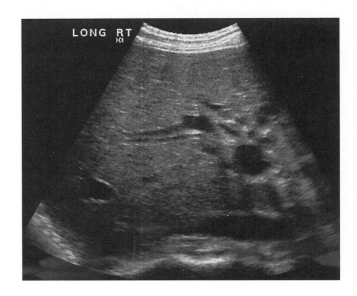

248. What does this image show?
    A. Light bulb sign
    B. Comet effect
    C. Parallel channel sign
    D. Dirty shadowing
    E. Mirror artifact

Question 249

This unhappily married 45-year-old woman wears her sunglasses during the ultrasound examination. She presents with weight loss, increased bilirubin, and a history of lung cancer. The following image is obtained:

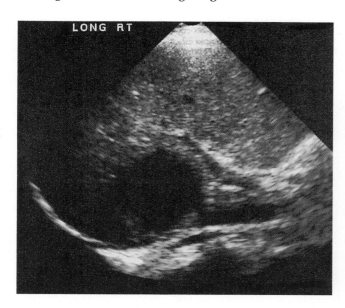

249. Which of the following possibilities seems **MOST** appropriate?
    A. Hemangioma
    B. Metastasis
    C. Liver cyst
    D. Renal tumor
    E. Domestic violence injury

Question 250

A patient with end-stage liver disease presents with hepatic encephalopathy. Using color flow Doppler, the following transverse image is obtained:

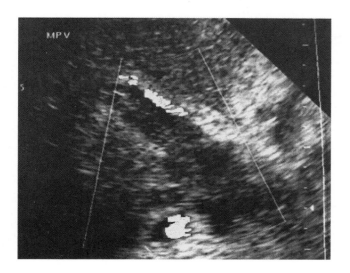

250. Which of the following is the **MOST** likely diagnosis?
    A. Budd-Chiari syndrome
    B. Cavernous transformation
    C. Portal vein thrombosis
    D. Portal vein aneurysm
    E. Large portal vein caused by portal hypertension

Question 251

Refer to the sagittal view of the right upper quadrant below:

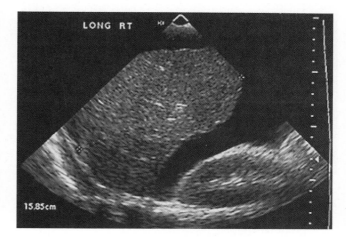

251. Which of the following is the **MOST** likely cause of the ascites seen on this image?
    A. Congestive heart failure
    B. Nephrotic syndrome
    C. Cirrhosis
    D. Malignancy
    E. Peritonitis

Question 252

A 40-year-old man presents to the emergency department with testicular pain. A testicular sonogram performed with a 5-MHz transducer yields the following image:

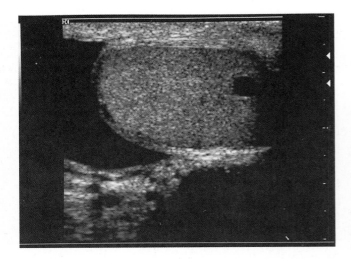

252. The surgeon was anxious to take this patient straight to the operating room. What does the sonologist suggest instead?
    A. Use color flow Doppler to see if the abnormal area is an aneurysm or an infarct
    B. Go ahead with the surgery
    C. Increase the transducer frequency because the lesion may be a cyst
    D. Biopsy the lesion percutaneously
    E. Decrease the transducer frequency because the lesion may be a cyst

Question 253

A patient was sent to ultrasound to evaluate a renal transplant complicated by hydronephrosis. The following image was obtained:

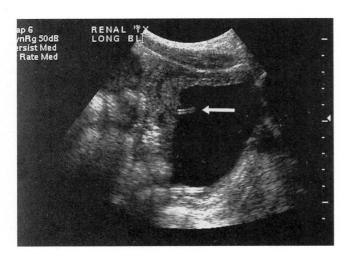

253. The arrow is pointing to
    A. a calcified distal ureter
    B. bladder calculi
    C. arterial calcification
    D. ring down artifact
    E. a renal stent

Questions 254 and 255

A 36-year-old man with a history of cocaine abuse presents with testicular pain. The following image is obtained:

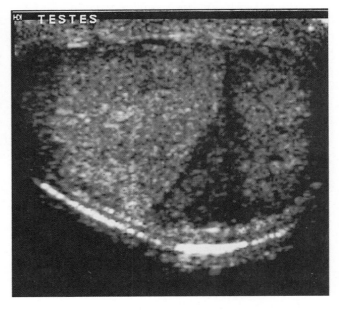

254. Which of the following is **MOST** consistent with the sonogram?
    A. Rete testis
    B. Cystic dysplasia
    C. Testicular abscess
    D. Testicular infarct
    E. Lymphoma

255. What additional technique will help confirm the diagnosis?
    A. Reexamination with Valsalva maneuver
    B. Color flow Doppler
    C. Standoff pad
    D. Needle aspiration
    E. Change in the patient's position

Question 256

A 17-year-old boy presented for a thyroid scan after a physical examination detected a questionable neck mass. A sagittal view of the left lobe of his thyroid is shown below:

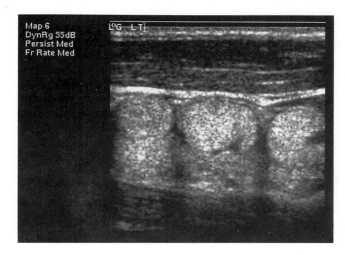

256. All of the following findings can be seen on the sonogram **EXCEPT**
A. the halo effect
B. multiple nodules
C. echogenic foci
D. cystic areas
E. a calcified center

Questions 257 and 258

A 56-year-old woman presents with congestive heart failure. The following oblique view of the liver is obtained:

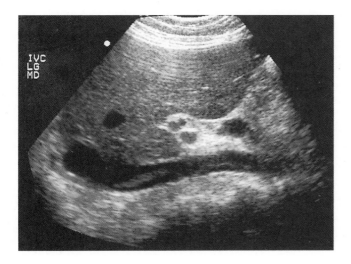

257. Which of the following is present on the sonogram?
A. Reverberation artifact
B. Inferior vena cava filter
C. Inferior vena cava thrombus
D. Extrinsic compression of the inferior vena cava
E. Normal inferior vena cava

258. Where else would you look after detecting this finding?
A. Parathyroid glands
B. Kidneys
C. Pancreas
D. Testicles
E. Spleen

Question 259

After a cadaveric renal transplant, a 26-year-old patient presented with hypertension. Doppler examination of the renal vessels showed the following image:

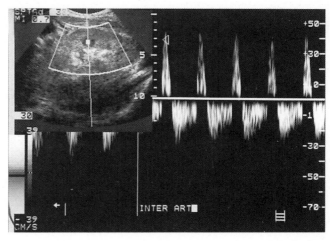

259. Which of the following flow patterns is seen on this image?
A. Normal flow
B. Triphasic flow
C. Reversed diastolic flow
D. Absent diastolic flow
E. Low-resistance flow

Question 260

A 52-year-old man presents with increasing right upper quadrant pain, splenomegaly, and fever. His liver sonogram is shown below:

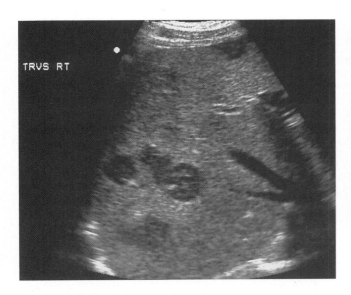

260. Which of the following is the **MOST** likely diagnosis?
    A. Cysts
    B. Liver laceration
    C. Hepatoma
    D. Lymphoma
    E. Hemangioma

Question 261

Refer to the transverse view of the kidneys below:

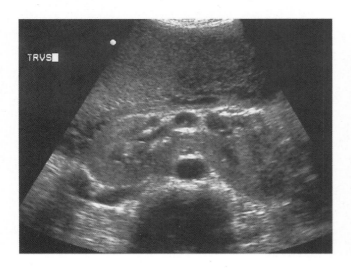

261. Which of the following abnormalities is present on this image?
    A. Column of Bertin
    B. Duplicated collecting system
    C. Crossed renal ectopia
    D. Horseshoe kidney
    E. Fetal lobulation

Question 262

A 34-year-old man presents with weight loss and testicular pain. The following image is obtained:

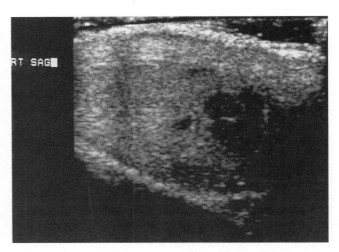

262. Which of the following is the **MOST** likely diagnosis?
    A. Undescended testicle
    B. Partial torsion
    C. Testicular cysts
    D. Malignant testicular mass
    E. Acute epididymitis

Question 263

A 60-year-old woman with known lung cancer and a history of recurrent urinary tract infections presents to ultrasound for a renal sonogram. Her blood pressure, recorded in the chart, is 120/74. Her renal sonogram is shown below:

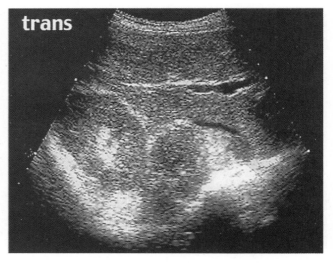

263. Which of the following is the **MOST** likely diagnosis?
    A. Chronic pyelonephritis
    B. Adrenal hemorrhage
    C. Pheochromocytoma
    D. Renal cell carcinoma
    E. Metastases to the adrenal gland

Question 264

Refer to the sagittal view of the hilum of the right testicle below:

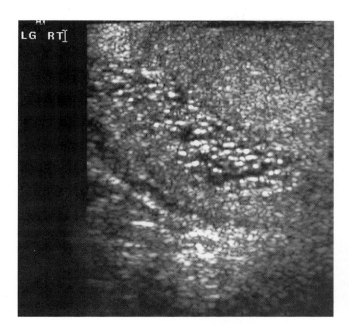

264. Which of the following is seen on this image?
A. Echopenic mass consistent with seminoma
B. Mass with varied echogenicity consistent with embryonal cell cancer
C. Rete testis
D. Mass with small cysts consistent with teratoma
E. Benign testicular cysts

Questions 265 and 266

Refer to the sagittal view of the left testicle below:

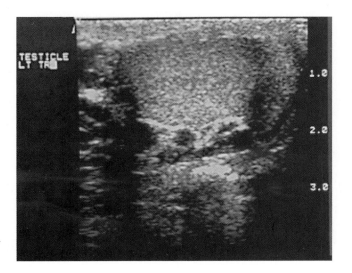

265. Which of the following is the **MOST** likely explanation for the finding seen on this image?
A. Epididymitis
B. Spermatocele
C. Hydrocele
D. Varicocele
E. Epididymal mass

266. Which additional technique would **NOT** clarify this finding?
A. Color flow Doppler
B. Pulsed Doppler
C. Valsalva maneuver
D. Trendelenburg position
E. Patient standing upright

Questions 267 and 268

Refer to the sagittal view of the testicle below:

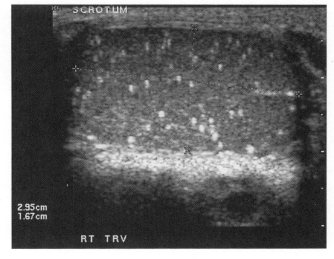

267. What does the image show?
A. Tuberculosis
B. Chronic infarcts
C. Scrotal pearls
D. Microlithiasis
E. Fungal balls

268. Which of the following is **TRUE** regarding this condition?
A. It is a cause of chronic pain
B. Underlying infection should be sought
C. There is an increased risk of malignancy
D. Patients should be advised to drink less milk
E. Infertility is more likely

Question 269

Refer to the transverse view of the testicle below:

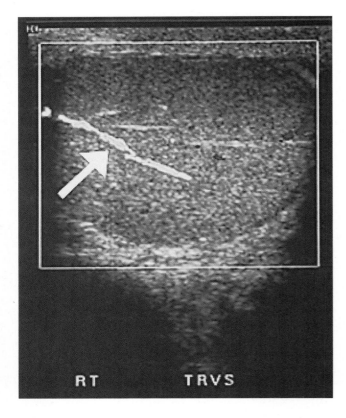

269. Which of the following is seen on this image?
    A. Linear testicular infarct
    B. Mediastinum testis
    C. Arterial calcification
    D. Calcified mass
    E. Gangrenous infection

Questions 270–274

For each of the following five questions, identify the corresponding numbered structure shown on the transverse view of the midabdomen below:

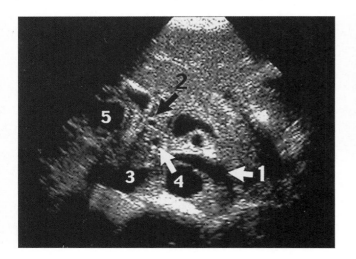

270. Number 1 is the
    A. left renal artery
    B. right renal vein
    C. splenic vein
    D. superior mesenteric vein
    E. left renal vein

271. Number 2 is the
    A. gastroduodenal artery
    B. common bile duct
    C. cystic duct
    D. sphincter of Oddi
    E. gastric artery

272. Number 3 is the
    A. main portal vein
    B. aorta
    C. inferior vena cava
    D. gallbladder
    E. duodenum

273. Number 4 is the
    A. gastric artery
    B. gastroduodenal artery
    C. cystic duct
    D. common bile duct
    E. common hepatic duct

274. Number 5 is the
    A. gastroduodenal artery
    B. duodenum
    C. main portal vein
    D. common bile duct
    E. gallbladder

Questions 275–278

Refer to the transverse view of the upper abdomen below:

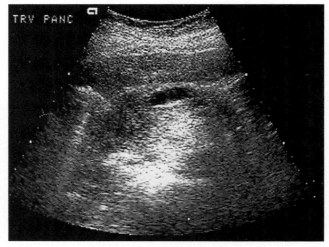

275. The cystic structure on this image **MOST** likely represents
    A. the portal confluence
    B. the pancreatic duct
    C. the common bile duct
    D. polycystic disease
    E. phlegmon

276. Which of the following is the **MOST** likely cause of the hypoechoic structure seen on this image?
    A. Gallstones
    B. Acute pancreatitis
    C. Lymphoma
    D. A mass in the head of the pancreas
    E. Hepatoma

277. The findings on this image should lead the sonographer to carefully examine all of the following **EXCEPT**
    A. the liver
    B. the intrahepatic biliary system
    C. the abdomen for intra-abdominal lymph nodes
    D. the common bile duct
    E. the ligamentum teres for recanalization

278. Which of the following clinical histories is consistent with the findings on this image?
    A. Decreased bilirubin
    B. A palpable mass in the right lower quadrant
    C. Severe epigastric pain
    D. Unexplained weight gain
    E. History of abdominal trauma

Question 279

Refer to the sagittal view of the left testicle below:

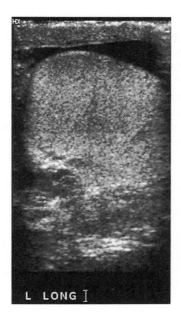

279. Which of the following histories best suits this patient?
    A. Longstanding chronic groin ache
    B. Wife felt a mass in the testicle
    C. Acute onset of tenderness in the groin
    D. Retroperitoneal nodes discovered with no clear source
    E. Low sperm count and infertility

Questions 280–283

Refer to the sagittal scrotal sonogram below:

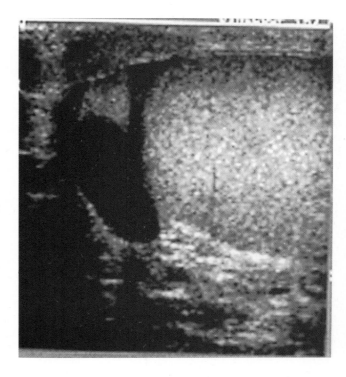

280. The abnormal finding on this image **MOST** likely originates in which structure?
    A. Mediastinum testis
    B. Rete testis
    C. Pampiniform plexus
    D. Epididymis
    E. Scrotal wall

281. The abnormal structure seen on this image is **MOST** likely composed of
    A. blood
    B. sperm
    C. bowel
    D. pus
    E. dilated veins

282. Which clinical history agrees with the findings on this image?
    A. One-year history of infertility
    B. A karate kick to the groin
    C. Elevated white blood cell count and low-grade fever
    D. Cryptorchidism
    E. Scrotal lump

283. Which course of management is **MOST** appropriate for this patient?
    A. No management
    B. Removal of the abnormal structure
    C. Orchidectomy
    D. Ten-day course of antibiotics
    E. Fine-needle aspiration

Questions 284 and 285

A 55-year-old man was referred for an abdominal ultrasound to rule out cholelithiasis, which was not present on the sonogram. Bilaterally, his kidneys measured approximately 7.5 cm in length. Transverse and sagittal views of the right renal region are shown below:

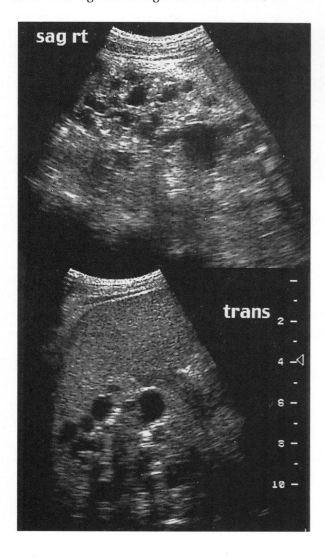

284. Which clinical history **MOST** likely belongs to this patient?
    A. Hematuria
    B. Flank pain
    C. Low-grade fever
    D. End-stage renal failure
    E. One of two brothers recently diagnosed with adult polycystic kidney disease

285. Which of the following is **TRUE** regarding the collecting system of this kidney?
    A. It is not seen well because of distortion by cysts
    B. It is filled with small calcifications, causing acoustic shadowing
    C. It is dilated because of obstruction from the cysts
    D. It is replaced by an abnormal amount of sinus fat
    E. It is duplicated

Questions 286–289

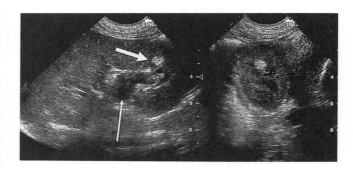

A 27-year-old diabetic patient with a history of recurrent fevers and urinary tract infections presents for a renal ultrasound. The following sagittal and transverse images were obtained:

286. All of the following methods would be helpful in identifying the structure indicated by the thin arrow **EXCEPT**
    A. standing the patient up to scan
    B. adjusting gain settings
    C. having the patient void
    D. using color flow Doppler

287. Given that the thin arrow points to a dilated collecting system, which of the following would **NOT** be helpful in determining the cause of this abnormality?
    A. Attempting to follow the ureter out of the kidney
    B. Looking for renal calculi
    C. Scanning the urinary bladder
    D. Checking the patient's chart for blood urea nitrogen and creatinine levels
    E. Examining the distal ureter at the posterior bladder

288. Which of the following is the **MOST** likely cause of the dilation?
  A. Lower pole calculus
  B. Pyonephrosis
  C. Diabetic nephropathy
  D. Ureterocele
  E. Angiomyolipoma

289. The structure identified by the thick arrow is **MOST** likely
  A. a renal calculus
  B. a hematoma
  C. an angiomyolipoma
  D. a fungal ball
  E. fibrolipomatosis

Questions 290–292

Refer to the renal sonogram below:

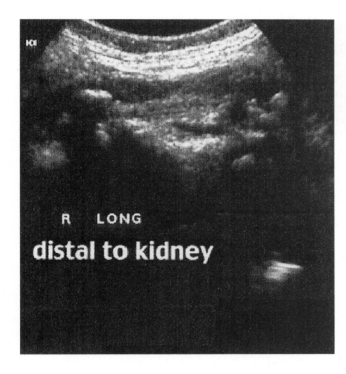

290. The structure identified by the arrow is the
  A. infundibulum
  B. hilum
  C. medulla
  D. pyramid
  E. calyx

291. Which of the following is the **MOST** likely cause of the pathology seen on this sonogram?
  A. Reflux
  B. Overly distended bladder
  C. Ureterocele
  D. Ureteral calculus
  E. Milk of calcium

292. Based on the sonogram, which of the following symptoms is this patient **MOST** likely experiencing?
  A. Pyuria
  B. Hematuria
  C. Anuria
  D. Oliguria
  E. Polyuria

Questions 293–296

A 29-year-old AIDS patient presents to the emergency room with persistent right upper quadrant and epigastric pain, especially after eating. Her bilirubin and liver function tests are normal. The following images of her pancreas are obtained:

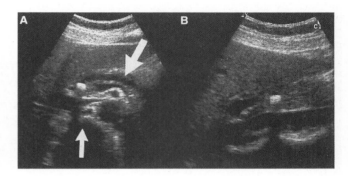

293. The large arrow is pointing to
  A. Wirsung's duct
  B. the splenic artery
  C. a collapsed stomach
  D. fluid in the lesser sac
  E. the cystic duct

294. If color flow Doppler is applied to the structure identified by the small arrow, the flow pattern will be
  A. triphasic
  B. monophasic
  C. absent
  D. biphasic
  E. turbulent

295. Which of the following statements is **MOST TRUE** concerning these images?
  A. The pancreatic duct is dilated secondary to the calcification in the common bile duct
  B. The gallbladder is contracted and full of stones
  C. The pancreatic duct is not visualized on these images
  D. Doppler flow in the portal vein would likely be absent
  E. The echogenicity of the pancreatic tissue is within normal limits

296. Image B was **MOST** likely produced using which of the following techniques?
    A. Transverse section
    B. After drinking water
    C. Longitudinal section
    D. After a fatty meal

Questions 297–299

A 62-year-old man was referred to the ultrasound department for a sonogram of his left groin after a femoral artery catheterization and subsequent pain and swelling at the catheter insertion site. The image below was taken with conventional color flow Doppler settings:

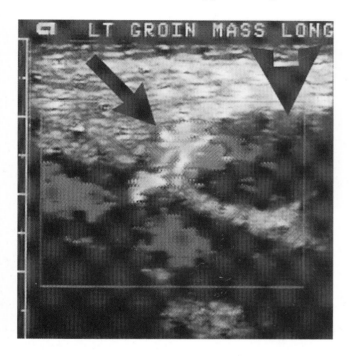

297. Given the patient's history and the appearance of the image, the arrow is pointing to
    A. turbulent flow in the femoral artery
    B. a thrombus
    C. an artifact secondary to incorrect transducer angle
    D. a false aneurysm
    E. the internal iliac vein

298. Which of the following statements is **TRUE** concerning the color flow Doppler pattern seen on this image?
    A. The blood flow in the femoral vein is moving away from the transducer and the blood flow in the femoral artery is moving toward the transducer
    B. The blood flow in the femoral artery is moving slower than normal
    C. A defect is present in the wall of the femoral artery
    D. There is evidence of retrograde flow in the femoral vein
    E. There is absence of flow in the femoral artery

299. The arrowhead is pointing to
    A. the common femoral vein
    B. dropout artifact
    C. the superficial femoral artery
    D. a plaque-filled vessel
    E. a thrombus

Questions 300–303

A 3-week-old male infant is brought to the emergency room with persistent projectile vomiting after feeding and excessive fussiness. Upon examination, a palpable mass is felt in the upper abdomen. The patient is sent for an abdominal sonogram. The following images are obtained:

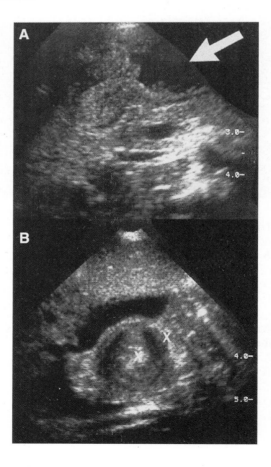

300. The sonographer should primarily focus on the
     A. stomach
     B. gallbladder
     C. liver
     D. pancreas
     E. jejunum

301. The arrow on image A is pointing to
     A. the gallbladder
     B. the duodenum
     C. a pancreatic pseudocyst
     D. an intrahepatic fluid collection
     E. a fluid-filled stomach

302. What is being measured on image B?
     A. Duodenal wall
     B. Ileum
     C. Stomach antrum
     D. Pyloric wall
     E. Uncinate process

303. Based on the images and the patient's history, what conclusion can be drawn?
     A. The sonogram is inconclusive; the patient should be referred to x-ray for a gastrointestinal study
     B. There is evidence of a stomach outlet obstruction; the patient should be referred to pediatric surgery
     C. The sonogram is normal
     D. The patient is most likely suffering from an allergy to his formula
     E. An intra-abdominal fluid collection is present that needs to be drained

Questions 304–306

A febrile patient with a high white blood cell count and right upper quadrant tenderness is referred for an ultrasound study. A transverse scan through the patient's liver is shown below:

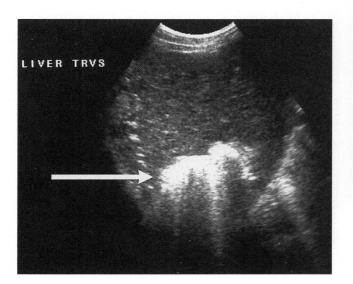

304. This image and the patient's history are **MOST** compatible with
     A. a staghorn calculus
     B. pneumobilia
     C. abscess formation
     D. an organized hematoma
     E. a porcelain gallbladder

305. The sonographer was able to better visualize the pathology by using a different technique than the one shown. Which of the following would be the **MOST** certain to yield better results?
     A. Scanning with a lower frequency transducer
     B. Scanning with a higher frequency transducer
     C. Scanning with the patient upright
     D. Scanning from the patient's right side with the patient in a supine position
     E. Scanning from the patient's right side with the patient in a right-side-up position

306. The bright echoes indicated by the arrow **MOST** likely represent
     A. fat
     B. gas
     C. lysed blood
     D. thickened pus
     E. granulomas

Questions 307 and 308

A 30-year-old febrile woman was admitted to the hospital with dehydration after a 1-week long episode of vomiting, flank pain, and microscopic hematuria. An abdominal/pelvic sonogram was performed. The following image was obtained:

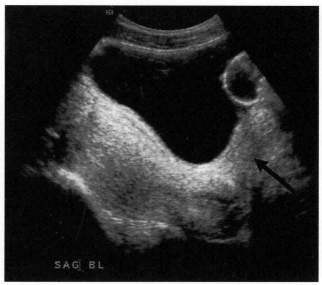

307. Which of the following is seen on this image?
    A. Transitional cell tumor
    B. Cystitis
    C. Ureterocele
    D. Ureteral stone
    E. There are no pathological findings on this sonogram

308. The arrow is pointing to the
    A. cervix
    B. vagina
    C. urethra
    D. bladder wall
    E. bowel

Questions 309 and 310

A 75-year-old man with urinary frequency is referred by his urologist for a renal sonogram because of an elevated laboratory value. His pelvic sonogram is shown below:

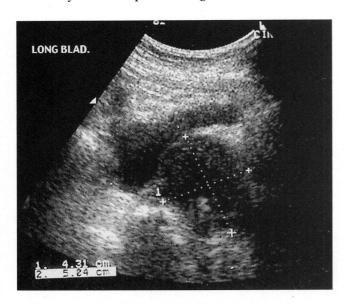

309. Based on the image, which of the following laboratory values is **MOST** likely to be elevated in this patient?
    A. Prostate-specific antigen (PSA)
    B. Aspartate aminotransferase (AST)
    C. White blood cells
    D. Phenolsulfotransferase (PST)
    E. α-Fetoprotein (AFP)

310. Based on the image, which of the following would be an appropriate next test?
    A. Color flow Doppler
    B. Cystoscopy
    C. Foley catheter insertion
    D. Colonoscopy
    E. Transrectal ultrasound

Questions 311 and 312

Refer to the transverse (A) and longitudinal (B) views of the pelvis below:

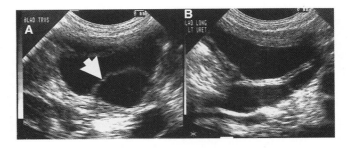

311. The arrow on image A is pointing to
    A. the bladder wall
    B. a mirror image
    C. the distal ureter
    D. the proximal urethra
    E. a Foley catheter

312. What additional finding would **MOST** likely be present in this patient?
    A. Retroperitoneal fibrosis
    B. Renal cell tumor
    C. Anuria
    D. Massive benign prostatic hypertrophy
    E. A duplicated collecting system

Questions 313 and 314

A premature, normal-appearing infant was admitted to the neonatal intensive care unit after a spontaneous vaginal delivery to a 17-year-old girl who had received no prenatal care. The baby was put on a respirator and a renal ultrasound was ordered 48 hours later for anuria. Both kidneys were very similar in appearance. The sonogram of the right kidney is shown below:

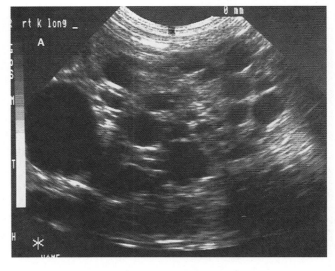

313. Which of the following is the **MOST** likely cause of the abnormality seen on the image?
    A. Meckel-Gruber syndrome
    B. Multicystic dysplastic kidney disease
    C. Infantile (autosomal recessive) polycystic kidney disease
    D. Trisomy 13 syndrome
    E. A genetic syndrome

314. Which of the following is the **BEST** management plan for this infant?
    A. Wait for resolution of the mass, which will occur with time
    B. Place a stent into the collecting system
    C. Start dialysis and continue until urine output improves
    D. Bilateral disease is incompatible with life
    E. Perform surgical resection

Questions 315–318

A 4-year-old girl was admitted to the hospital with a diagnosis of renal failure and was referred for a renal ultrasound. A longitudinal view of her kidney is shown below:

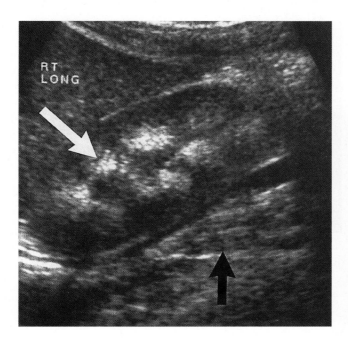

315. Which area of the kidney is indicated by the white arrow?
    A. Infundibulum
    B. Sinus fat
    C. Cortex
    D. Calyx
    E. Medulla

316. Which of the following findings is **MOST** likely to be seen in this patient?
    A. Hypercalciuria
    B. Serum creatinine value of 0.4
    C. Fever
    D. Renal vein thrombosis
    E. Pyuria

317. Which of the following is **NOT** a likely precursor to the pathology indicated in this case?
    A. Long-term furosemide (Lasix) administration
    B. Renal tubular acidosis
    C. Hypervitaminosis D
    D. Hypercalcemia
    E. Milk of calcium

318. Which structure is indicated by the black arrow?
    A. Gerota's fascia
    B. Perinephric space
    C. Crus of the diaphragm
    D. Psoas muscle
    E. Glisson's capsule

Questions 319–322

A 4-year-old girl is referred by her pediatric nephrologist to the ultrasound department for her annual abdominal ultrasound. Her renal function has slightly decreased since her last sonogram. The longitudinal image of her liver and kidney is shown below:

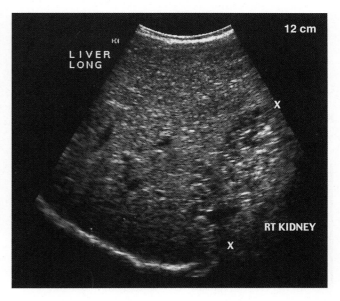

319. Which of the following is **TRUE** concerning the echogenicity of the kidney as compared to the liver?
    A. The kidney is too echogenic
    B. The kidney is not echogenic enough
    C. The kidney is appropriately echogenic
    D. An accurate comparison cannot be made because the liver is abnormal
    E. An accurate comparison cannot be made because the gain is set incorrectly

320. What can be assumed about the contralateral kidney in this patient?
    A. It has the same appearance as the kidney in this image
    B. No assumption can be made without scanning the opposite kidney
    C. It is most likely normal in appearance
    D. It is small and echogenic
    E. It is hydronephrotic

321. Taking into consideration the appearance of the kidney, what conclusion can be drawn about the condition of the liver on this image?
    A. The liver is sonographically normal
    B. The liver is fibrotic in association with the disease process of the kidney
    C. The liver is affected with the same disease process as the kidney in 40% of cases
    D. The liver cannot be accurately evaluated because of improper gain settings
    E. The appearance of the liver is abnormal but not associated with the disease process of the kidney

322. Which of the following is **TRUE** concerning possible future pregnancies in this patient?
    A. A future child has a 25% chance of being affected
    B. A future child has a 50% chance of being affected
    C. A future child will not be affected
    D. A future child has a 100% chance of being affected
    E. Only future children that are female will be affected

Questions 323 and 324

Refer to the sagittal view of the right renal region below:

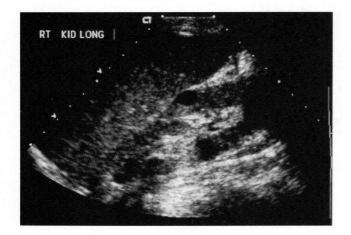

323. The arrowheads are pointing to
    A. an area of dropout
    B. acoustic shadowing
    C. slice thickness artifact
    D. acoustic enhancement
    E. reverberation artifact

324. The pathology seen on the image has a very characteristic appearance. Which of the following will **NOT** help to confirm the diagnosis?
    A. Absence of internal echoes
    B. A smooth outline
    C. Good through transmission
    D. Fluid-filled appearance
    E. Size of the entity

Question 325

Refer to the sagittal view of the right upper quadrant below:

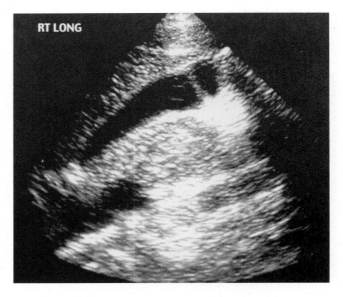

325. Which of the following is seen on the sonogram?
    A. Fundal fenestration
    B. Hartmann's pouch
    C. Septal defect
    D. Phrygian cap
    E. Colonic bulb

Question 326

An efficient sonographer put her next patient on the table before the receptionist had the paperwork ready. She scanned around quickly to get an overview of the abdomen, and froze the image as shown below:

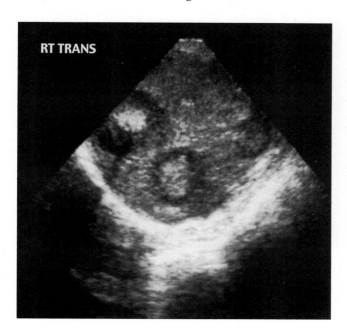

326. When the sonographer went to the desk to get the chart, she realized she did not know the patient's name. She chose the correct chart based on the patient's indication for the examination. What did it say on the requisition?
    A. Liver sonogram—decreased carcinoembryonic antigen (CEA)
    B. Liver sonogram—primary breast cancer
    C. Liver sonogram—primary brain cancer
    D. Liver sonogram—decreased α-fetoprotein (AFP)
    E. Liver sonogram—history of alcohol abuse

Questions 327–330

Refer to the sonogram of the gallbladder below:

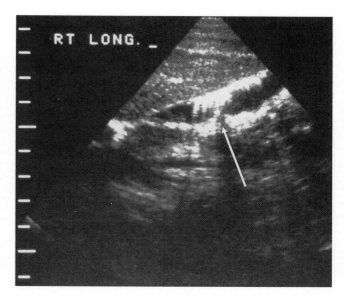

327. Which of the following **BEST** describes the finding in the anterior aspect of this gallbladder?
    A. Diffuse shadowing
    B. Reverberation artifact
    C. Debris
    D. Organizing hematoma
    E. Comet tail artifact

328. The appearance of the finding on this sonogram is pathognomonic for
    A. sludge in the Rokitansky-Aschoff sinuses
    B. cholesterol crystals in the Rokitansky-Aschoff sinuses
    C. air in the Rokitansky-Aschoff sinuses
    D. stones in Hartmann's pouch
    E. air in Hartmann's pouch

329. This sonogram demonstrates the classic ultrasound appearance of
    A. stellate artifact
    B. a porcelain gallbladder
    C. adenomyomatosis
    D. staghorn calculus
    E. adenomyosis

330. The region marked by the arrow represents
    A. shadowing from a gallstone
    B. acoustic enhancement from a Rokitansky-Aschoff sinus
    C. acoustic impedance from fibrosis
    D. shadowing from fat in the gallbladder mucosa
    E. shadowing from a polyp

Question 331

A 53-year-old man was sent to ultrasound with the following indications: no pain or jaundice, weight loss, increased aspartate aminotransferase (AST), a long history of smoking, and shortness of breath. A transverse section through the left lobe of the liver was taken (see below). The right lobe of the liver, the gallbladder, and the common bile duct were well visualized and appeared completely normal.

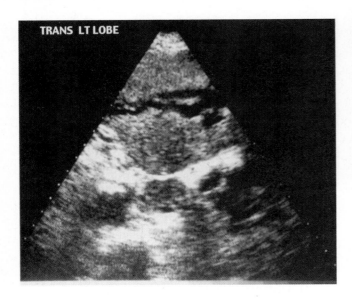

331. Which of the following statements is **NOT** true?
    A. The patient's bilirubin is increased
    B. The patient needs a chest x-ray
    C. The sonogram demonstrates the parallel channel sign
    D. There is another abnormality in the left lobe of the liver not shown on this image
    E. The great vessels should be carefully examined for lymphadenopathy and the abdomen for ascites

Questions 332 and 333

The patient is a white male from Oklahoma with no history of alcohol abuse. The following transverse view of the liver is obtained:

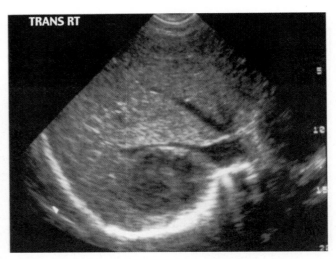

332. A biopsy of the pathology seen on the sonogram would take place in the
    A. superior portion of the left medial lobe of the liver
    B. inferior portion of the left medial lobe of the liver
    C. superior portion of the right anterior lobe of the liver
    D. inferior portion of the right anterior lobe of the liver
    E. superior portion of the right posterior lobe of the liver

333. Based on the patient's history and the sonogram, the **MOST** likely diagnosis is
    A. a metastatic lesion
    B. hepatocellular disease
    C. a hemangioma
    D. hepatocellular carcinoma
    E. Kaposi's sarcoma

Questions 334 and 335

Refer to the oblique sagittal view of the liver below:

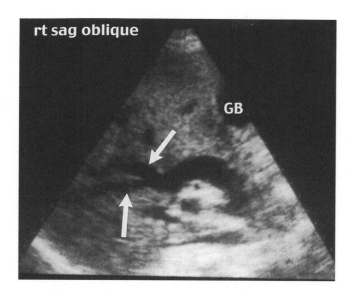

334. The anatomy marked by the arrows represents
   A. the main and right portal veins
   B. the right and left portal veins
   C. prominent hepatic veins
   D. the right and left bile ducts
   E. the common hepatic duct and common bile duct

335. The pathology shown on the sonogram is
   A. choledocholithiasis
   B. portal vein hypertension
   C. portal vein thrombosis
   D. a biliary duct obstruction
   E. a Klatskin tumor

Question 336

Refer to the gallbladder sonogram below:

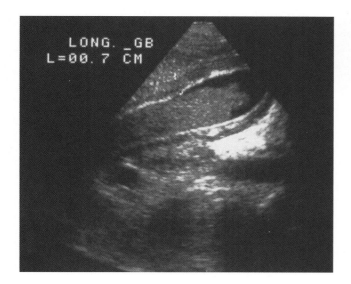

336. The abnormality seen on the sonogram could be caused by any of the following **EXCEPT**
   A. AIDS cholangiopathy
   B. hepatitis
   C. ascites
   D. portal hypertension
   E. testicular torsion

Questions 337 and 338

A 14-year-old boy was being treated for infectious mononucleosis. After taking his pitbull for a walk, he experienced sharp pain in his left shoulder. His anxious mother took him immediately to the emergency room where an efficient resident ordered an abdominal ultrasound study. The sonographer scanned the right and left upper quadrants, finding no abnormalities except the splenic enlargement that had been noted during his original work-up. Content to let this finding explain his shoulder pain, the resident sent him home only to have an anxious and now angry mother bring him back 2 days later. The resident, now nervous, ordered a repeat sonogram. This time the left upper quadrant showed a subtle, hypoechoic line that demonstrated no flow with color Doppler and an anechoic space below the left diaphragm, all of which can be seen on the image below:

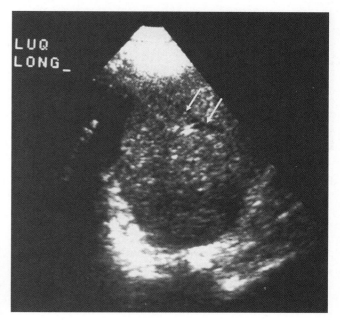

337. What is the **MOST** reasonable differential diagnosis for the hypoechoic line indicated by the small arrows?
   A. Scarring from the infection in the spleen
   B. A dilated venous structure in the spleen
   C. A splenic fracture
   D. A normal variant
   E. Interface between splenic lobes

338. What is the **MOST** reasonable differential diagnosis for the anechoic space?
    A. A subphrenic or subcapsular splenic abscess
    B. A subphrenic or subcapsular splenic hematoma
    C. Ascites
    D. Left pleural effusion
    E. Splenic infarct

Questions 339 and 340

A cardiac patient being treated with antibiotics for subacute bacterial endocarditis presented to her internist with a fever of unknown origin. Left upper quadrant pain prompted the doctor to order an abdominal sonogram to locate the source of the fever. The requisition simply stated, "Fever of unknown origin (FUO)." The sonogram of her left upper quadrant is shown below:

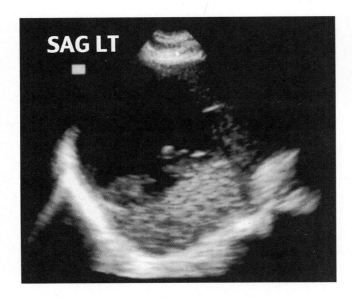

339. This patient was correctly diagnosed with a splenic abscess. Which of the following features was **NOT** helpful in making this diagnosis?
    A. Size
    B. Acoustic enhancement
    C. Debris in an irregularly shaped collection
    D. Fever and a high leukocyte count
    E. Location

340. Which of the following techniques would help the sonographer to differentiate this mass from an organizing hematoma?
    A. A lower frequency transducer
    B. Doppler
    C. A needle inserted under ultrasound control
    D. A higher frequency to demonstrate the splenic capsule
    E. Scanning at a different level of inspiration or expiration

Questions 341 and 342

A patient experiencing right upper quadrant pain is referred for an ultrasound examination. The patient's history is otherwise normal. The left sagittal view taken through the spleen and left kidney is shown below:

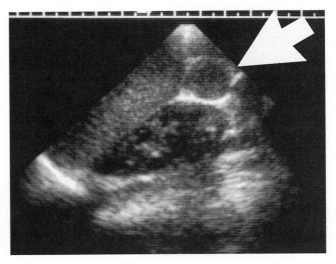

341. The round area indicated by the white arrow is most compatible with
    A. renal cell carcinoma
    B. a splenic metastatic lesion
    C. an enlarged lymph node
    D. a splenule
    E. a hypernephroma

342. The vascular supply for the abnormal area comes from
    A. branches of the left testicular or ovarian artery
    B. branches of the splenic artery
    C. accessory vessels directly from the aorta
    D. branches of the iliac artery
    E. branches of the diaphragmatic artery

Questions 343–345

Refer to the sagittal view taken coronally through the spleen below (note that there is no left kidney on this image):

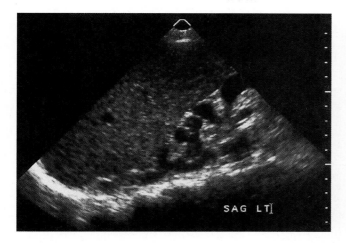

343. Given the pathology demonstrated on this image, which of the following is the **MOST** logical primary diagnosis?
    A. Abdominal aortic aneurysm
    B. Large pelvic mass
    C. Portal hypertension
    D. Metastatic adenocarcinoma
    E. Lymphadenopathy

344. Which of the following techniques would **NOT** be useful in assessing this condition?
    A. Pulsed Doppler
    B. Color flow Doppler
    C. A decubitus view of the gallbladder
    D. Ingestion of water
    E. Examination of the ligamentum teres

345. Which of the following would **NOT** be expected in a severe example of this condition?
    A. Echogenic liver texture
    B. Splenomegaly
    C. Ascites
    D. Hepatopetal flow
    E. Hepatofugal flow

Questions 346 and 347

A patient being evaluated for metastatic disease was found to have metastases in his liver, lymphadenopathy, and the lesions in his spleen that are demonstrated on the image below:

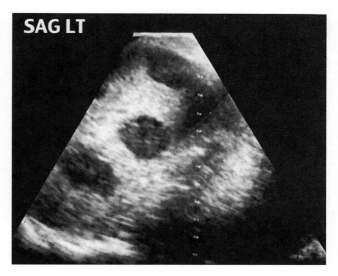

346. The sonologist diagnosed the splenic lesions as metastases based on all of the following criteria **EXCEPT**
    A. the cystic contents of the lesions
    B. the fact that the lesions are multifocal
    C. the lack of increased acoustic enhancement
    D. the lack of air in the lesions
    E. patient history

347. The primary malignancy eventually found in this patient proved to be the one **MOST** likely to metastasize to the spleen, which is
    A. lung cancer
    B. colon cancer
    C. breast cancer
    D. kidney cancer
    E. melanoma

Questions 348–353

Refer to the diagram below:

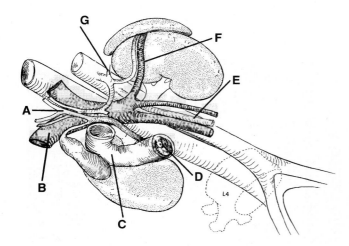

348. The structure labeled C is the
    A. common bile duct
    B. pancreatic head
    C. C-loop of the duodenum
    D. right portal vein
    E. gastroduodenal artery

349. The structure labeled B is the
    A. common bile duct
    B. hepatic artery
    C. gastroduodenal ligament
    D. right portal vein
    E. left portal vein

350. The structure labeled D is the
    A. ampulla of Vater
    B. hepatic artery
    C. gastroduodenal artery
    D. gastroduodenal ligament
    E. right portal vein

351. The structure labeled G is the
    A. common bile duct
    B. left renal artery
    C. left renal vein
    D. gastric artery
    E. splenic hilum

352. The structure labeled A is the
    A. common hepatic duct
    B. left renal artery
    C. cystic duct
    D. second portion of the duodenum
    E. common bile duct

353. The structure labeled E is the
    A. common bile duct
    B. splenic vein
    C. superior mesenteric vein
    D. second portion of the duodenum
    E. inferior vena cava

Questions 354–356

Refer to the sagittal image of the liver below:

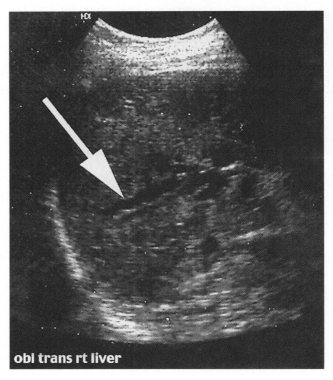

obl trans rt liver

354. This image demonstrates the classic appearance of
    A. a dilated common duct
    B. polycystic liver disease
    C. portal vein thrombosis
    D. peripheral duct dilation
    E. normal liver parenchyma

355. The more anterior of the two structures indicated by the arrow is **MOST** likely a
    A. portal vein
    B. biliary radicle
    C. recanalized paraumbilical vein
    D. hepatic vein
    E. Kupffer tubule

356. The quickest, most efficient way to prove that something is part of the biliary tree is to
    A. use color flow Doppler
    B. trace structures back to their origin
    C. turn the patient into a decubitus position
    D. check the portal vein velocity
    E. guess

Questions 357–359

A right sagittal scan through the liver in a patient with a history of alcohol abuse is shown below:

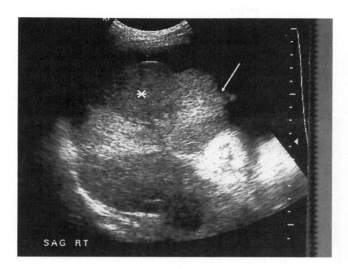

357. Which of the following entities **MOST** likely describes the overall diagnosis in this patient?
    A. Acute hepatitis
    B. Multiple metastases
    C. Hepatic infarction
    D. Chronic hepatitis
    E. Chronic cirrhosis

358. The area indicated by the asterisk appears to be
    A. normal parenchyma
    B. metastases
    C. fibrosis caused by hepatocellular destruction
    D. a hepatoma
    E. acoustic enhancement from ascites

359. All of the following features often accompany the condition shown on the image **EXCEPT**
    A. surface nodularity changes
    B. ascites
    C. prominent borders to portal vasculature
    D. regenerating nodules
    E. portal hypertension

Questions 360–362

A 30-year-old woman was scanned for pain in the right upper quadrant. Everything was found to be normal except for gallstones and the pathology shown on the image below:

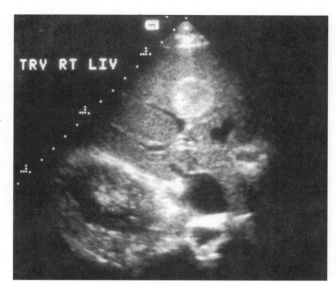

360. Based on the information available, the first differential diagnosis for this lesion is
    A. an adenoma
    B. metastasis
    C. fatty infiltration
    D. a hemangioma
    E. a hepatoma

361. All of the following are typical characteristics of this lesion **EXCEPT**
    A. it shows flow on conventional color flow Doppler
    B. it is often an isolated finding
    C. it has an echogenic appearance
    D. it may exhibit central necrosis or thrombosis
    E. it is more common in women

362. If left untreated, how will this lesion **MOST** likely appear on serial ultrasound examinations?
    A. Increased in size
    B. Increased in number
    C. Decreased in size
    D. Decreased in number
    E. Unchanged

Questions 363–365

A 62-year-old man is referred to ultrasound to evaluate a midabdominal mass found during physical examination. The following image is obtained:

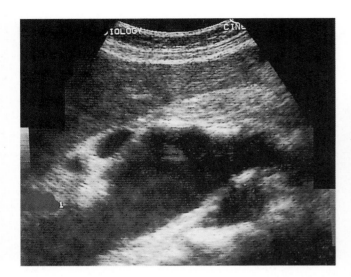

363. To ensure proper management of this patient, it is important to image all of the following **EXCEPT**
    A. the renal arteries
    B. the celiac axis
    C. the inferior vena cava
    D. the superior mesenteric artery
    E. the iliac bifurcation

364. The low-level echoes in the mass seen on the image **MOST** likely represent
    A. slow blood flow
    B. the intima of the aorta
    C. gas
    D. reverberation artifact
    E. a thrombus

365. Which of the following would be **MOST** helpful in further evaluating the mass?
    A. Compression
    B. A change in the patient's position
    C. Color flow Doppler
    D. Adjustment of the gain settings
    E. Spectral analysis

Questions 366–368

A 2-year-old girl toddled into the corner of a coffee table, which protruded well up under her costal margin. A large bruise resulted, but the child remained quiet and became pale, with a rapid pulse. By the time she arrived in the emergency room she was lethargic, stirring only to ask for water. An abdominal CT scan was ordered to assess the trauma. The next day a baseline sonogram was ordered so the pathology could be followed without radiation. The following image was obtained:

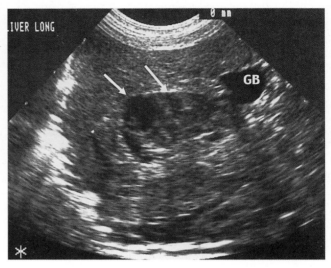

366. Based solely on the patient's history, which of the following is the correct diagnosis?
    A. Hepatic infarct
    B. Biloma
    C. Hematoma
    D. Caroli's disease
    E. Hepatic abscess

367. Based solely on the sonographic criteria, which of the following could be the correct diagnosis?
    A. Hepatic abscess
    B. Hemorrhagic cyst
    C. Degenerating hepatoblastoma
    D. Any of the above
    E. None of the above

368. If the sonogram had been performed as soon as the child came into the emergency room, what would the ultrasound appearance have been in comparison with the image obtained?
    A. Exactly the same
    B. Same texture, only smaller
    C. More hyperechoic
    D. More hypoechoic

Questions 369–372

A 42-year-old, mildly obese mother of five presents with colicky right upper quadrant pain. A sonogram of her liver, bile ducts, and gallbladder is shown below. She does not have a positive sonographic Murphy's sign. Decubitus views of her gallbladder show no change in the location of the echogenic region marked by arrows in the following image:

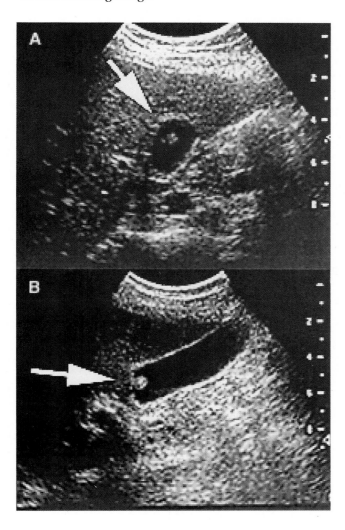

369. Based solely on the patient's history, which of the following conditions will her clinician **MOST** likely expect?
    A. Sclerosing cholangitis
    B. Biliary atresia
    C. Acute acalculous cholecystitis
    D. Renal colic
    E. Cholelithiasis

370. Based on the patient's history and both images, the diagnosis could be all of the following **EXCEPT**
    A. gallbladder cancer
    B. cholesterolosis
    C. a cholesterol polyp
    D. a small, adherent gallstone
    E. a floating gallstone

371. Based on image A only, the **MOST** likely diagnosis is
    A. gallbladder cancer
    B. cholesterolosis
    C. a cholesterol polyp
    D. a small, adherent gallstone
    E. a floating gallstone

372. All of the following techniques are useful in distinguishing between floating gallstones and gallbladder polyps **EXCEPT**
    A. a lower frequency transducer
    B. decubitus views of the gallbladder
    C. prone views of the gallbladder
    D. checking the chart to see if the patient has had any oral cholecystographic agents
    E. erect views of the gallbladder

373. A 22-year-old man presents with an elevated human chorionic gonadotropin (HCG) level. The sonographer should scan the
    A. breast
    B. pancreas
    C. scrotum
    D. thyroid
    E. prostate

374. Which of the following areas of the prostate gland has the most peripheral zone tissue?
    A. Base
    B. Apex
    C. Periurethral area
    D. Anterior aspect
    E. Superior aspect

375. Thermal effects can be caused by a change in the
    A. near field
    B. far field
    C. power
    D. gain
    E. transducer frequency

376. A palpable "olive" sign is one of the common criteria used by clinicians to request which of the following ultrasound examinations?
    A. Renal sonogram on a patient with a history of adult polycystic kidney disease
    B. Sonogram of the pancreas on a patient with an elevated amylase
    C. Sonogram of the groin after femoral catheterization and subsequent swelling
    D. Sonogram of the aorta on an elderly patient with epigastric pain
    E. Sonogram of the stomach on an infant with persistent projectile vomiting

377. Time gain compensation (TGC), depth gain compensation (DGC), or swept gain compensates for sound
    A. reflection
    B. refraction
    C. focusing
    D. attenuation
    E. propagation speed

378. A cirrhotic liver is hyperechoic, which means
    A. there are no reflectors
    B. there are few echoes
    C. there are high-impedance interfaces
    D. there are many reflectors
    E. there is decreased echogenicity

379. A patient with an abdominal aortic aneurysm of 3.1 cm has a follow-up scan done, which reveals an increase in diameter to 5.0 cm. However, surgical intervention shows no change in diameter. What could be a reasonable explanation for this discrepancy in size?
    A. The last quality assurance was performed 5 years ago
    B. It is a variable aneurysm
    C. The patient position was different on the follow-up scan
    D. A different transducer was used for the follow-up scan
    E. The patient ate immediately before the follow-up scan

380. In patients with Budd-Chiari syndrome, which lobe of the liver is spared?
    A. Right
    B. Left
    C. Caudate
    D. Quadrate
    E. Medial

381. Which of the following abnormalities **MOST** often complicates intercostal percutaneous liver biopsy?
    A. Pneumothorax
    B. Retroperitoneal bleeding
    C. Pancreatitis
    D. Bowel perforation
    E. Liver abscess

382. On a transverse image of the abdomen, at the level of the hepatic veins, a fluid collection was found posterior but not superior to the liver, extending from the lateral margin of the trunk to the spine. A decision was made to culture the fluid. How should the patient be positioned for the puncture?
    A. Left lateral decubitus position, with wedges or pillows to stabilize the patient
    B. Supine position, to keep the patient steady and allow the needle to be inserted perpendicular to the table
    C. Sitting position
    D. Prone position, with a pillow under the abdomen to spread the ribs
    E. Trendelenburg position

383. Pneumothorax is routinely ruled out after a pleurocentesis by
    A. auscultating the lungs
    B. injecting contrast before the needle is removed and obtaining a chest x-ray
    C. obtaining a posteroanterior chest x-ray taken on inspiration
    D. obtaining a posteroanterior chest x-ray taken on expiration
    E. looking for pneumothorax with ultrasound

384. A patient recently diagnosed with AIDS is sent for a baseline sonogram. All of the following are related to AIDS and could be found on an abdominal ultrasound study **EXCEPT**
    A. multiple abscesses in the liver or spleen
    B. flukes in the gallbladder
    C. a thick-walled gallbladder
    D. lymphadenopathy
    E. enlarged, echogenic kidneys

385. Six days after a cesarean section, a patient develops a fever and has a drop in her hemoglobin level. She is referred to ultrasound for a careful examination of all the following areas **EXCEPT**
    A. anterior to the rectus muscles
    B. posterior to the rectus muscles
    C. posterior to the sacrum
    D. posterior to the bladder
    E. the uterine wall

386. One year after surgery, a patient presents complaining of tenderness deep to the incision. The 3-cm long incision is directly below the umbilicus and has healed nicely. The patient has a slight fever and a mildly elevated white blood cell count. His hematocrit is normal. On ultrasound, a dense, linear echo with well-defined shadowing is seen in the midline, posterior to the incision within the mesentery. The diagnosis is confirmed with a CT scan. Which of the following is the **MOST** likely differential diagnosis?
    A. Lymphocele
    B. Calculus
    C. Hematoma
    D. Gossyphiboma
    E. Postoperative air

387. A 35-year-old man has irregularly thickened mucosa in dilated bile ducts. This finding is indicative of
    A. primary biliary cirrhosis
    B. a choledochal cyst
    C. AIDS cholangitis
    D. biliary atresia
    E. Heister's biliary hypertrophy

388. An elderly patient is referred for an ultrasound study by her surgeon. The sonographer spends most of the scanning time imaging the renal and superior mesenteric arteries and the celiac axis. The patient had surgery the following week for her
    A. osteoporosis
    B. abdominal aortic aneurysm
    C. hydronephrosis
    D. glomerulonephritis
    E. renal calculi

389. A 13-year-old girl was referred for a pelvic ultrasound 2 days after she underwent surgery for a ruptured appendix. She was febrile and had leukocytosis. The surgeon was looking for a postoperative abscess. Trying to scan around a gas pocket without disturbing the incision, the sonographer asked the patient to turn up toward her right side. The patient complained that her right shoulder hurt too much to turn. Given that all of the patient's history is relevant, what did the sonogram show?
    A. An abscess in the right paracolic gutter
    B. A hematoma in the right shoulder
    C. A right subphrenic abscess
    D. Enlarged lymph nodes
    E. An ovarian cyst

390. A patient fell on the ice and hit his back on the edge of a step. He was bruised but did not have pain unless he was walking or climbing stairs, in which case he had pain in his right lower back. He was febrile, but his urinalysis and white blood cell count were normal. He was referred for an ultrasound study, which revealed a
    A. hematoma in the iliopsoas muscle
    B. fracture in the kidney
    C. retroperitoneal abscess
    D. ruptured spleen

391. In a patient recently diagnosed with lymphoma, the sonographer discovered a 5-cm mass in the porta hepatis on the initial abdominal survey. The mass was probably enlarged lymph nodes. For which of the following indications was this patient **MOST** likely referred to ultrasound?
    A. Epigastric pain
    B. Jaundice
    C. Weight loss
    D. Flank pain
    E. Fever

392. A 30-year-old man is referred to ultrasound for generalized right upper quadrant tenderness and early signs of jaundice. His gallbladder appears normal, but there are bright focal areas without shadowing scattered throughout his liver. On close inspection, these areas are seen to be the walls of the portal vein branches. What is first in the list of differential diagnoses?
    A. Choledocholithiasis
    B. Multiple focal abscesses
    C. Metastatic lesions
    D. Hepatitis
    E. Pneumobilia

393. An 82-year-old man with a 10-year history of alcohol abuse is admitted with abdominal pain. His amylase and lipase levels are normal, as is the configuration of his pancreas. However, an abdominal sonogram shows that his pancreas is markedly less echogenic than his liver and is difficult to see. Which of the following transducers would provide the **BEST** image of this patient's right hemidiaphragm?
    A. Sector transducer (2 MHz)
    B. Curved array transducer (3.5 MHz)
    C. Vector transducer (3.5 MHz)
    D. Annular array transducer
    E. Linear array transducer (5 MHz)

394. A preoperative ultrasound study reveals a solitary liver mass displacing two structures in the liver. The surgeon is told he can confine his operation to the medial segment of the left lobe. Which two structures are being displaced?
    A. Ligamentum teres and gallbladder
    B. Fissure for the ligamentum venosum and left portal vein
    C. Main portal vein and hepatic duct
    D. Left hepatic vein and middle hepatic vein

395. The right and left lobes of the liver are separated by all of the following **EXCEPT**
    A. the falciform ligament
    B. the gallbladder
    C. the interlobar fissure
    D. the middle hepatic vein

396. A patient with end-stage cirrhosis exhibits hepatofugal portal flow, making the presence of collateral vessels likely. A close look at which of the following will **MOST** easily demonstrate collateral flow?
    A. Gallbladder region
    B. Ligamentum teres
    C. Spleen
    D. Ligamentum venosum
    E. Renal hilum

397. A casual reading of an abdominal sonogram in a patient with a Riedel's lobe could result in which of the following misdiagnoses?
    A. A mass in the head of the pancreas
    B. Hepatomegaly
    C. A mass in the spleen
    D. Hypernephroma
    E. Hepatoma

398. On an otherwise routine abdominal survey, a vessel is seen arising from the superior mesenteric artery and heading toward the porta hepatis. Color flow Doppler demonstrates hepatopetal flow. The vessel is **MOST** likely
    A. a portosystemic collateral
    B. the coronary artery
    C. a replaced right hepatic artery
    D. the gastric artery
    E. the gastroduodenal artery

399. An inexperienced sonography student was unable to visualize a patient's gallbladder. The patient had no incisions and assured the sonographer that she had fasted as instructed. Knowing that the clinician suspected gallstones, the sonographer decided to take enough images so as not to miss the gallbladder. Without realizing it, the sonographer demonstrated the gallbladder filled with stones on which of the following views?
    A. Transverse view, including the long axis of the right portal vein
    B. Longitudinal view at the level of the duodenum
    C. Left lateral decubitus view at the level of the pancreas
    D. Longitudinal view, including the right portal vein and the main lobar fissure
    E. Longitudinal view through the liver and right kidney

400. A patient is sent to ultrasound for an "abdominal survey" with no history. Questioning the patient produces vague, unsatisfactory answers. The sonographer looks in the patient's chart and decides to focus the study on the liver and biliary system. Which of the following laboratory results did the sonographer **MOST** likely find in the patient's chart?
    A. Decreased α-fetoprotein
    B. Low hematocrit
    C. Elevated alkaline phosphatase
    D. Elevated amylase
    E. Elevated creatinine

401. In a patient with a highly echogenic liver, all of the following laboratory values can help distinguish between cirrhosis and a normal liver **EXCEPT**
    A. acetylcholinesterase
    B. aspartate aminotransferase (AST)
    C. gamma-glutamyltransferase (GGT)
    D. alanine aminotransferase (ALT)
    E. liver function tests (LFTs)

402. A patient had laboratory data and clinical symptoms suggesting stones in the gallbladder or biliary tree. The sonographer felt he had ruled out these diagnoses by demonstrating a normal gallbladder, a 4-mm common duct anterior to the right portal vein, and no peripheral duct dilation. The sonologist sent him back for additional views of the
    A. main lobar fissure
    B. ligamentum teres
    C. pancreas and right kidney
    D. common bile duct in the head of the pancreas
    E. portal vein

403. Although there are many variations in normal anatomy, the usual site for the bifurcation of the common hepatic duct into the right and left hepatic ducts takes place
A. posterior and medial to the hepatic artery
B. anterior to the portal vein bifurcation
C. in the lateral portion of the head of the pancreas
D. anterior and superior to the right hepatic artery

404. A 16-year-old boy was being scanned for right upper quadrant pain. There was no evidence of stones in the intrahepatic ducts or gallbladder, but the common duct was 6.5 mm at the level of the right portal vein. Soon after the sonographer was called away to assist with an emergency, the bored and hungry patient ate a Snickers bar. When the common duct was scanned 40 minutes later, it measured 8.5 mm at the same level. Which of the following is the **MOST** likely explanation for the increased measurement?
A. A gallstone was recently passed
B. There is a stone in the distal common duct that is at least partially obstructing the biliary system
C. The fat in the candy bar decreased the release of cholecystokinin
D. There is obstruction caused by hepatocellular disease
E. This is the normal response to the ingestion of a candy bar

405. An asymptomatic, 80-year-old woman is having her abdominal aortic aneurysm scanned to follow the size. The alert sonographer finds a gallstone and a 7-mm common bile duct in the porta hepatis. Which of the following statements is **TRUE?**
A. The patient needs surgery to prevent possible obstructive jaundice
B. The patient recently passed a gallstone
C. The gallstone is incidental; the duct is normal in size for her age
D. The patient is asymptomatic because the duct is obstructed from her aneurysm
E. The patient has a positive Murphy's sign

406. A sagittal view at the level of the common duct reveals multiple bright, linear echoes scattered throughout the liver. The echoes exhibit "dirty" shadowing and, in one area, a ring down artifact. Which of the following situations could **NOT** be responsible for the bright echoes disseminated in the liver?
A. Surgical clips from a cholecystectomy
B. A choledochojejunostomy
C. A sphincterotomy
D. Gallbladder ileus

407. A sonogram on a patient referred for right upper quadrant pain shows an enlarged gallbladder and dilated peripheral ducts with no evidence of calculi. The extrahepatic common bile duct is normal in caliber; the only evidence of a stone is just proximal to Hartmann's pouch, complete with shadowing, but it does not change position on a left lateral decubitus view. This condition is **MOST** likely
A. Mirizzi syndrome
B. *Ascaris lumbricoides*
C. Caroli's disease
D. Sclerosing cholangitis
E. Klatskin tumor

408. A 23-year-old college student is referred by the university health clinic because of diffuse abdominal and right upper quadrant pain. There is some free fluid in her abdomen and an encapsulated mass in her liver that is solid but contains complex cystic components. The sonologist, quite correctly, makes hepatic adenoma the first differential diagnosis for all of the following reasons **EXCEPT** one. Which is it?
A. Upon questioning, the patient reported having been on oral contraceptives since her freshman year
B. Metastatic lesions in her liver would have a "bull's eye" appearance
C. The cystic areas are compatible with bleeding inside the mass, as hepatic adenomas are prone to do
D. While ultrasound features are variable, hepatic adenomas often appear encapsulated

409. A focal mass that does not appear to be a regenerating nodule is seen on ultrasound in a patient with end-stage cirrhosis. The mass should be considered malignant until proved otherwise. This statement is **TRUE** because
A. there is no completely solid hepatic tumor that is benign
B. the histology of a mass cannot be proved until a biopsy is performed
C. malignant tumors in cirrhosis are always vascular, which can always be proved with color flow Doppler
D. it is unusual to see regenerating nodules in cirrhosis
E. cirrhosis is strongly associated with hepatocellular carcinoma

410. Which of the following statements concerning metastatic lesions to the liver is **TRUE?**
    A. Metastases in the gallbladder are from melanoma
    B. Metastases from the colon invariably appear as "bull's eye" lesions
    C. Color flow Doppler demonstrates if a tumor or metastatic lesion is vascular
    D. Lymphoma causes hypoechoic lesions in the liver
    E. One can never make a tissue-specific diagnosis from the sonographic appearance of a lesion

411. A branching tubular structure in the liver is either an intrahepatic portal vein or a dilated bile duct. All of the following criteria would identify it as a bile duct **EXCEPT**
    A. through transmission
    B. a tortuous course
    C. a monophasic Doppler signal
    D. being adjacent to a larger portal vein
    E. echogenic walls

412. A child with known medullary sponge kidney presents with hematuria and is sent to ultrasound to look for nephrocalcinosis. The sonographer sees rounded, echo-free structures in the liver with good acoustic enhancement. The structures vary in size and some appear to be connected by thinner tubular structures. What is the first differential diagnosis?
    A. Autosomal recessive polycystic disease
    B. Caroli's disease
    C. Autosomal dominant polycystic disease
    D. Meckel-Gruber syndrome
    E. Biliary duct dilation

OBSTETRICS AND GYNECOLOGY COMPREHENSIVE EXAMINATION

Each numbered statement or question is followed by a minimum of four options. Select the ONE that is BEST.

1. Which of the following does **NOT** cause endometrial thickening after menopause?
   A. Benign endometrial hyperplasia
   B. Endometrial cancer
   C. Estrogen therapy
   D. Multiple endometrial polyps
   E. Atrophy of the endometrium

2. Which of the following is **NOT** a feature of ectopic pregnancy?
   A. Adnexal ring sign
   B. Fluid in the cul-de-sac
   C. Decidual thickening
   D. Adnexal mass
   E. Broad ligament hypertrophy

3. A sonographer was scanning a new patient for unknown dates when he learned from the patient that she was a poorly controlled insulin-dependent diabetic. He was especially careful to look for neural tube defects, because the incidence in diabetes is increased
   A. two times
   B. three times
   C. four times
   D. five times
   E. ten times

Questions 4 and 5

Refer to the image of the fetus below:

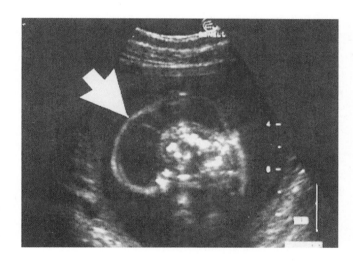

4. The arrow is pointing to
   A. an amniotic band
   B. a membrane between twin sacs
   C. a cystic hygroma
   D. an amniotic sheet
   E. the borders of a bleed

5. This image was obtained at which of the following levels?
   A. Neck
   B. Leg
   C. Sacrum
   D. Kidney
   E. Chest

Questions 6–8

Refer to the endovaginal sagittal view of the uterus below:

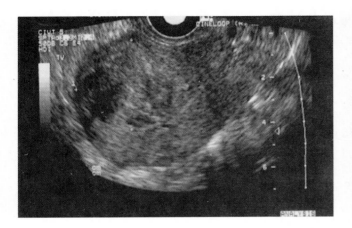

6. Which of the following is the **MOST** likely cause of the pathology measured on this image?
   A. Partial mole
   B. Choriocarcinoma
   C. Fibroid
   D. Endometrial mass
   E. Uterine cancer

7. Where is this process?
   A. Submucosal
   B. Pedunculated
   C. Subserosal
   D. Intramural
   E. Intracavitary

8. Which of the following may be caused by this entity?
   A. Vaginal discharge
   B. Pain on intercourse
   C. Menorrhagia
   D. Colicky local tenderness
   E. Leg pain

Questions 9–12

Refer to the obstetric sonogram below:

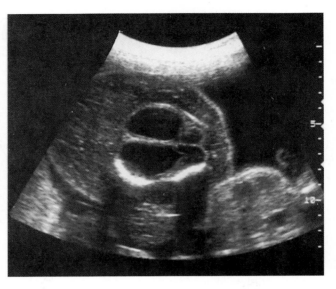

9. Which of the following conditions does this image **MOST** likely represent?
   A. Stuck twin syndrome
   B. Twin-to-twin transfusion syndrome
   C. A normal twin and a twin with intrauterine growth restriction (IUGR)
   D. An acardiac twin with a "pump" twin
   E. A rudimentary twin and a normal-sized twin

10. Which of the following conditions is seen in the brain of the more anterior twin?
    A. Alobar holoprosencephaly
    B. Hydranencephaly
    C. Severe ventriculomegaly
    D. Dandy-Walker syndrome

11. What other abnormality would you expect to find in the anterior fetus with the gross abnormality?
    A. Cystic hygroma
    B. Omphalocele
    C. Immobile legs
    D. Pleural effusion
    E. Polydactyly

12. What may happen to the posterior twin when this abnormality is present?
    A. Macrosomia may develop
    B. Hydrops may develop
    C. Intrauterine growth restriction (IUGR) may occur
    D. Fetal death is inevitable without treatment
    E. Oligohydramnios may develop around it

13. Which of the following muscles is longitudinally oriented and located in the midline of the anterior body wall?
    A. Piriformis muscle
    B. Levator ani muscle
    C. Rectus abdominis muscle
    D. Latissimus dorsi muscle
    E. Psoas major muscle

14. A monozygotic monochorionic monoamniotic pregnancy can result in
    A. fraternal twins
    B. identical twins in two sacs
    C. a singleton pregnancy
    D. an ectopic pregnancy
    E. stuck twins

15. The lecithin:sphingomyelin ratio is used to determine
    A. cardiac output
    B. fetal weight
    C. fetal malformations
    D. fetal lung maturity
    E. the presence of infection

16. All of the following conditions can cause dilation of the fallopian tube **EXCEPT**
    A. an ectopic pregnancy
    B. endometriosis
    C. pelvic inflammatory disease
    D. tubal ligation
    E. an endometrial polyp

Questions 17–20

Refer to the endovaginal sagittal and transverse views of the pelvis below:

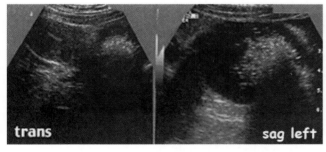

17. Endovaginal sagittal and transverse views of the pelvis are seen. What is visible?
    A. Solid mass on the left
    B. Left adnexal simple cyst
    C. Left ovarian cancer
    D. Left complex mass
    E. Loop of bowel on the left

18. Which of the following is the **MOST** likely cause of this mass?
    A. Dermoid cyst
    B. Ovarian cancer
    C. Ovarian cystadenoma
    D. Corpus luteum
    E. Dominant follicle

19. What alternative approach could be used to confirm the diagnosis?
    A. White blood cell count
    B. CT scan
    C. Percutaneous biopsy
    D. Dilation and evacuation
    E. Liver scan

20. Associated pathology is **MOST** likely to be found in the
    A. liver
    B. para-aortic nodes
    C. pancreas
    D. other ovary
    E. cul-de-sac

Questions 21 and 22

Refer to the image of a fetus below:

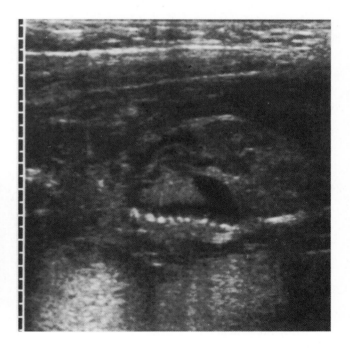

21. What is seen on this view of a fetus?
    A. Pleural effusion
    B. Pericardial effusion
    C. Mass in the fetal chest
    D. Spinal anomaly
    E. Placental mass

22. What is the **MOST** appropriate next step in the management of this fetus?
    A. Perform an amniocentesis for chromosomes
    B. Drain the fluid under ultrasound control
    C. Perform a triple screen blood test
    D. Repeat the sonogram in 4 weeks
    E. Perform the Wassermann test for syphilis

Questions 23–25

Refer to the abdominal circumference view of a fetus below:

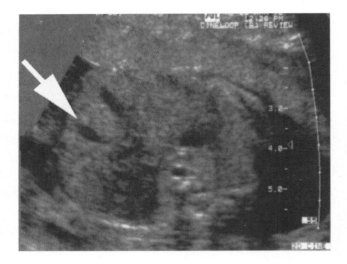

23. Which of the following organs is seen on this sonogram?
    A. Kidneys
    B. Lungs
    C. Spleen
    D. Heart
    E. Bladder

24. The white arrow is pointing to the
    A. umbilical vein
    B. right portal vein
    C. stomach
    D. right renal pelvis
    E. gallbladder

25. Which of the following is **MOST** responsible for the poor quality of this abdominal circumference view?
    A. The kidneys are seen, so the view was taken at too low a level
    B. A portion of lung is seen, so the view was taken at too high a level
    C. The view is oblique
    D. The heart is visible on the image

26. The phase of the endometrial cycle from days 14–28 is the
    A. menstrual phase
    B. proliferative phase
    C. secretory phase
    D. follicular phase
    E. luteal phase

27. Fetal death *in utero* that reveals overlapping of the calvarial bones is referred to as
    A. the lemon sign
    B. the banana sign
    C. Spalding's sign
    D. Murphy's sign
    E. Chiari sign

Questions 28 and 29

Refer to the sagittal endovaginal view of a uterus below:

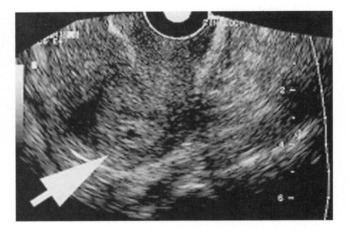

28. The arrow is pointing to
    A. an interstitial pregnancy
    B. a choriocarcinoma
    C. an intrauterine pregnancy
    D. an intracavitary fibroid
    E. an intracavitary bleed

29. Which of the following **BEST** accounts for the findings on this sonogram?
    A. A pregnancy at 3 weeks' gestation
    B. A pregnancy at 4.5 weeks' gestation
    C. A pregnancy at 8 weeks' gestation
    D. A missed abortion
    E. A 12-week blighted ovum

30. A patient at 32 weeks' gestation becomes pale and sweaty during the course of a prolonged obstetric sonogram. The patient is in the standard examination position. What should you do?
    A. Call a doctor and discontinue the examination
    B. Ask the patient to come back another day
    C. Ask the patient to walk around to get the fetus in another position
    D. Put the patient in the Trendelenburg position
    E. Turn the patient on her side

Questions 31 and 32

Refer to the transverse endovaginal view of two ovaries below:

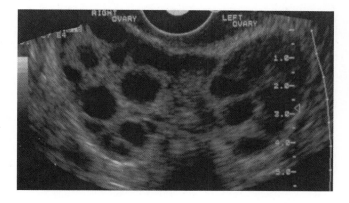

31. Which of the following associated findings might be present in the uterus of this patient?
    A. Endometrial polyp
    B. Endometrial cancer
    C. Hydatidiform mole
    D. Multiple fibroids
    E. Pyometra

32. Based on the findings on this image, which of the following blood tests should be performed?
    A. [alpha]–Fetoprotein level
    B. CA125 test
    C. Erythrocyte sedimentation rate
    D. White blood cell count
    E. Human chorionic gonadotropin level

Questions 33 and 34

Refer to the transverse image of a fetal abdomen below:

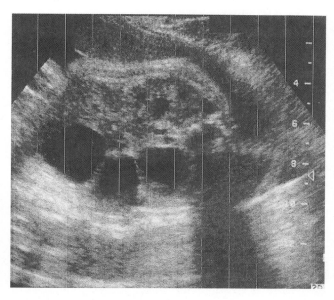

33. This fetal abdomen contains
    A. distended bowel
    B. a cystic tumor
    C. a dilated stomach and duodenum consistent with duodenal atresia
    D. a severely dilated kidney with ureteropelvic junction obstruction
    E. a multicystic, dysplastic kidney

34. Which of the following statements is **TRUE** regarding the mildly dilated renal pelvis seen on this image?
    A. It is unusual
    B. It suggests posterior urethral valves with consequent bilateral obstruction
    C. It is of no clinical significance
    D. It may be related to a ureteropelvic junction obstruction
    E. It is unlikely to be the result of reflux

35. Which of the following muscles is a hammock-like muscle that stretches between the pubis and coccyx and aids in holding the pelvic organs in place?
    A. Iliopsoas muscle
    B. Obturator internus muscle
    C. Piriformis muscle
    D. Levator ani muscle
    E. Psoas major muscle

36. Ovulation induction that leads to hyperstimulation can present with all of the following **EXCEPT**
    A. ascites
    B. hydronephrosis
    C. enlarged ovaries
    D. cervical canal thickening
    E. a pleural effusion

37. Delayed postpartum hemorrhage can be caused by all of the following **EXCEPT**
    A. retained products of conception
    B. placenta percreta
    C. a retained placenta
    D. cesarean incision hematoma
    E. endometritis

38. At what gestational age can the biparietal diameter first be measured?
    A. 10 weeks
    B. 12 weeks
    C. 16–18 weeks
    D. 20 weeks

Questions 39–41

These endovaginal sagittal views of the uterus were taken before and during a procedure. The consequences of the procedure can be seen on the image to the left:

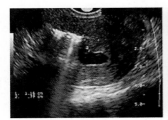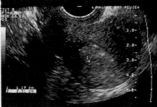

39. All of the following could explain the appearance of the endometrium on the image to the right **EXCEPT**
    A. endometrium in the secretory phase
    B. localized thickening of the endometrium
    C. an intracavitary mass
    D. a polyp
    E. endometrium in the proliferative phase

40. Which of the following procedures was performed?
    A. Hysterosonogram (saline infusion study)
    B. Dilation and curettage
    C. Cone biopsy
    D. Percutaneous biopsy
    E. Voiding cystogram

41. What does the procedure show (see the image above)?
    A. Calcification in the endometrium
    B. Shadowing from a metallic instrument in the endometrium
    C. Air trapped in front of a mass
    D. A polyp on a stalk
    E. A well-defined fibroid

42. All of the following statements describe the vagina **EXCEPT**
    A. it is 8–10 cm in length
    B. it is a collapsible muscular tube
    C. it extends from the external genitalia to the external os
    D. it may contain nabothian cysts
    E. Gartner's duct cysts lie anterior to it

Questions 43 and 44

Refer to the view of the fetal head below:

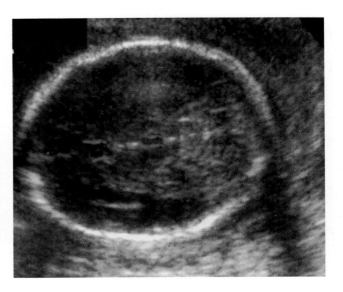

43. All of the following findings make this head circumference unsatisfactory for biparietal diameter and head circumference measurements **EXCEPT**
    A. presence of the cavum septum pellucidum
    B. presence of the cerebral peduncles
    C. presence of the cerebellar vermis
    D. absence of the thalamus

44. The shape of the skull is indicative of
    A. dolichocephaly
    B. frontal bossing
    C. a skull fracture
    D. brachycephaly
    E. a normal skull

Questions 45 and 46

A localized view of a portion of a 17-week-old fetus is shown below:

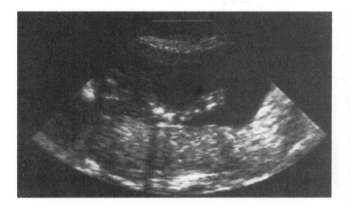

45. Which of the following anatomical structures is being examined?
    A. Ribs
    B. Face and skull
    C. arm
    D. Pelvis

46. Which of the following is the **MOST** likely diagnosis?
    A. Thanatophoric dwarfism
    B. Achondrogenesis
    C. Osteogenesis imperfecta
    D. Achondroplasia
    E. Diastrophic dwarfism

47. The classic symptoms of placental abruption include
    A. painless bleeding in the first trimester
    B. painless bleeding in the second trimester
    C. pain and bleeding in the third trimester
    D. painless bleeding in the third trimester
    E. pain and bleeding in the first trimester

48. Which of the following findings would **NOT** support the diagnosis of ectopic pregnancy?
    A. Fluid in the cul-de-sac
    B. A decidual reaction
    C. Local tenderness over the mass
    D. A pseudogestational sac
    E. An increased hematocrit level

49. Before a gynecologic sonogram, which of the following is **NOT** a standard practice in an outpatient clinic?
    A. Greeting the patient using her first name and taking her into the examination room
    B. Explaining the procedure to the patient
    C. Examining the patient requisition and chart for details of the case
    D. Explaining that the use of the endovaginal probe is standard practice and is usually painless
    E. Inserting the patient name and number onto the ultrasound system

Questions 50 and 51

Refer to the image of the endometrial cavity below:

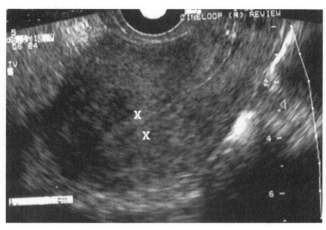

50. Based on the endometrial cavity shown, this patient is in what phase of the menstrual cycle?
    A. Menstruation
    B. Luteal phase
    C. Ovulation
    D. Proliferative phase

51. Assuming this patient's ovaries are normal, which of the following statements about her ovary at the time this image was obtained is **TRUE**?
    A. A dominant follicle is present
    B. A calcified corpus luteum is present
    C. Multiple small follicles are present
    D. There is no ovarian activity
    E. Several large follicles are present

Questions 52 and 53

Refer to the view of the fetus below:

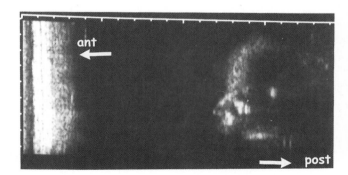

52. The amount of amniotic fluid present is
    A. less than normal
    B. normal
    C. slightly more than normal
    D. significantly more than normal

53. The portion of the fetus shown is a
    A. normal profile view
    B. profile view showing micrognathia
    C. chest view showing an anterior chest mass
    D. prone view showing a distorted spine

54. Which of the following is a reactive result for a non-stress test?
    A. A maternal heart rate of 65–70 bpm after a 10-minute walk on a treadmill
    B. At least one 2-cm pocket of amniotic fluid
    C. A consistent fetal heart rate for the duration of the examination
    D. Two or more fetal heart rate accelerations in 20 minutes
    E. Sustained fetal breathing

Questions 55–57

Refer to the transabdominal sagittal view of the pelvis below:

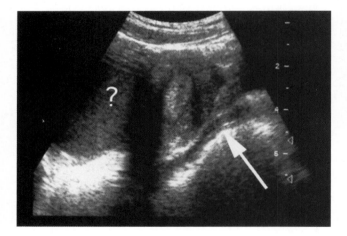

55. The arrow is pointing to
    A. a ureter
    B. the rectum
    C. the vagina
    D. a loop of bowel
    E. the sacrum

56. Which of the following is the **MOST** likely explanation for the area indicated by the question mark?
    A. Large fibroid
    B. Large simple cyst
    C. Endometrioma
    D. Echogenic amniotic fluid
    E. Fluid-filled bowel

57. Which of the following techniques would **NOT** be helpful in confirming the diagnosis?
    A. Using an endovaginal probe
    B. Filling the bladder
    C. Observing the contents of the mass for movement when the maternal abdomen is manually compressed
    D. Using color flow
    E. Changing the transducer frequency

Questions 58–60

Refer to the view of a fetal face below:

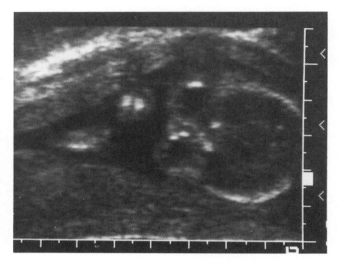

58. What abnormality does this view show?
    A. Hypertelorism
    B. Cleft lip
    C. Hypotelorism
    D. Micrognathia
    E. Proboscis

59. What measurement is useful in the diagnosis of this abnormality?
    A. Interocular distance
    B. Ocular measurement
    C. Binocular distance
    D. Nasal length
    E. Lens distance

60. What other structure should be examined in detail?
    A. Kidneys
    B. Stomach
    C. Brain
    D. Limbs
    E. Liver

61. The type of intrauterine growth retardation (IUGR) in which the head grows at a normal rate but the abdomen does not is
    A. symmetrical IUGR
    B. asymmetrical IUGR
    C. femur-sparing IUGR
    D. none of the above

62. Bilateral partial agenesis of the genitourinary system in a 13 year old is **MOST** likely to cause
    A. a septate uterus
    B. uterus didelphys
    C. uterine aplasia
    D. a bicornuate uterus
    E. a T-shaped uterus

63. The outer walls of the blastocyst are covered by
    A. decidua
    B. chorionic villi
    C. decidua capsularis
    D. mesoderm
    E. ectoderm

Question 64

Refer to the view of a fetus below:

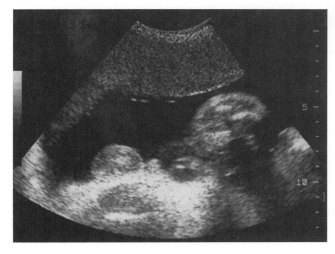

64. Which of the following structures is seen on this sonogram?
    A. Extremity mass
    B. Male genitalia
    C. Female genitalia
    D. Chorioangioma
    E. Facial mass

Question 65

Refer to the image of a twin pregnancy below:

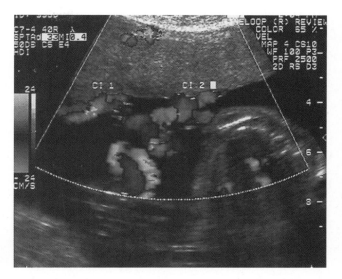

65. Which of the following is seen on this sonogram?
    A. Two-vessel cord
    B. Very long cord
    C. Cord entanglement
    D. Cord knot
    E. Vasa previa

66. Ovarian cancer will **MOST** likely metastasize to the
    A. kidneys
    B. liver
    C. breasts
    D. brain
    E. colon

Questions 67 and 68

An image of a small-for-dates fetus is shown below:

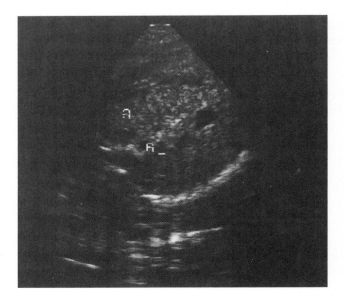

67. What is demonstrated on this image?
    A. Placentomegaly
    B. Cervical incompetence
    C. Two-vessel cord
    D. Anhydramnios
    E. Rudimentary twin

68. The letter "A" represents
    A. a double aorta
    B. normally placed adrenal glands
    C. the appendices
    D. absence of the kidneys
    E. laterally displaced adrenal glands

Question 69

Refer to the transverse view of the pelvis below:

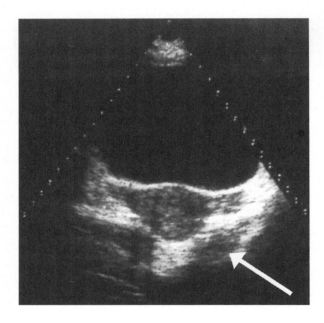

69. The arrow is pointing to
    A. the left ovary
    B. a hydrosalpinx
    C. a rectal neoplasm
    D. the piriformis muscle
    E. the sacrum

70. Which of the following pelvic muscles cannot be seen with ultrasound?
    A. Obturator internus muscle
    B. Psoas muscle
    C. Iliacus muscle
    D. Levator ani muscle
    E. Piriformis muscle

Questions 71 and 72

Refer to the view of the fetal pelvis below:

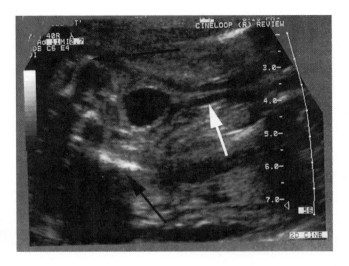

71. The white arrow is pointing to
    A. a small bowel loop
    B. a dilated ureter
    C. the aortic bifurcation
    D. an umbilical artery
    E. the psoas muscle

72. The black arrow is pointing to which of the following structures?
    A. Lumbar spine
    B. Femoral head
    C. Pubic symphysis
    D. Iliac crest
    E. Osteochondroses

73. A second trimester fetal ultrasound is ordered secondary to a rapidly increasing fundal height. Polyhydramnios is found on the ultrasound, as well as a femoral length that falls in the 5th percentile. Which of the following measurements would **NOT** be helpful in this case?
    A. Chest:abdomen ratio
    B. Head:abdomen ratio
    C. Renal length
    D. Humerus length
    E. Fibula length

74. The lateral ventricular width in the fetus should be measured using
    A. an axial view close to the posterior end of the choroid plexus in the atrium of the ventricle
    B. a coronal view of the anterior horn of the ventricle
    C. a sagittal view of the temporal horn of the ventricle
    D. an axial view of the anterior horn of the ventricle
    E. a coronal view of the head showing the largest portion of the body of the ventricle

Questions 75 and 76

Refer to the coronal view of a fetal brain below:

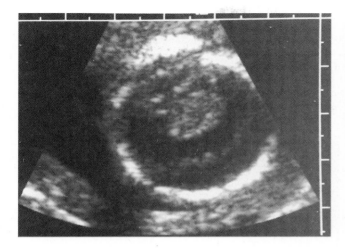

75. Which of the following structures is seen on this image?
    A. Normal thalamus
    B. Normal third ventricle
    C. Two lateral ventricles
    D. Fused thalamus
    E. Cavum septum pellucidum

76. Which of the following entities is often associated with the abnormality seen on this image?
    A. Omphalocele
    B. Gastroschisis
    C. Ureteropelvic junction obstruction
    D. Cataract
    E. Short femur

77. In GIFT procedures, conception occurs in
    A. a test tube
    B. the uterus
    C. a surrogate
    D. the ovary
    E. the fallopian tube

Question 78

Refer to the obstetric sonogram below:

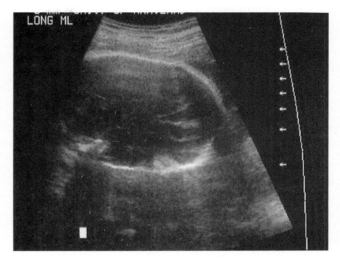

78. This view of a fetal cranium shows
    A. two small, calcified intracranial tumors
    B. evidence of cytomegalic inclusion disease
    C. changes compatible with toxoplasmosis
    D. the petrous and sphenoid ridges
    E. *in utero* fracture of the skull

Questions 79–82

Refer to the transverse image of the fetal abdomen below:

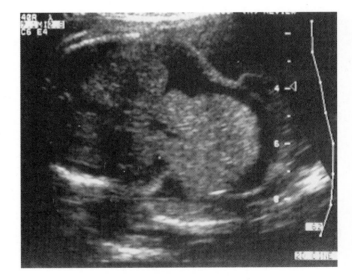

79. This view of the fetal abdomen shows
    A. gastroschisis
    B. bladder extrophy
    C. limb/body wall complex
    D. an omphalocele
    E. pentalogy of Cantrell

80. Which of the following are in the abdominal wall defect?
    A. Liver, ascites, and gut
    B. Liver and gut
    C. Gut and ascites
    D. Liver and ascites
    E. Liver, ascites, and stomach

81. Based on the contents of this abdominal wall defect, the chance of a chromosomal anomaly is
    A. 0%
    B. 20%
    C. 60%
    D. 80%
    E. 100%

82. What other organ is **MOST** likely to show anomalies in association with this defect?
    A. Kidneys
    B. Brain
    C. Heart
    D. Digits
    E. Lungs

83. A single cyst seen outside of the ovary in the adnexa is **MOST** likely a
    A. follicular cyst
    B. corpus lutein cyst
    C. serous cystadenoma
    D. paraovarian cyst
    E. nabothian cyst

84. Which of the following is **NOT** a characteristic of monochorionic monoamniotic twins?
    A. Late division occurs at 7–13 days
    B. There is a shared amniotic and chorionic sac
    C. There are four membranes in the intersac septum
    D. It is a rare occurrence
    E. It raises the risk of perinatal mortality

85. The potential space between the posterior bladder wall and the fundus of the uterus is the
    A. fornix
    B. space of Retzius
    C. pouch of Douglas
    D. anterior cul-de-sac
    E. posterior cul-de-sac

86. The **LEAST** accurate measurement in the estimation of gestational age of a dolichocephalic fetus is
    A. cephalic index
    B. biparietal diameter
    C. head circumference
    D. intraocular distance
    E. transcerebellar diameter

87. In a hypoxic fetus, the last parameter to decline in the biophysical profile is
    A. amniotic fluid volume
    B. fetal heart rate
    C. fetal breathing
    D. fetal movement
    E. fetal tone

Questions 88–90

Refer to the endovaginal sagittal view of the pelvis in a 60-year-old woman below:

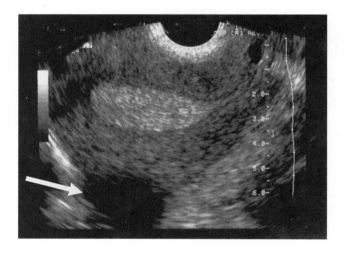

88. Regarding the endometrial echoes, it is **MOST** likely that
    A. this is a normal secretory phase of the menstrual cycle
    B. an intracavitary polyp is present
    C. benign endometrial hyperplasia is present
    D. endometrial cancer is present
    E. an intracavitary fibroid is present

89. Which of the following is the **MOST** likely explanation for the black area indicated by the arrow?
    A. Ascitic fluid
    B. Ovarian cyst
    C. Dermoid
    D. Degenerating fibroid
    E. Uterine cancer

90. To determine the origin of the black area indicated by the arrow, all of the following techniques would be of value **EXCEPT**
    A. trying to go between the mass and the uterus with the endovaginal probe
    B. using color flow to see if vessels in the uterus connect to the mass
    C. using the transrectal probe to get another angle on the interface between the uterus and the mass
    D. pushing on the abdomen manually to see if the mass changes position relative to the uterus
    E. using MRI

Questions 91–93

Refer to the transabdominal transverse view of the uterus below:

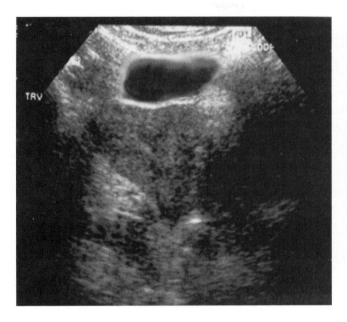

91. Which of the following is present on this image?
    A. Uterine fibroid
    B. Intrauterine pregnancy
    C. Uterus didelphys
    D. Subseptate uterus
    E. Bicornuate uterus

92. This patient would **MOST** likely present with
    A. vaginal bleeding
    B. pelvic pain
    C. repeated miscarriages
    D. vaginal discharge
    E. an inability to get pregnant

93. The sonographer should also scan the
    A. pancreas
    B. liver
    C. para-aortic nodes
    D. kidneys
    E. adrenal glands

Questions 94 and 95

A patient with a history of multiple abdominal and pelvic operations presents for a pelvic sonogram. A transverse view through her pelvis is shown below (Ut = uterus):

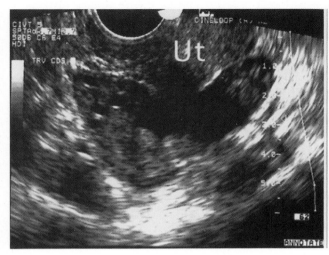

94. Which of the following entities is present on this image?
    A. Ovarian cyst
    B. Dermoid
    C. Dilated bowel
    D. Fluid in the cul-de-sac
    E. Dilated ureter

95. All of the following symptoms are related to the sonographic findings **EXCEPT**
    A. infertility
    B. chronic lower abdominal pain
    C. pain on intercourse
    D. constipation
    E. metromenorrhagia

96. Most gynecologic neoplasms occur
    A. before puberty
    B. during puberty
    C. during menopause
    D. after menopause
    E. during the childbearing years

97. Which of the following techniques **BEST** shows a two-vessel cord?
    A. Transverse view of the cord using pulsed Doppler
    B. Transverse oblique color flow view of the bladder showing the one artery alongside
    C. Cord insertion view
    D. Transverse view of the cord using color flow

Questions 98 and 99

Refer to the combined image of the ovary and an associated Doppler pattern below:

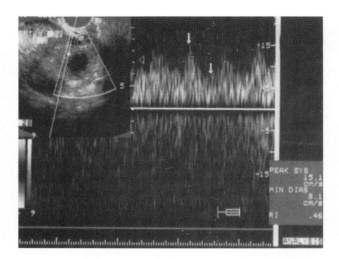

98. Judging from the Doppler pattern, this patient is **MOST** likely in which of the following phases of the menstrual cycle?
    A. Secretory phase
    B. Proliferative phase
    C. Follicular phase
    D. Menstruation
    E. Three-line phase

99. The structure in the ovary is **MOST** likely
    A. a follicle
    B. a cystadenoma
    C. ovarian cancer
    D. a corpus luteum
    E. a dermoid

Questions 100 and 101

Refer to the transverse view through a fetal chest below:

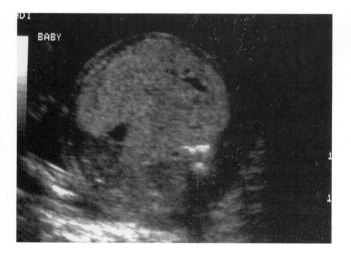

100. Which of the following is seen on this image?
    A. Large hemothorax
    B. Teratoma of the lung
    C. Large cystic adenomatoid malformation of the lung
    D. Rhabdomyoma of the heart

101. Based on the abnormal finding on this image, what complication should be sought?
    A. Oligohydramnios
    B. Placental atrophy
    C. Hydrops
    D. Vein of Galen malformation
    E. Nuchal thickening

102. All of the following are unsatisfactory sites for intrauterine contraceptive devices **EXCEPT**
    A. at the cornu
    B. partially in the myometrium
    C. at the cervix
    D. at the fundus of the uterus
    E. in the body of the uterus

Questions 103 and 104

Refer to the image of a fetal cranium below:

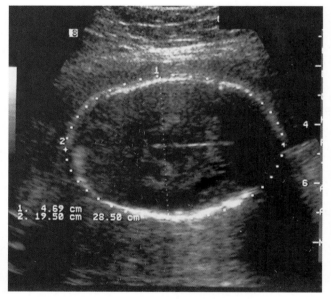

103. Which of the following measurement techniques would you use to quantify the abnormality on this sonogram?
    A. Biparietal diameter
    B. Head circumference
    C. Intraorbital distance
    D. Cephalic index
    E. Ventricular width

104. The abnormality seen on this sonogram is associated with
    A. polyhydramnios
    B. lethal dwarfism
    C. breech presentation
    D. undue transducer pressure
    E. osteogenesis imperfecta

Questions 105 and 106

Refer to the sagittal view of the pregnant uterus shown below:

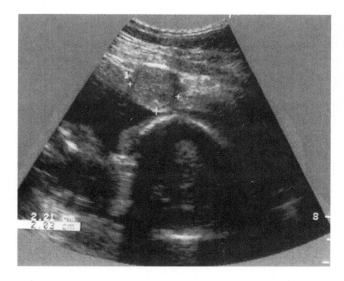

105. What is being measured on this image?
    A. Myometrial contraction
    B. Fetal arm width
    C. Cesarean section incision scar
    D. Fibroid
    E. Cervical width

106. Which of the following complications is **NOT** associated with this finding in a pregnant woman?
    A. Difficulty clinically dating the pregnancy because the pregnancy feels larger than it is by dates
    B. Prolonged labor due to incoordinate contractions
    C. Pain if "red degeneration" occurs
    D. Obstruction of delivery with a large cervical mass
    E. Early placental maturation

Questions 107 and 108

Refer to the transverse view of a female pelvis below:

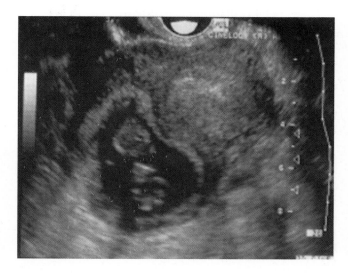

107. Which of the following is the **MOST** likely diagnosis?
    A. Normal intrauterine pregnancy
    B. Eight-week pregnancy with an intrasac bleed
    C. Interstitial pregnancy
    D. Bicornuate pregnancy
    E. Eight-week pregnancy with a fibroid

108. What findings in association with this type of pregnancy would compel immediate surgery?
    A. High diastolic flow on Doppler
    B. Adnexal ring sign
    C. Extrauterine adnexal mass
    D. High [beta]-human chorionic gonadotropin level
    E. Free fluid with internal echoes in the cul-de-sac

109. Ultrasound is performed before chorionic villi sampling to determine all of the following **EXCEPT**
    A. that the fetus is alive
    B. the date of the pregnancy
    C. the fetal number
    D. the position of the placenta
    E. the status of fetal breathing

110. A cesarean section was performed on a 29-year-old postdates patient. After the procedure, the patient developed a low-grade fever and leukocytosis. The differential diagnosis includes all of the following **EXCEPT**
    A. a hematoma
    B. an infected hematoma
    C. jaundice
    D. an abscess
    E. a wound infection

111. All of the following conditions cause fixation of the pelvic structures so that they do not move when examined with the vaginal probe **EXCEPT**
    A. metastases
    B. pelvic inflammatory disease
    C. endometriosis
    D. pelvic surgery
    E. dermoids

Questions 112 and 113

Refer to the transverse endovaginal view of the right adnexa below:

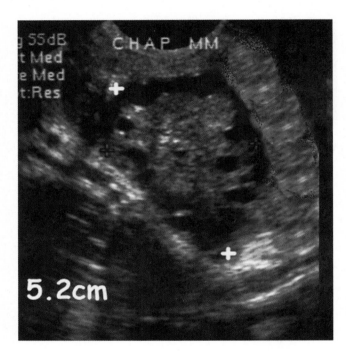

112. Which of the following findings is present on this image?
    A. Dermoid
    B. Dominant follicle
    C. Ovarian neoplasm
    D. Polycystic ovary syndrome
    E. Pelvic inflammatory disease

113. Which of the following symptoms is typical of this condition?
    A. Vaginal discharge
    B. Pelvic pain
    C. Infrequent, light periods
    D. Anorexia nervosa
    E. Diarrhea

114. Which of the following is helpful in the treatment of stuck twin syndrome?
    A. Prolonged bed rest
    B. Placing the mother in the left-side-down position
    C. Removing fluid from the amniotic sac around the larger twin
    D. A high-protein diet
    E. Early delivery when the condition is first seen

Questions 115 and 116

Refer to the transverse and sagittal views of the pelvis in an elderly woman below (Ut = uterus):

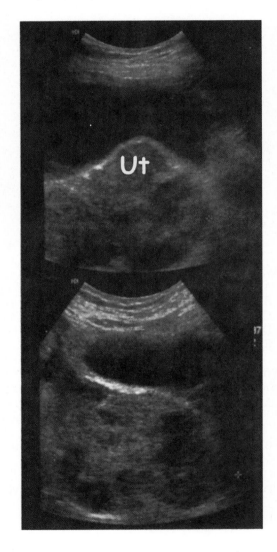

115. In addition to the pelvis, scanning this patient should include all of the following **EXCEPT**
    A. the kidneys
    B. the liver
    C. the para-aortic nodes
    D. the peritoneum
    E. the gallbladder

116. An endovaginal examination would be **MOST** valuable for determining if
    A. the mass is mobile
    B. there is gut involvement
    C. the ovaries are part of the mass
    D. there is hydronephrosis
    E. the para-aortic nodes are involved

Question 117

Refer to the lateral view of a fetal foot below:

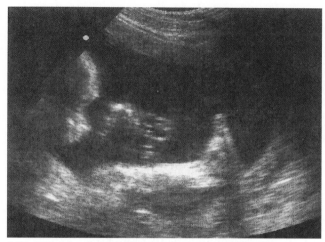

117. Which of the following is seen on this image?
    A. Rocker-bottom foot
    B. Clubfoot
    C. A normal foot
    D. A foot affected by lethal dwarfism
    E. Polyhydramnios

Question 118

Refer to the transverse view of the left adnexa below:

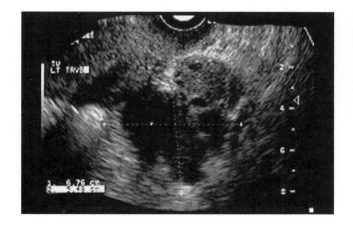

118. The measured structure is **MOST** likely
    A. an ovarian cystadenoma
    B. a dermoid
    C. a dominant follicle
    D. hydrosalpinx
    E. a cystic fibroid

119. A 6-day-old infant presents for a pelvic sonogram. The parents are distraught because they have been told that the baby has ambiguous genitalia. The sonogram is ordered to
    A. define internal anatomy
    B. confirm hermaphroditism
    C. confirm labioscrotal fusion
    D. confirm micropenis
    E. confirm clitoral hypertrophy

120. The muscle that lines the side wall of the pelvis is the
    A. levator ani muscle
    B. obturator internus muscle
    C. iliopsoas muscle
    D. rectus abdominis muscle
    E. latissimus dorsi muscle

Questions 121 and 122

Refer to the image of a fetal head below:

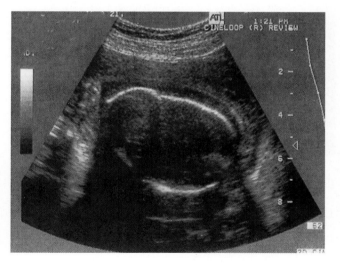

121. What is the **MOST** likely cause of the skull changes seen on this image?
    A. Thanatophoric dwarfism
    B. Osteogenesis imperfecta
    C. Diabetes mellitus
    D. Hydrops
    E. Fetal death

122. Which of the following abnormalities would **NOT** be helpful in supporting the diagnosis?
    A. Absence of fetal heart motion on M-mode
    B. Crunched up fetal shape
    C. Amniotic fluid echoes
    D. Loss of visualization of internal fetal structures
    E. Increased resistance in the umbilical cord on Doppler

123. Visualization of which of the following structures in the fetal brain indicates that the level is too low for an accurate measurement of the biparietal diameter?
    A. Interhemispheric fissure
    B. Cavum septum pellucidum
    C. Cerebral peduncles
    D. Choroid plexus
    E. Temporal horns of the lateral ventricle

Questions 124 and 125

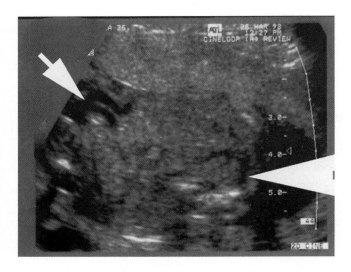

Refer to the transverse view of the fetal abdomen below:

124. The arrowhead is pointing to
    A. the kidneys
    B. the adrenal glands
    C. the psoas muscle
    D. a mesoblastic nephroma
    E. the colon

125. The arrow is pointing to
    A. the cord insertion
    B. an allantoic cyst
    C. the portal vein
    D. an omphalocele
    E. gastroschisis

Questions 126 and 127

Refer to the obstetric sonogram below:

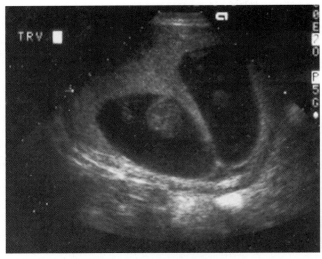

126. What does this image show?
    A. Monochorionic monoamniotic twins
    B. Monochorionic diamniotic twins
    C. Dichorionic diamniotic twins
    D. Singleton pregnancy with a large perisac bleed
    E. Twins with fetal death in one sac

127. This diagnosis is **BEST** confirmed by
    A. counting the components of the membrane
    B. finding the twin peak sign
    C. identifying different fetal genitalia
    D. evaluating during the first trimester
    E. identifying two placentas

Question 128

Refer to the two transverse views of the pelvis in the same patient, one with color flow and one without, below:

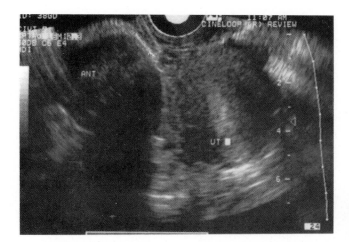

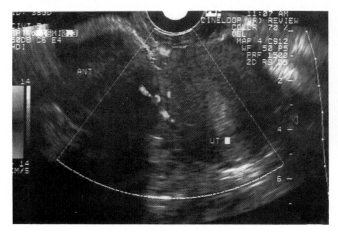

128. What additional information does color flow provide about the pelvic mass?
   A. The mass is malignant
   B. There is increased vascularity, indicating infection
   C. Vessels extend from the uterus to the mass, indicating a fibroid
   D. The color flow pattern confirms an endometrioma

129. Which of the following is the **MOST** reliable indicator of a poor fetal prognosis in the first trimester?
   A. Large yolk sac
   B. One-week fetal growth delay
   C. Fetal heart rate of 50
   D. Perisac bleed
   E. Minimal fetal limb movement

130. An asymptomatic patient at 18 weeks' gestation presents for a sonogram. A placenta previa is seen overlapping the internal os by 3 cm. Which of the following statements is **TRUE**?
   A. The placenta will most likely move toward the fundus within the next 6–8 weeks
   B. The patient should be put on bed rest until delivery
   C. A cesarean section should be performed
   D. Vaginal bleeding will occur over the remainder of the pregnancy
   E. This is a normal variant

Questions 131–134

Refer to the transverse view of the left adnexa below:

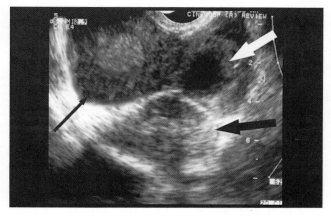

131. Which of the following structures is marked by the thick black arrow?
   A. Posterior fibroid
   B. Left ovarian process
   C. Pelvic kidney
   D. Ovarian cancer
   E. Endometrioma

132. The endometrial echoes on this image are
   A. normal for the proliferative phase
   B. consistent with atrophy
   C. much thicker than normal
   D. normal for the secretory phase

133. The thin black arrow points to the uterus. What might such an endometrial appearance signify?
   A. An intracavitary fibroid
   B. A decidual reaction related to ectopic pregnancy
   C. Heavy menstruation
   D. An intrauterine contraceptive device
   E. Normal proliferative endometrium

134. The white arrow points to left adnexal pathology. This structure appears to be outside of the ovary. Which of the following maneuvers could be used to discover the nature of the structure?
    A. Pushing against it with the endovaginal probe to see if it is tender
    B. Using a water enema
    C. Filling the bladder and looking at the structure on a transabdominal view
    D. Using color flow to see vascularity
    E. Using an endovaginal probe to look for heart motion

135. Which of the following structures is **NOT** seen when measuring the abdominal circumference at the proper level?
    A. Umbilical artery
    B. Aorta
    C. Stomach
    D. Fetal adrenal glands
    E. Transverse spine

Question 136

Refer to the profile view below:

136. Which of the following statements about this image is **TRUE**?
    A. It is technically unsatisfactory
    B. It shows micrognathia
    C. It shows frontal bossing
    D. It shows a proboscis
    E. It is normal

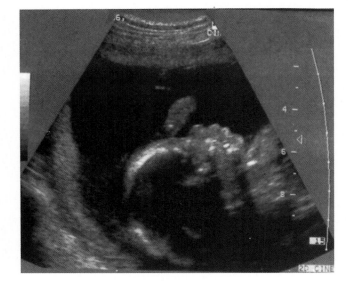

Questions 137 and 138

Refer to the transverse view of a fetal trunk below:

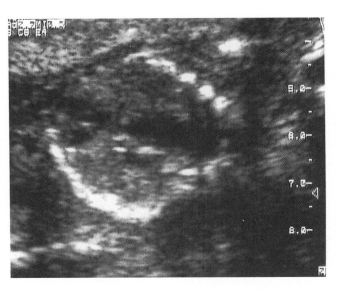

137. What does this image show?
    A. A type III cystic adenomatoid malformation of the lung
    B. Teratoma of the lung
    C. A diaphragmatic hernia
    D. A vascular malformation
    E. Situs inversus

138. What additional finding would support this diagnosis?
    A. No stomach on a view of the abdomen
    B. A large fetal abdomen
    C. A cardiac abnormality
    D. A dilated large bowel

139. All of the following statements describe hydrosalpinx **EXCEPT**
    A. hypoechoic with shadowing artifact
    B. anechoic and tubular
    C. multiple tubular, anechoic adnexal structures
    D. easily mistaken for a dilated ureter
    E. extraovarian cystic process

140. Demise of a twin in the second trimester with maceration is called
    A. a vanishing twin
    B. a fetus papyraceous
    C. an acardiac twin
    D. twin-to-twin transfusion syndrome
    E. a conjoined twin

141. All of the following may result in an inaccurate biophysical profile score **EXCEPT**
    A. fasting state of the mother
    B. an overactive fetus
    C. a resting fetus
    D. fetal hiccups
    E. premature rupture of membranes

Questions 142 and 143

A 17-year-old girl presents with intermittent lower abdominal pain. An endovaginal sagittal view of her uterus is shown below:

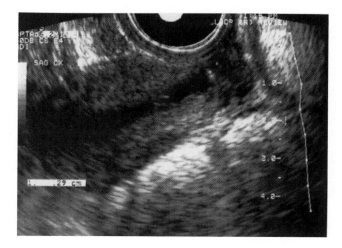

142. Which of the following histories is **MOST** likely in this patient?
    A. Pelvic inflammatory disease
    B. Amenorrhea
    C. Vaginal discharge
    D. Sexual assault
    E. Positive pregnancy test

143. The obstruction is located at the
    A. hymen
    B. middle of the uterus
    C. external os
    D. internal os
    E. transverse vaginal septum

Question 144

Refer to the view of an early pregnancy below:

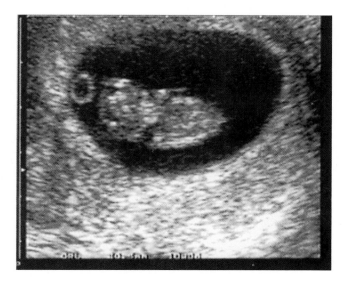

144. This image shows
    A. a fetal halo
    B. an intrasac bleed
    C. a normal yolk sac
    D. a large yolk sac
    E. nuchal edema

145. In a postmenopausal patient with vaginal bleeding, what is the advantage of finding an endometrial cavity less than 5 mm thick?
    A. No fibroids are present
    B. An ovarian mass can be excluded
    C. Endometrial atrophy is present
    D. Endometrial cancer cannot be present
    E. A polyp cannot be present

Question 146

Refer to the image of a fetal thorax below:

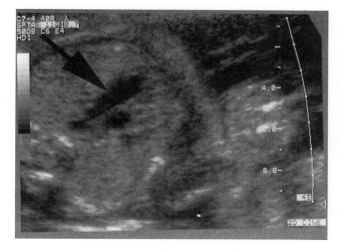

146. The arrow is pointing to the
    A. left ventricular outflow tract
    B. right ventricular outflow tract
    C. left ventricle
    D. right ventricle
    E. transverse aortic arch

147. A third trimester sonogram revealing polyhydramnios and macrosomia should raise the question of
    A. preeclampsia
    B. maternal hypertension
    C. placental insufficiency
    D. maternal diabetes
    E. fetal hypertension

148. Which of the following techniques is **MOST** accurate for measuring femoral length in a second trimester fetus?
    A. Measure the lateral surface of the femur that lies in the far field
    B. Use a sector scanner, being sure to scan at right angles to the shaft of the bone
    C. Measure the femoral shaft from the distal epiphysis to the femoral head
    D. Measure the medial surface of the femur in the near field, perpendicular to the ultrasound beam

Questions 149 and 150

Refer to the transverse view of the fetal trunk below:

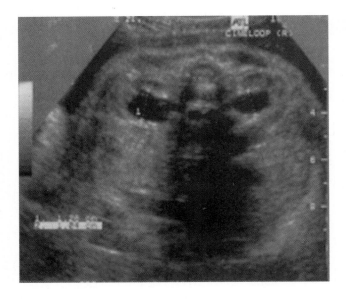

149. The two measured structures represent
    A. loops of distended small bowel
    B. loops of distended large bowel
    C. bilateral ovarian cysts
    D. bilateral distended renal pelves
    E. the gallbladder and the stomach

150. Which of the following does **NOT** require a detailed assessment?
    A. The gender of the fetus
    B. The echogenicity of the renal parenchyma
    C. The ureters for possible dilation
    D. The bladder for possible enlargement
    E. The liver

Questions 151–153

Refer to the adjacent sagittal image, of the uterus below:

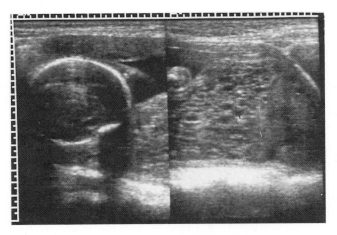

151. The appearances on this image are **MOST** consistent with
    A. a placental infarct
    B. diabetes mellitus
    C. an intraplacental bleed
    D. TORCH infection
    E. a partial mole

152. Which of the following investigations should be performed next?
    A. Amniocentesis
    B. Urinary [beta]-human chorionic gonadotropin levels
    C. Serum [alpha]-fetoprotein analysis
    D. Dilation and curettage
    E. Serum estriol levels

153. What adnexal finding is often associated with this entity?
    A. Corpus luteum cysts
    B. Follicular cysts
    C. Thecalutein cysts
    D. Endometrioma
    E. Hydrosalpinx

Questions 154 and 155

Refer to the transverse view of the left adnexa with the uterus (not seen on this image) to the left:

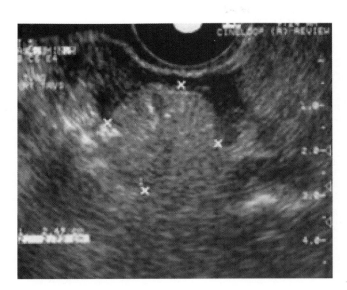

Questions 157–162

Refer to the diagram below:

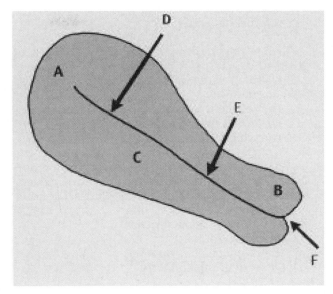

154. Which of the following is the **MOST** likely explanation for the structure being measured?
    A. Pedunculated fibroid
    B. Bowel mass
    C. Ovarian dermoid
    D. Endometrioma
    E. Peritoneal inclusion cyst

155. Which of the following is **NOT** a sonographic appearance associated with the entity seen on this image?
    A. An echo-free cyst
    B. A cyst containing areas of shadowing
    C. A cyst with multiple thick septa
    D. A mass with echogenic material on the anterior aspect forming a fluid level
    E. A hypoechoic, solid mass

156. Which of the following chart segments is **NOT** relevant to a gynecologic sonogram performed on a 70-year-old woman?
    A. History of abdominal surgery
    B. Date of her last normal menstrual period
    C. History of tuberculosis and diabetes mellitus
    D. Complaints of abdominal pain
    E. History of vaginal bleeding

157. The letter "A" represents the
    A. fundus
    B. cervix
    C. corpus
    D. internal os
    E. external os

158. The letter "B" represents the
    A. cervix
    B. corpus
    C. internal os
    D. external os
    E. endometrium

159. The letter "C" represents the
    A. fundus
    B. cervix
    C. corpus
    D. internal os
    E. external os

160. The letter "D" represents the
    A. fundus
    B. corpus
    C. internal os
    D. external os
    E. endometrium

161. The letter "E" represents the
    A. fundus
    B. cervix
    C. corpus
    D. internal os
    E. external os

162. The letter "F" represents the
    A. fundus
    B. cervix
    C. corpus
    D. internal os
    E. external os

163. Which of the following is **NOT** a characteristic of twin-to-twin transfusion syndrome?
    A. There are large intraplacental arterial-arterial anastamoses
    B. The recipient twin is large and edematous
    C. The donor twin is small and anemic
    D. The recipient twin is small

164. A 7-year-old girl presents for a pelvic sonogram. She has developed breasts and pubic and axillary hair. Which of the following **BEST** describes her condition?
    A. Adult sexual characteristics
    B. Precocious puberty
    C. Pseudoprecocious puberty
    D. Onset of normal puberty

165. Nabothian cysts
    A. cause repeated miscarriages
    B. are part of pelvic inflammatory disease
    C. are a normal variant finding
    D. become larger during the menstrual cycle
    E. are painful during intercourse

166. Which of the following does **NOT** cause fluid in the endometrial cavity?
    A. Radiation to cervical cancer
    B. Imperforate hymen
    C. Menstruation
    D. Hysterosonogram
    E. Bicornuate uterus

Questions 167 and 168

Refer to the image of the fetus below:

167. Which of the following abnormalities is seen on this image?

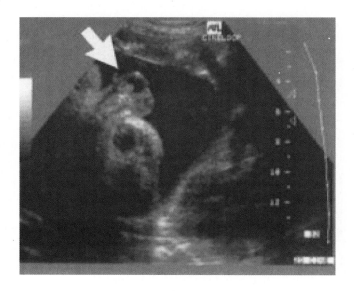

    A. Abnormal nasal mass
    B. Hypertelorism
    C. Small hydrocele
    D. Mass at the cord insertion

168. Based on the abnormal finding, which of the following statements is **TRUE**?
    A. Fetal hydrops will always be present also
    B. There will be atrophy of the testicle after birth
    C. This finding is a common normal variant
    D. This finding is associated with an undescended testicle
    E. The processus vaginalis has fused prematurely

Questions 169 and 170

Refer to the sagittal image of the fetus below (Bl = bladder):

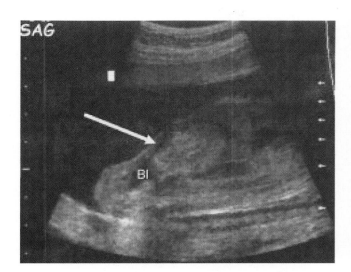

169. The structure indicated by the arrow is **MOST** likely
    A. a urachal remnant
    B. dilated small bowel
    C. an umbilical artery
    D. a vascular malformation
    E. the border of an abdominal mass

170. What additional technique would be **MOST** useful in confirming the nature of this structure?
    A. Coronal view
    B. Transverse view
    C. Color flow analysis
    D. Harmonics analysis
    E. Repeat sonogram after an interval to see changes in bladder size

171. All of the following are sonographic features of agenesis of the corpus callosum **EXCEPT**
    A. colpocephaly
    B. vertically aligned gyri
    C. a high-riding third ventricle
    D. a third ventricle cyst
    E. cerebellar hypoplasia

172. Curvilinear structures seen in the gestational sac in the first trimester include all of the following **EXCEPT**
    A. the amniotic membrane
    B. the vitelline duct
    C. the yolk sac
    D. a nuchal line less than 3 mm thick
    E. the chorionic membrane

Questions 173 and 174

Refer to the transverse view of a heart below:

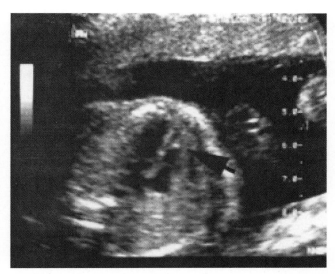

173. The arrow is pointing to
    A. Ebstein's anomaly
    B. coarctation of the aorta
    C. an echogenic focus in the heart
    D. an abnormal tricuspid valve

174. Based on the finding on this image, a special effort should be made to detect findings associated with
    A. osteogenesis imperfecta
    B. trisomy 21
    C. Arnold-Chiari II malformation
    D. an omphalocele
    E. renal anomalies

Question 175

Endovaginal views on the left were obtained from a 28-year-old, sexually active patient with pelvic pain. The images are shown below:

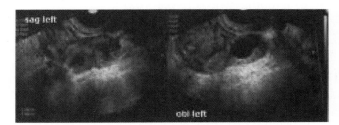

175. Which of the following components of this patient's history is **MOST** important in arriving at a diagnosis?
    A. The date of her last pregnancy
    B. Her history of stillborn children
    C. The date of her last period
    D. The characteristics of her periods
    E. A history of pain with intercourse

176. Follicle-stimulating hormone and luteinizing hormone are produced by
    A. the ovaries
    B. graafian follicles
    C. the corpus albicans
    D. the anterior lobe of the pituitary gland
    E. proliferation of the endometrial lining

Question 177

Refer to the fetal head below:

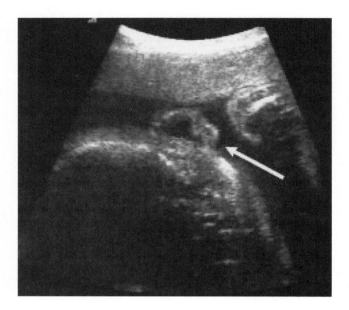

177. The structure indicated by the arrow represents
    A. an encephalocele
    B. a normal nose
    C. a fetal limb
    D. a fetal ear
    E. a cranial tumor

178. Which of the following pregnancies is **NOT** at risk for intrauterine growth restriction?
    A. A mother who eats a steady diet of fast food
    B. A mother who is 15 years old
    C. A mother who is a 40-year-old vegan
    D. A pregnancy with a two-vessel cord
    E. A mother who lives 10,000 feet above sea level

179. An infertile patient with a 28-day cycle is monitored with ultrasound to determine the ideal time of conception. On day 18 of her cycle, a single echo-free cyst measuring 3.5 cm is found in her right ovary. Which of the following conclusions can be drawn?
    A. Intercourse should be expeditiously performed
    B. A corpus luteum has developed
    C. An endometrioma has developed
    D. A luteinized, unruptured follicle is present
    E. An intraovarian pregnancy is developing

Questions 180 and 181

Two sonograms were taken approximately 5 minutes apart using an endovaginal probe. The results are shown below:

180. The two sonograms show
    A. posterior placenta previa
    B. cervical incompetence
    C. premature labor
    D. premature labor or cervical incompetence
    E. bleed adjacent to the cervix

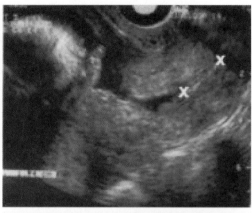

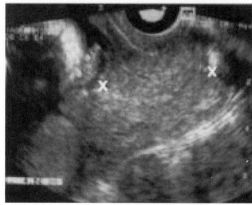

181. What pathologic condition is present on the lower image?
    A. Abruptio placenta
    B. Total placenta previa
    C. Partial placenta previa
    D. Placental infarct
    E. A low-lying placenta

Questions 182 and 183

Refer to the transabdominal sagittal view of the uterus below:

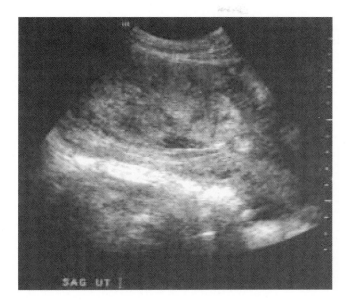

182. Which of the following is the **MOST** likely diagnosis?
    A. Multiple fibroids
    B. Hematocolpos
    C. Adenomyosis
    D. Choriocarcinoma
    E. Partial mole

183. Where else would sonographically visible complications arise with this process?
    A. Kidneys
    B. Liver
    C. Para-aortic nodes
    D. Pancreas

Question 184

Neither ovary is seen on the endovaginal transverse view of the pelvis below (Ut = uterus):

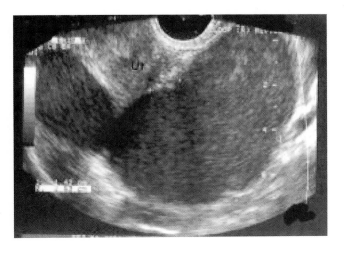

184. Which of the following histories would you expect to obtain from this patient?
    A. Prior pelvic surgery
    B. Cervical tenderness and vaginal discharge
    C. Malignant disease elsewhere
    D. Pelvic pain and infertility
    E. Asymptomatic

Questions 185–187

Refer to the sagittal and transverse images of the fetal trunk below:

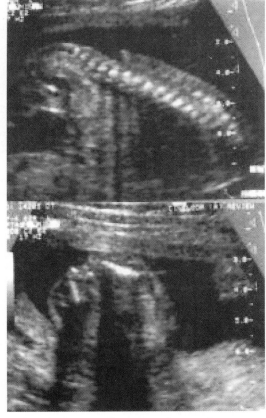

185. What is seen on these two images?
    A. Normal lumbar and sacral spine
    B. Spina bifida
    C. Dwarfism
    D. Midabdominal mass
    E. Hypoplastic bladder

186. Based on the abnormal finding on these images, evaluation of the amniotic fluid would reveal abnormal levels of
    A. maternal serum α-fetoprotein
    B. estriol
    C. human chorionic gonadotropin
    D. acetylcholinesterase
    E. triglyceride

187. What is the approximate spinal level at which the abnormality begins?
    A. S1
    B. T5
    C. T10
    D. L3
    E. C5

Question 188

Refer to the endovaginal view of the right adnexa below:

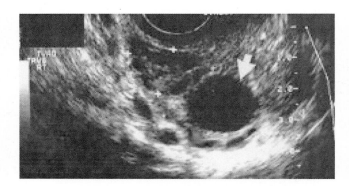

188. The white arrow is pointing to
    A. a dominant follicle
    B. a paraovarian cyst
    C. a dermoid
    D. the iliac artery
    E. the bladder

189. Estrogen is mainly secreted by
    A. graafian follicles
    B. the corpus luteum
    C. the anterior lobe of the pituitary gland
    D. the corpus albicans
    E. the thyroid gland

190. An abnormal head:abdomen ratio may be caused by all of the following **EXCEPT**
    A. microcephaly
    B. macrosomia
    C. symmetrical intrauterine growth restriction
    D. hydrocephalus
    E. gastroschisis

Questions 191 and 192

Refer to the image of a fetus and placenta below:

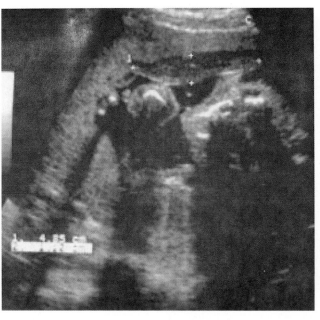

191. What is the nature of the area outlined by the crosses?
    A. Separation of the amniotic and chorionic membranes
    B. Marginal bleed
    C. Amniotic bands
    D. Amniotic sheet
    E. Remnants of a resorbed twin

192. Which of the following techniques would be **MOST** helpful in showing this abnormality?
    A. Use Doppler
    B. Increase the gain
    C. Use color flow
    D. Turn the patient in the decubitus position and rescan
    E. Change transducer frequency

Questions 193 and 194

Refer to the obstetric sonogram below:

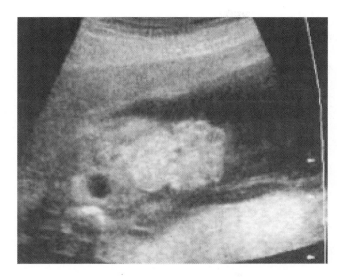

193. What fetal abnormality is seen on this image?
    A. Liver-containing omphalocele
    B. Gut-containing omphalocele
    C. Gastroschisis
    D. Umbilical hernia
    E. Sacrococcygeal teratoma

194. Common associations of this condition include
    A. cardiac abnormalities
    B. pentalogy of Cantrell
    C. karyotypic abnormalities
    D. bowel distention
    E. hydronephrosis

Questions 195–198

Refer to the transabdominal sagittal view of the pelvis in the midline below:

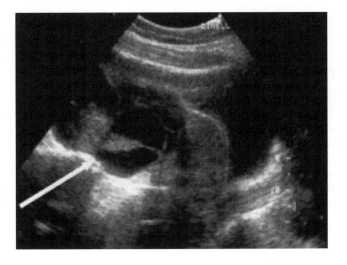

195. Which of the following terms **BEST** describes the area indicated by the arrow?
    A. Cystic
    B. Echogenic
    C. Solid
    D. Partially cystic and partially solid
    E. Echopenic

196. The mass is located
    A. in the uterus
    B. in the left ovary
    C. in the right ovary
    D. in the cul-de-sac
    E. superior to the uterus

197. Which of the following pathologies is **MOST** likely present on this image?
    A. Uterine fibroid
    B. Endometrioma
    C. Ovarian cancer
    D. Ovarian cystadenoma
    E. Inflammatory mass

198. All of the following techniques could be used to help in the diagnosis **EXCEPT**
    A. using Doppler to assess vascularity
    B. looking for metastases to the liver and para-aortic nodes
    C. assessing the kidneys for secondary hydronephrosis
    D. using an endovaginal probe to determine if the ovaries can be seen separate from the mass
    E. looking in the endometrial cavity for polyps

199. A 23-year-old patient presenting for an outpatient gynecologic sonogram has had amenorrhea for 8 years. She complains of chest pain and coughing up blood. She has been living in Liverpool, England for the last 3 years and has a Native-American boyfriend. She smokes three packs of cigarettes a day and has a foul-smelling vaginal discharge. She is a heavy marijuana user and drinks a six-pack of beer a day. Which of the following would you note in this patient's record?
    A. The heavy marijuana and cigarette use
    B. The history of amenorrhea
    C. That her boyfriend is Native American
    D. The history of coughing up blood
    E. That she has been living in Liverpool, England for 3 years

Questions 200 and 201

Refer to the image of a fetus below:

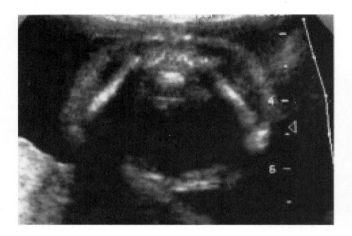

200. Which of the following is seen on this image?
    A. Both iliac crests and the spine
    B. Hypotelorism with holoprosencephaly
    C. A low spina bifida
    D. Hydrocephalus with skin thickening
    E. An enlarged bladder with posterior urethral valves

201. Which of the following entities **CANNOT** be assessed using this sonographic view?
    A. Spina bifida
    B. Down syndrome
    C. Bladder extrophy
    D. Sacrococcygeal teratoma
    E. Cord tethering

202. Why is defining the level of the uppermost extension of spina bifida important?
    A. It determines if hydrocephalus will occur
    B. It helps predict the severity of urinary tract abnormalities
    C. It helps predict the severity of rectal problems
    D. It helps predict the chance of limited leg motion

Question 203

The following sonogram shows a twin pregnancy, with twin A to the left and twin B to the right. The white arrow is pointing to an intersac membrane between the twins. Doppler flow patterns were obtained from twin A at the site indicated by the square:

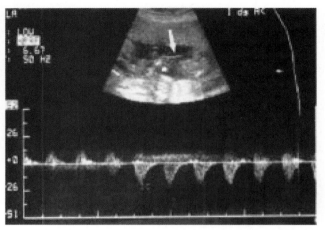

203. Which of the following is the **MOST** likely explanation for the Doppler flow pattern seen in twin A?
    A. Absent diastolic flow due to stuck twin syndrome
    B. Normal umbilical artery flow
    C. Normal umbilical vein flow
    D. Fetal death *in utero* in one twin
    E. Absent diastolic flow due to atrial septal defect

Questions 204 and 205

Refer to the transverse image of the pregnant uterus below:

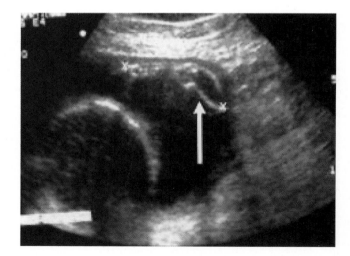

204. What is the **MOST** likely explanation for the measured structure?
    A. Cord calcification
    B. Blood clot
    C. Dead twin
    D. Rudimentary twin
    E. Grade 3 placenta

205. What α-fetoprotein level would be expected with this sonographic finding?
    A. 8 multiples of the mean (MoM)
    B. 4 MoM
    C. 2 MoM
    D. 1 MoM
    E. 0.5 MoM

Questions 206–208

Refer to the view of the fetal head below:

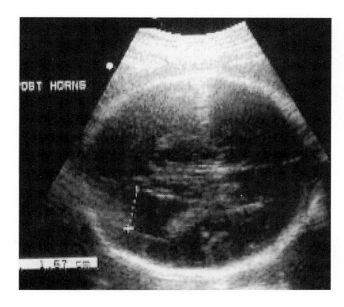

206. What abnormality is seen on this image?
    A. Choroid plexus cyst
    B. Ventriculomegaly
    C. Intracranial mass
    D. Arachnoid cyst
    E. Dandy-Walker syndrome

207. Which feature of agenesis of the corpus callosum is seen on this image?
    A. Colpocephaly
    B. Vertically aligned gyri
    C. High-riding third ventricle
    D. Third ventricle cyst
    E. No corpus callosum

208. In agenesis of the corpus callosum, which additional view would be helpful in the detection of radiating gyri?
    A. Axial view
    B. Coronal view
    C. Oblique view
    D. Transverse view
    E. Sagittal view

Questions 209 and 210

Refer to the saggital view of the left adnexa below:

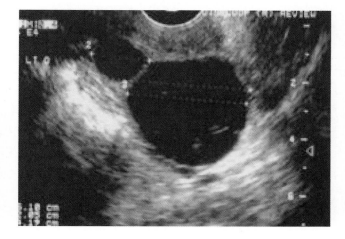

209. Which of the following entities is present in the ovary?
    A. Two simple cysts
    B. A complex cyst and a simple cyst
    C. Two follicles
    D. A dermoid and a cyst
    E. A neoplasm and a cyst

210. Which of the following additional techniques would be **MOST** useful in determining if the mass contains complex material?
    A. Using pulsed Doppler
    B. Examining the other ovary
    C. Increasing the gain
    D. Pushing the ovary with an endovaginal probe
    E. Looking from another axis

211. A grade 3 placenta is an acceptable normal variant at
    A. 20 weeks
    B. 28 weeks
    C. 32 weeks
    D. 36 weeks
    E. 45 weeks

212. Which of the following is **NOT** a cause of an intraperitoneal cystic mass?
    A. Duplication cyst
    B. Mesenteric cyst
    C. Meconium cyst
    D. Pericardial cyst
    E. Ovarian cyst

Question 213

Refer to the view of the fetus below:

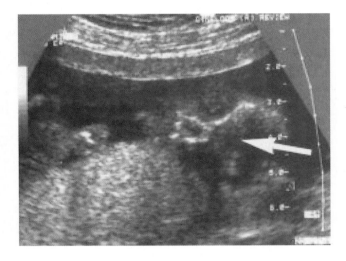

213. The arrow is pointing to the
    A. chin
    B. forehead
    C. pubic symphysis
    D. sternum
    E. occiput

Questions 214 and 215

Refer to the endovaginal longitudinal view of the uterus below:

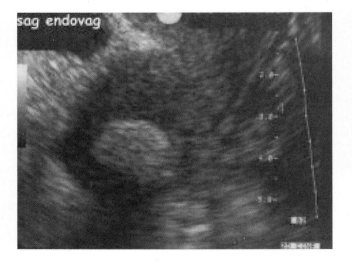

214. The mass is
    A. submucosal
    B. intracavitary
    C. subserosal
    D. pedunculated
    E. intramural

215. The echotexture of the mass is due to the fact that the mass contains
    A. gas
    B. calcium
    C. fat
    D. many interfaces
    E. pus

216. Pulsed Doppler is routinely used in a fetus with intrauterine growth restriction to assess
    A. chorioangioma
    B. placenta abruptio
    C. fetal breathing
    D. fetal tone
    E. physiologic status

217. A lateral ventricle is considered dilated if it is more than
    A. 6 mm wide
    B. 10 mm wide
    C. 14 mm wide
    D. 17 mm wide
    E. 20 mm wide

Questions 218 and 219

Refer to the sagittal view of the uterus below:

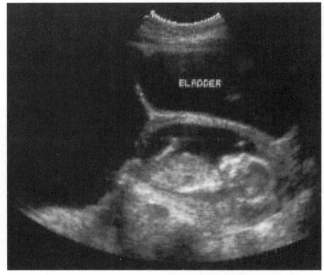

218. What abnormality is seen on this image?
    A. Overdistended maternal bladder
    B. Overdistended fetal bladder
    C. Cyst superior to the uterus
    D. Fundal fibroid
    E. Twin pregnancy

219. What is the **MOST** likely cause of the finding on this sonogram?
    A. Dermoid cyst
    B. Cystadenoma of the ovary
    C. Corpus luteum cyst
    D. Mesenteric cyst
    E. Liver cyst

Question 220

Refer to the transverse view through the abdomen of a fetus below:

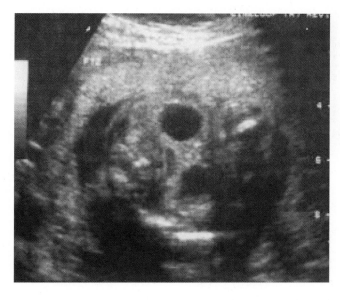

220. Which of the following is the **MOST** likely explanation for the appearances on this sonogram?
    A. Hydronephrosis
    B. A multicystic, dysplastic kidney
    C. A renal cyst
    D. An enlarged gallbladder
    E. An ovarian cyst

221. A graafian follicle
    A. is a primary follicle
    B. supports the growth of the ovum
    C. is a secondary follicle
    D. is the remnant of the corpus luteum
    E. is too large and will not rupture

Questions 222 and 223

Refer to the right transabdominal oblique view showing the uterus and an ovary below:

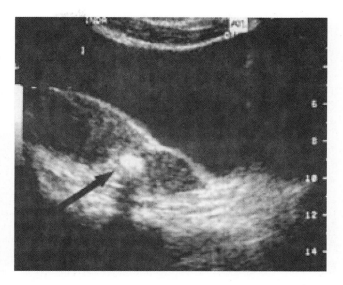

222. The arrow is pointing to
    A. an area of calcification in the ovary
    B. a portion of gut containing gas
    C. a fat- and hair-filled dermoid
    D. an intrauterine contraceptive device
    E. tubal ligation clips

223. Which of the following is **MOST** likely to be responsible for the appearances on this image?
    A. Dermoid
    B. Hemorrhage
    C. Recent corpus luteum
    D. Ovarian cancer
    E. Hydrosalpinx

Questions 224 and 225

Refer to the coronal view of a fetal trunk in a 28-week pregnancy below:

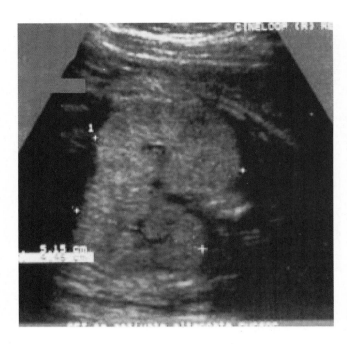

224. What abnormality is seen on this image?
    A. Large echogenic kidneys consistent with medical renal disease
    B. Bilateral intra-abdominal masses
    C. Large echogenic kidneys consistent with infantile polycystic kidney disease
    D. Large echogenic kidneys consistent with dysplastic renal disease
    E. Bilateral adrenal masses consistent with neuroblastoma

225. The condition seen on this image is
    A. autosomal dominant
    B. autosomal recessive
    C. always lethal *in utero*
    D. associated with intracranial aneurysms
    E. associated with cysts in the pancreas and liver

226. Which of the following processes does **NOT** involve the liver?
    A. Pelvic inflammatory disease
    B. Ovarian cancer
    C. Choriocarcinoma
    D. Ovarian dermoid
    E. Breast cancer

227. The first structure visible with ultrasound in the embryo, when it is 3 mm long, is the
    A. heart
    B. head
    C. spine
    D. gut

Questions 228–231

Refer to the two views of the fetal skull and brain below:

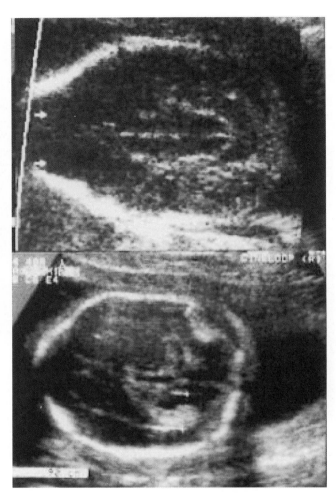

228. Which of the following findings is seen on these images?
    A. Strawberry-shaped skull
    B. Orange-shaped skull
    C. Lemon-shaped skull
    D. Skull fracture
    E. Changes consistent with osteogenesis imperfecta

229. Which of the following findings is seen in the fetal brain?
    A. Banana-shaped cerebellum
    B. Ventriculomegaly
    C. Enlarged cisterna magna
    D. Enlarged third ventricle
    E. Fused thalamus

230. What other pathology is commonly associated with this malformation?
    A. Sacrococcygeal teratoma
    B. Myelomeningocele
    C. Ovarian cyst
    D. Cardiac anomaly
    E. Klippel-Feil syndrome

231. The sonographer should also look in detail at the
    A. hands
    B. lower extremities
    C. heart
    D. kidneys
    E. eyes

Questions 232–237

Refer to the pelvic diagram below:

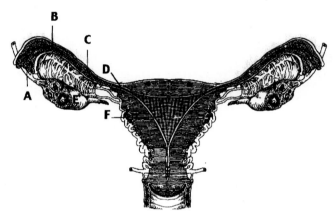

232. The letter "A" represents the
    A. fimbriae
    B. isthmus
    C. ampulla
    D. ovary
    E. cornu

233. The letter "B" represents the
    A. fimbria
    B. isthmus
    C. ampulla
    D. ovary
    E. cornu

234. The letter "C" represents the
    A. fimbria
    B. isthmus
    C. ampulla
    D. ovary
    E. cornu

235. The letter "D" represents the
    A. endometrial cavity
    B. fimbria
    C. isthmus
    D. ampulla
    E. cornu

236. The letter "E" represents the
    A. fimbria
    B. isthmus
    C. ampulla
    D. ovary
    E. cornu

237. The letter "F" represents the
    A. endometrial cavity
    B. fimbria
    C. isthmus
    D. ampulla
    E. cornu

238. A 55-year-old postmenopausal woman presents with vaginal bleeding. Her clinical history includes the use of sequential hormone replacement therapy. When is it **BEST** to perform endovaginal sonography in this patient?
    A. During bleeding
    B. At the beginning of the hormonal cycle
    C. At the end of the hormonal cycle
    D. At any time in the cycle

239. A hypoechoic mass that is 4 cm by 2 cm and has moving structures within is seen on the surface of the placenta. Color Doppler shows no flow. Which of the following is the **MOST** likely diagnosis?
    A. Wharton's jelly deposition
    B. Chorioangioma
    C. Placental cyst
    D. Venous lake
    E. Marginal bleed

Questions 240–242

Refer to the image of the fetal brain below:

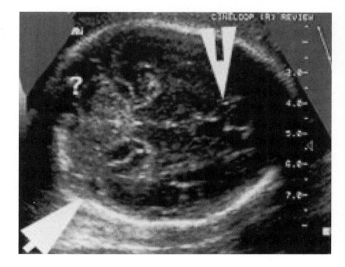

240. The arrowhead is pointing to
    A. the anterior (frontal) horn of the lateral ventricle
    B. the cavum septum pellucidum
    C. a cyst in the third ventricle
    D. the temporal horn of the lateral ventricle
    E. the thalamus

241. The question mark relates to the
    A. cisterna magna
    B. cerebellum
    C. ambient cistern
    D. tentorium
    E. vermis

242. The arrow is pointing to the
    A. cavum septum pellucidum
    B. lateral (cerebral) ventricle
    C. third ventricle
    D. dura mater
    E. thalamus

Question 243

Refer to the image of the fetal brain below:

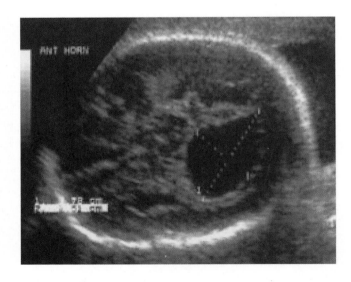

243. What finding is seen on this image?
    A. Choroid plexus cyst
    B. Dilated lateral ventricles
    C. Arachnoid cyst
    D. Dilated third ventricle
    E. Enlarged cisterna magna

Questions 244–246

Refer to the view of the pregnant uterus below:

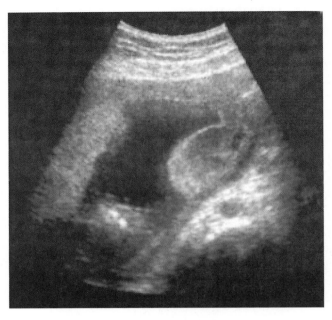

244. Which of the following is seen on this image?
    A. Venous lake
    B. Grade 3 placenta
    C. Molar pregnancy
    D. Succenturiate lobe
    E. Placenta previa

245. Which of the following techniques is useful when this finding is suspected?
    A. Using the endovaginal probe
    B. Placing the patient in the Trendelenberg position
    C. Turning the patient on her side
    D. Using color flow Doppler
    E. Using the transrectal probe

246. All of the following may be clinically significant concerning this entity **EXCEPT**
    A. it may remain *in utero* when the main portion of the placenta delivers
    B. the connecting vessel may run across the internal os of the cervix and rupture at delivery
    C. the condition is associated with more bleeding at delivery than the usual placental sites
    D. the sequestrated portion can be a placenta previa when the main portion is at the fundus
    E. it may cause premature labor

247. All of the following are included in the standard obstetric system for recording parity **EXCEPT**
    A. number of full-term pregnancies
    B. number of pregnancies
    C. number of miscarriages or abortions
    D. number of premature pregnancies
    E. number of adoptions

248. Which of the following is **NOT** true about tamoxifen?
    A. Prolonged use after breast cancer reduces the risk of recurrence
    B. There is an increased risk of endometrial cancer
    C. Prolonged use causes endometrial polyps
    D. Prolonged use causes subendometrial endometriosis deposits
    E. It can be used for hormone replacement therapy

Questions 249 and 250

Refer to the image of a fetal face showing the orbits below:

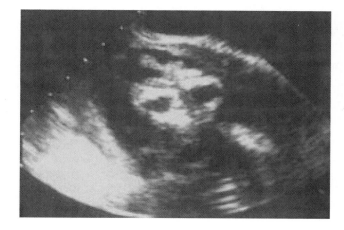

249. What abnormality is present on this image?
    A. Proboscis
    B. Cleft lip and palate
    C. Hypertelorism of the orbits
    D. Cataract
    E. Anencephaly

250. All of the following may be present with this anomaly **EXCEPT**
    A. polyhydramnios
    B. iniencephaly
    C. myelomeningocele
    D. meningocele
    E. hydrocephalus

251. A 42-year-old patient has bilateral hydronephrosis and hydroureter. Which of the following pelvic problems might be responsible?
    A. Corpus luteum cyst
    B. Dermoid
    C. Pelvic lymphoma
    D. Endometrial hyperplasia
    E. Endometrial polyp

Questions 252 and 253

Refer to the image of the fetal chest below:

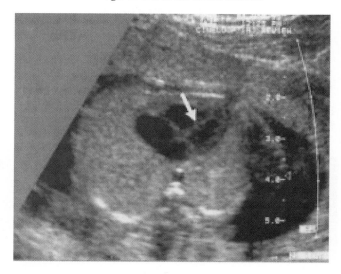

252. The arrow is pointing to
    A. the left ventricular wall
    B. the right ventricular wall
    C. the interventricular septum
    D. the atrial septum
    E. a ventriculoseptal defect

253. What is this view called?
    A. Left ventricular outflow tract (LVOT) view
    B. Four-chamber view
    C. Right ventricular outflow tract (RVOT) view
    D. Short-axis view
    E. Ductus arch view

Question 254

Sonograms of a 30-week pregnancy were obtained. This image shows the right renal fossa (B1 = bladder):

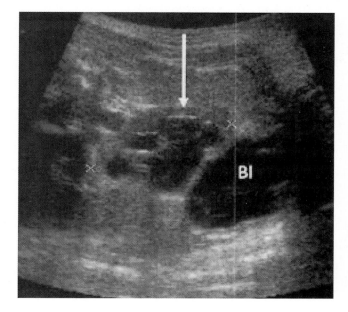

254. What is the **MOST** likely explanation for the structure indicated by the arrow?
    A. Complex ovarian cyst
    B. Tortuous ureter with ureterocele
    C. Pelvic multicystic kidney
    D. Pelvic hydronephrotic kidney
    E. Hydrometrocolpos

Question 255

The image below was taken in the fetus from question #254, but in the other flank:

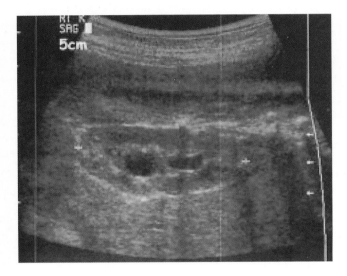

255. Which of the following is seen on this image?
    A. Multiple central cysts in the kidney
    B. Tortuous, dilated ureter
    C. Mild hydronephrosis with compensatory hypertrophy
    D. A horseshoe kidney with mild hydronephrosis
    E. A pancake kidney with mild hydronephrosis

256. Which of the following is **NOT** a cause of skin thickening in a 30-week-old fetus?
    A. Macrosomia
    B. Fetal death
    C. Hydrops
    D. Spina bifida
    E. Cystic hygroma

257. What structures should be seen at the level at which the biparietal diameter is measured?
    A. Cavum septum pellucidum, lateral ventricle, and cisterna magna
    B. Thalamus, third ventricle, and cerebellum
    C. Thalamus, third ventricle, and cavum septum pellucidum
    D. Lateral ventricle, thalamus, and cavum vergae
    E. Third ventricle, cavum septum pellucidum, and cisterna magna

Questions 258–263

Refer to the diagram of hormonal changes related to the menstrual cycle below:

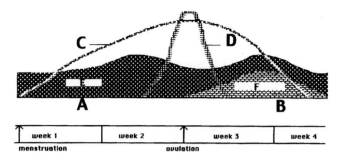

258. The letter "A" represents which of the following phases of the menstrual cycle?
    A. Secretory phase
    B. Luteal phase
    C. Proliferative phase
    D. Menstrual phase
    E. Three-line phase

259. The letter "B" represents which of the following phases of the menstrual cycle?
    A. Secretory phase
    B. Proliferative phase
    C. Follicular phase
    D. Menstrual phase
    E. Three-line phase

260. The letter "C" represents which of the following hormones?
    A. Follicle-stimulating hormone
    B. Luteinizing hormone
    C. Estrogen
    D. Progesterone
    E. Thyroid-stimulating hormone

261. The letter "D" represents which of the following hormones?
    A. Follicle-stimulating hormone
    B. Luteinizing hormone
    C. Estrogen
    D. Progesterone
    E. Thyroid-stimulating hormone

262. The letter "E" represents which of the following hormones?
    A. Follicle-stimulating hormone
    B. Luteinizing hormone
    C. Estrogen
    D. Progesterone
    E. Thyroid-stimulating hormone

263. The letter "F" represents which of the following hormones?
    A. Follicle-stimulating hormone
    B. Luteinizing hormone
    C. Estrogen
    D. Progesterone
    E. Thyroid-stimulating hormone

264. In which of the following conditions is the cisterna magna small or absent?
    A. Dandy-Walker syndrome
    B. Hydranencephaly
    C. Holoprosencephaly
    D. Arnold-Chiari II malformation
    E. Anencephaly

Questions 265 and 266

Refer to the image of the fetal brain below:

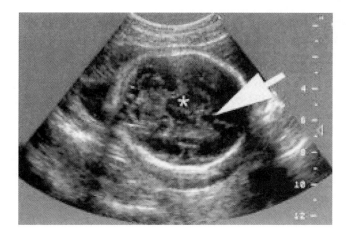

265. The arrow is pointing to the
    A. lateral ventricle
    B. cavum septum pellucidum
    C. falx
    D. interhemispheric fissure
    E. cisterna magna

266. The star indicates the
    A. cerebellum
    B. internal capsule
    C. temporal horn
    D. thalamus
    E. third ventricle

267. Which of the following is a known side effect of prolonged use of diagnostic Doppler ultrasound?
    A. Tissue freezing
    B. Tissue explosions
    C. Tissue heating
    D. Induced abortions
    E. Macrosomia

Question 268

Refer to the transverse view of the adnexa taken with an endovaginal probe below (Ut = uterus):

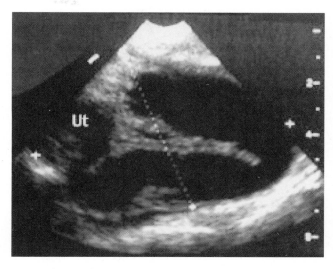

268. Which of the following is the **MOST** likely diagnosis?
    A. Ovarian cancer
    B. Simple cyst of the ovary
    C. Paraovarian cyst
    D. Hydrosalpinx
    E. Endometrioma

Question 269

Refer to the image of a fetal limb below:

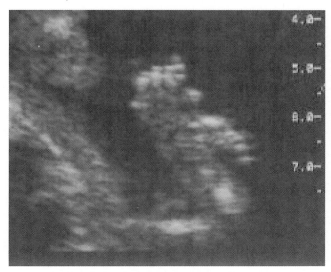

269. Which of the following abnormalities is seen on this image?
    A. A mass growing on the foot
    B. Osteogenesis imperfecta
    C. Polydactyly of the hand
    D. A proboscis
    E. Thanatophoric dwarfism

Questions 270–276

Refer to the diagram of the pregnant uterus below:

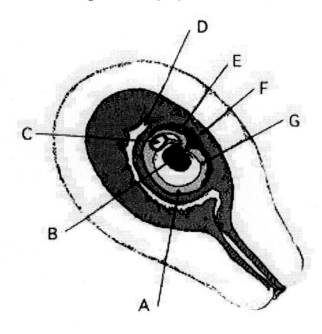

270. The letter "A" indicates the
    A. chorion frondosum
    B. amniotic membrane
    C. extraembryonic coelom
    D. decidua basalis
    E. yolk sac

271. The letter "B" indicates the
    A. chorion frondosum
    B. embryo
    C. extracelomic space
    D. decidua basalis
    E. yolk sac

272. The letter "C" indicates the
    A. chorion frondosum
    B. amniotic membrane
    C. extracelomic space
    D. embryo
    E. yolk sac

273. The letter "D" indicates the
    A. chorion frondosum
    B. amniotic membrane
    C. extracelomic space
    D. endometrial cavity
    E. decidua basalis

274. The letter "E" indicates the
    A. chorion frondosum
    B. amniotic membrane
    C. extracelomic space
    D. endometrial cavity
    E. decidua basalis

275. The letter "F" indicates the
    A. chorion frondosum
    B. amniotic membrane
    C. extracelomic space
    D. endometrial cavity
    E. decidua basalis

276. The letter "G" indicates the
    A. chorion frondosum
    B. amniotic membrane
    C. extracelomic space
    D. decidua basalis
    E. yolk sac

277. Which of the following is the **MOST** accurate way of estimating gestational age in the first trimester?
    A. Crown-rump length
    B. Femur length
    C. Biparietal diameter
    D. Gestational sac size
    E. Head circumference

278. A 43-year-old woman has a long history of infertility and has recently had rectal bleeding once a month. Which of the following is **MOST** likely to be found on a pelvic sonogram?
    A. A mass with calcification and high-level echoes
    B. Bilateral dilated tubular structures
    C. A solid ovarian mass with ascites
    D. Masses containing even, echogenic material inside and outside of the ovaries
    E. Hydronephrotic pelvic kidneys

279. Fluid containing internal echoes is seen in the cul-de-sac. All of the following are potential causes **EXCEPT**
    A. normal ovulation
    B. a ruptured ovarian cyst
    C. a ruptured ectopic pregnancy
    D. a solid mass in the ovary
    E. a dermoid

280. The arterial supply to the ovary is directly from the
    A. pudendal artery
    B. iliac artery
    C. ovarian artery
    D. uterine artery
    E. uterine and ovarian arteries

Questions 281 and 282

Refer to the sagittal image of the pregnant uterus below:

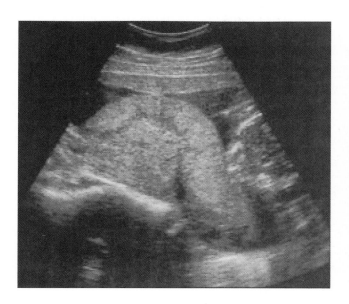

281. Which of the following is the **MOST** likely cause of the appearances on this image?
    A. Myometrial contraction
    B. Leiomyoma
    C. Chorioangioma
    D. Bicornuate uterus
    E. Severe spinal deformity

282. What additional procedure or technique would be appropriate to further evaluate this patient?
    A. Using the endovaginal probe
    B. Placing the patient erect
    C. Reexamining the patient after 20 minutes
    D. Having the patient return another day

283. Which of the following is **NOT** a neural crest anomaly?
    A. Cleft lip
    B. Anencephaly
    C. Spina bifida
    D. Iniencephaly
    E. Encephalocele

Question 284

Refer to the transverse view of an early intrauterine pregnancy below:

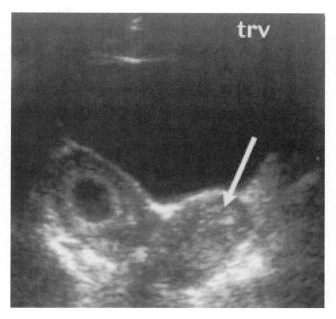

284. Which of the following is the **MOST** likely explanation for the structure indicated by the arrow?
    A. Twin ectopic pregnancy
    B. Uterus didelphys with a decidual reaction
    C. Ovarian mass
    D. Dilated ureter
    E. Fibroid with calcific degeneration

Question 285

Refer to the view of the fetal brain below:

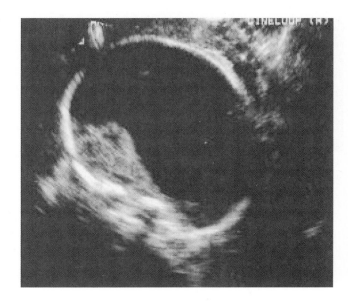

285. Which of the following abnormalities is seen on this image?
    A. Anencephaly
    B. Holoprosencephaly
    C. Hydranencephaly
    D. Acrania
    E. Severe hydrocephalus

286. Which of the following components of the brain is easily visible at 9 weeks?
    A. Primitive lateral ventricles
    B. Primitive third ventricle
    C. Primitive fourth ventricle
    D. Primitive thalamus
    E. Primitive cerebellum

287. Which of the following **BEST** describes the ovarian artery Doppler flow pattern in the secretory phase of the menstrual cycle?
    A. High-resistance flow pattern
    B. Low diastolic flow pattern
    C. Decreased
    D. Low-resistance flow pattern
    E. Varied with respiration

Questions 288–290

Refer to the transverse transabdominal view of the pelvis below:

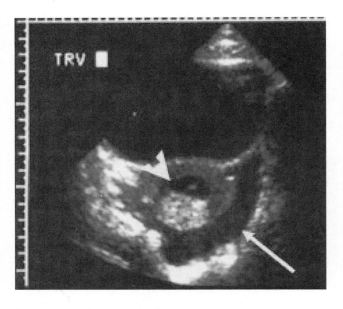

288. Which of the following is the **MOST** likely explanation for the structure indicated by the arrow?
    A. Fluid in the cul-de-sac
    B. Dilated loop of sigmoid colon
    C. Dilated fallopian tube
    D. Paraovarian cyst
    E. Ovarian cyst

289. Which of the following techniques would **NOT** be helpful in further assessing the findings?
    A. Taking a history
    B. Performing a water enema
    C. Placing the patient in the Trendelenburg position
    D. Using color flow Doppler
    E. Performing a culdocentesis

290. The arrowhead is pointing to
    A. a uterine fibroid
    B. an adnexal mass
    C. fluid in the endometrial cavity
    D. endometrial cancer
    E. the psoas muscle

291. Which of the following is the **MOST** accurate pregnancy test?
    A. Frog assay of β-human chorionic gonadotropin (β-HCG)
    B. α-Fetoprotein measured in IU/L
    C. Radioimmune assay of β-HCG
    D. Monoclonal enzyme-linked assay of urinary β-HCG
    E. Radioimmune assay of carcinoembryonic antigen

Questions 292 and 293

Refer to the transverse view of a pelvis below (Ut = uterus):

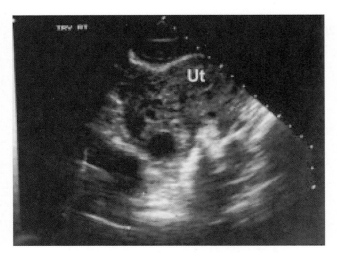

292. Which of the following is the **MOST** likely history for this patient?
    A. A 90-year-old woman with a palpable right adnexal mass
    B. A 25-year-old woman with a family history of ovarian cancer
    C. A 60-year-old man with a family history of prostate cancer
    D. A 25-year-old woman with a positive pregnancy test and abdominal pain
    E. A 25-year-old woman with a history of intercourse with numerous partners

293. Which of the following tests or procedures is the obstetrician **MOST** likely to order?
    A. Transrectal sonogram
    B. β-Human chorionic gonadotropin levels
    C. α-Fetoprotein levels
    D. CAT scan
    E. Laparotomy

Question 294

Refer to the transverse view of the female pelvis below:

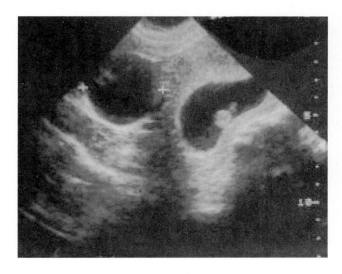

294. Which of the following entities is **MOST** likely being measured?
    A. Renal cyst
    B. Bladder
    C. Corpus luteum cyst
    D. Mesenteric cyst
    E. Ectopic pregnancy

295. β-Human chorionic gonadotropin (β-HCG) levels
    A. are greatest 1 month after conception
    B. gradually increase throughout the first trimester in a normal pregnancy
    C. take 6 months to return to normal after delivery
    D. continue to rise at a normal rate with ectopic pregnancy
    E. may be used to monitor fetal health in the second trimester

296. All of the following impair fertility **EXCEPT**
    A. a submucosal fibroid
    B. pelvic inflammatory disease
    C. endometrial implants in the adnexa
    D. membership in a Catholic order of nuns
    E. a burst appendix

Question 297

Refer to the midline sagittal transabdominal view of the pelvis below:

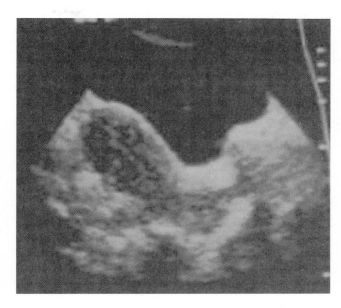

297. Which of the following is present on this image?
    A. Normal appearances
    B. Rectal mass
    C. Vaginal mass
    D. Bladder mass
    E. Prepubertal uterus

Question 298

The following image of twins was obtained with the mother on her right side:

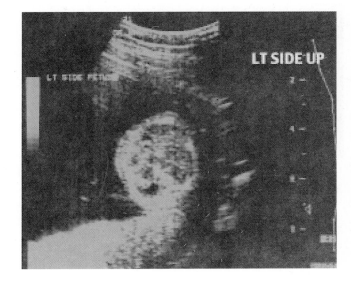

298. Which of the following conditions is present on this image?
    A. Twin-to-twin transfusion syndrome
    B. Acardiac twin
    C. Stuck twin syndrome
    D. Intrauterine growth restriction of one twin
    E. Conjoined twins

299. A sonogram shows an empty uterus, but the patient has a positive pregnancy test and reports that she is 5 weeks pregnant. Which of the following diagnoses is **NOT** possible?
    A. Ectopic pregnancy
    B. Early intrauterine pregnancy
    C. Complete spontaneous abortion
    D. False-positive pregnancy test
    E. Blighted ovum

300. Which of the following is the **MOST** likely cause of decreased amniotic fluid at 13 weeks?
    A. Severe bilateral hydronephrosis
    B. Renal agenesis
    C. Premature rupture of membranes
    D. Infantile polycystic kidney disease
    E. Intrauterine growth restriction

Questions 301 and 302

Refer to the transverse transabdominal image of the pelvis below:

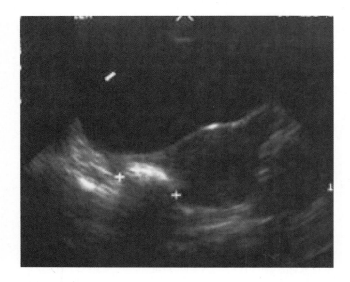

301. Which of the following is being measured on this image?
    A. Right ovary
    B. Dermoid
    C. Loop of bowel
    D. Extraovarian endometrioma
    E. Extraovarian paraovarian cyst

302. Which of the following techniques would you use to refine the diagnosis?
    A. Color flow
    B. Power Doppler
    C. Pulsed Doppler
    D. Real-time imaging

Questions 303–306

Refer to the image of an early pregnancy below:

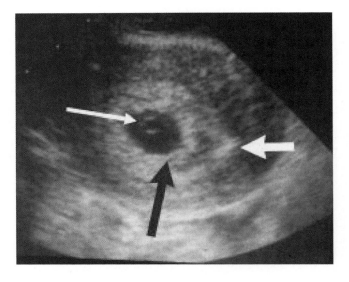

303. What is seen on this image?
    A. Intrauterine pregnancy at 3 weeks postconception
    B. Intrauterine pregnancy at 5 weeks postconception
    C. Extrauterine pregnancy at 5 weeks gestational age
    D. Intrauterine pregnancy at 7 weeks gestational age
    E. Intrauterine pregnancy at 3 weeks gestational age

304. The large white arrow is pointing to
    A. the chorion frondosum
    B. an early placenta
    C. the decidua basalis
    D. a decidual reaction of the endometrium
    E. a perisac bleed

305. The small white arrow is pointing to
    A. the chorionic membrane
    B. an intrasac bleed
    C. the secondary yolk sac
    D. the primary yolk sac
    E. the amniotic membrane

306. The black arrow is pointing to
    A. a decidual reaction of the endometrium
    B. the chorion frondosum
    C. the decidua basalis
    D. an early placenta

307. Multiple large echo free cysts are seen in both ovaries of a patient with a positive pregnancy test. Unfortunately, a tantalum mesh in the abdominal wall for treatment of a hernia prevents views of the uterus. Possible explanations for the changes in the ovaries include all of the following **EXCEPT**
    A. bilateral intraovarian endometrioma
    B. hyperstimulation syndrome
    C. hydatidiform mole
    D. partial mole
    E. twins

308. An 8-year-old girl is suspected of having precocious puberty. Which of the following ultrasonic findings supports this diagnosis?
    A. A 1-cm cyst in the right ovary
    B. A tube-shaped uterus
    C. A pear-shaped uterus with a thick endometrial lining
    D. A 2-cm, echogenic focus in the left ovary
    E. Height above the 90th percentile

Questions 309–311

Refer to the transverse transabdominal view of the pelvis in a 35-year-old patient showing an extraovarian left adnexal mass (Ut = uterus; B = bladder):

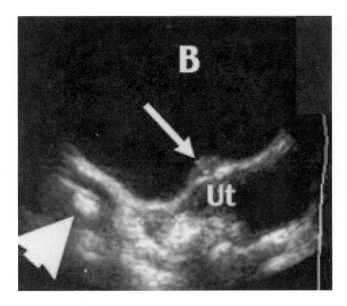

309. The arrow is pointing to
    A. an adnexal mass
    B. a bladder wall mass
    C. sediment in the bladder
    D. a bladder stone
    E. a uterine mass

310. The mass indicated by the arrow is related to the left adnexal mass. Which of the following is the **MOST** likely explanation for the mass indicated by the arrow?
    A. Fungal infection on the bladder wall
    B. Ovarian cancer metastasis to the bladder
    C. Bladder wall endometrioma
    D. Trauma to the bladder wall and left adnexa
    E. Technical artifact

311. The arrowhead is pointing to
    A. a right ovarian mass
    B. a bowel mass
    C. the sciatic nerve in the psoas muscle
    D. the piriformis muscle
    E. the obturator muscle

312. Fluid in the cul-de-sac may be secondary to all of the following **EXCEPT**
    A. a ruptured ectopic pregnancy
    B. a ruptured ovarian cyst
    C. pelvic inflammatory disease
    D. ovulation
    E. a urinary tract infection

Question 313

Refer to the image of the pregnant uterus below:

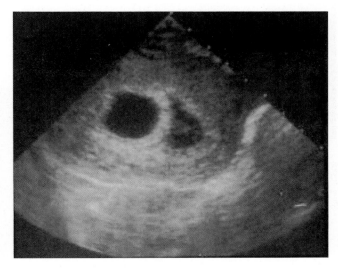

313. What is seen on this image?
    A. A normal twin pregnancy
    B. An intrasac bleed
    C. A subchorionic bleed
    D. A bleed between the gestational sac and endometrial lining
    E. An intraplacental bleed

314. Which of the following is **NOT** associated with hydatidiform moles?
    A. Hyperemesis gravidarum
    B. Vaginal bleeding
    C. Decreased human chorionic gonadotropin
    D. Hypertension prior to 20 weeks
    E. Asian origin

315. The **BEST** time for conception is when
    A. the endometrium is 3 mm thick
    B. the endometrium is 10 mm thick
    C. there is a follicle of 9 mm in the ovary
    D. a corpus luteum has developed
    E. the three-line pattern is seen in the endometrium

Question 316

Refer to the transabdominal longitudinal view of the pelvis below:

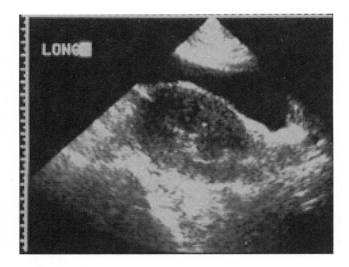

316. Which of the following is present on this image?
    A. Subserosal lipoma
    B. Intracavitary fibroid
    C. Cystic degeneration of a fibroid
    D. Endometrial cancer
    E. Pedunculated fibroid

317. At which of the following gestational ages is it **MOST** dangerous for the mother to take antiepileptic drugs?
    A. 4–10 weeks
    B. 11–18 weeks
    C. 19–26 weeks
    D. 27–34 weeks
    E. 35–40 weeks

318. On a profile view, information can be obtained about which of the following structures?
    A. Eyes
    B. Nostrils
    C. Ears
    D. Chin
    E. Cheeks

Questions 319 and 320

A sonogram performed at 32 weeks and confirmed by earlier sonogram and last menstrual period shows the following measurement data:

   Biparietal diameter = 7.1 cm = 32 weeks
   Head circumference = 27 cm = 32 weeks
   Abdominal circumference = 24 cm = 28 weeks
   Femoral length = 6.1 cm = 32 weeks

Based on these findings, the composite gestational age is 31 weeks.

319. Which of the following would you conclude is present?
    A. A normal fetus
    B. A small normal fetus
    C. An intrauterine growth restricted fetus
    D. A large fetus
    E. A macrosomic fetus

320. Based on the measurement data, which of the following amniotic fluid index (AFI) measurements would you expect?
    A. AFI = 5
    B. AFI = 10
    C. AFI = 15
    D. AFI = 20
    E. AFI = 25

321. Which of the following anomalies can be detected in the first trimester?
    A. Acrania anencephaly complex
    B. Duodenal stenosis
    C. Achondroplasia
    D. Osteogenesis imperfecta

Question 322

Refer to the image of an 8-week intrauterine pregnancy below:

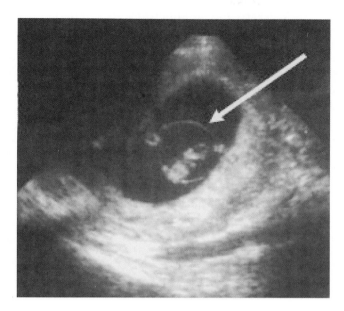

322. The arrow is pointing to
    A. the amniotic membrane
    B. the chorionic membrane
    C. nuchal thickening
    D. the vitelline duct
    E. an intra-amniotic bleed

Question 323

Refer to the sagittal midline transabdominal image below:

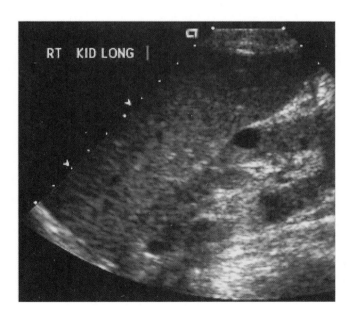

323. This uterus is
    A. anteverted and retroflexed
    B. retroverted
    C. retroverted and retroflexed
    D. normoverted
    E. anteflexed and normoverted

324. Which of the following fluids is **LEAST** echogenic?
    A. Amniotic fluid in the first trimester
    B. Extracelomic fluid
    C. Amniotic fluid in the third trimester
    D. Fluid in the yolk sac
    E. Intra-amniotic blood

325. The normal postmenopausal uterus is
    A. pear shaped and approximately $9 \times 6 \times 4$ cm
    B. tube shaped and approximately $9 \times 6 \times 4$ cm
    C. pear shaped and approximately $6 \times 4 \times 3$ cm
    D. tube shaped and approximately $6 \times 4 \times 3$ cm
    E. too small to find

326. All of the following signify a poor prognosis in the first trimester **EXCEPT**
    A. a small, calcified yolk sac
    B. a large yolk sac
    C. an embryo pulse rate of less than 80
    D. good 5.5 weeks dates with no embryo visible
    E. a perisac bleed that is 3 cm with a viable embryo

327. Blood can accumulate in all of the following areas **EXCEPT**
    A. in the amniotic cavity
    B. in the extracelomic space
    C. around the gestational sac
    D. in the intrauterine cavity
    E. in the yolk sac

Questions 328–330

A female patient has a β-human chorionic gonadotropin level of 80,000. A sagittal view of her pelvis is shown below:

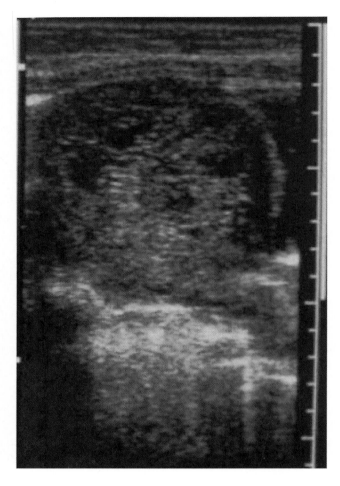

328. What is occurring in this patient's uterus?
    A. Large fibroid
    B. Missed abortion
    C. Hydatidiform mole
    D. Placenta accreta
    E. Placenta previa

329. This patient would be expected to have which of the following symptoms?
    A. Vaginal bleeding
    B. Abdominal pain
    C. Leg swelling
    D. Urinary frequency

330. Statistically, this patient is **MOST** likely to be
    A. Egyptian
    B. Russian
    C. Japanese
    D. English
    E. American

331. What is the effect of postmenopausal hormone replacement therapy on the endometrium?
    A. No effect
    B. Thins the endometrium to less than 4 mm
    C. Thickens the endometrium to 5 mm
    D. Thickens the endometrium to a variable degree
    E. Thickens the endometrium to more than 8 mm

332. The successful fertilization of the sperm and the ovum directly results in a
    A. blastocyst
    B. morula
    C. zygote
    D. oocyte
    E. fimbria

333. A gestational sac is eccentrically located toward the left at the fundus. All of the following could be responsible for this eccentric position **EXCEPT**
    A. a normal variant
    B. right-sided fibroids
    C. a bicornuate uterus
    D. a cornual pregnancy
    E. a missed abortion

334. What is the principal benefit of prolonged administration of estrogen to menopausal women?
    A. Decreases heart disease and osteoporosis
    B. Decreases cancer and lymphoma
    C. Decreases infection
    D. Prevents hot flashes
    E. Improves sexual drive

Questions 335 and 336

A mother whose blood group is O negative and who has a history of a previous stillbirth presents for a sonogram at 28 weeks. Fetal ascites and a large placenta are seen on the sonogram.

335. What additional findings are commonly associated with these findings?
    A. Duodenal atresia
    B. Clubfeet
    C. Pleural effusion
    D. Hydrocephalus
    E. Hydronephrosis

336. Which of the following is the **MOST** likely underlying diagnosis?
    A. Rubella
    B. Down syndrome
    C. Rh incompatibility
    D. Neural crest anomaly
    E. Prune-belly syndrome

337. A patient had intercourse on only one occasion and is now 5 weeks pregnant. A transabdominal sonogram shows a gestational sac measuring 1.2 cm. No fetal pole or yolk sac is visible. All of the following may be present **EXCEPT**
    A. a blighted ovum
    B. an early, normal pregnancy
    C. a twin pregnancy with early demise of the second twin
    D. a heterotopic pregnancy
    E. a missed abortion

338. A procedure used in the first trimester to obtain villi from the developing fetus for a karyotype is
    A. Percutaneous umbilical blood sampling
    B. Amniocentesis
    C. Gamete intrafallopian transfer
    D. Chorionic villi sampling
    E. Zygote intrafallopian tube transfer

339. Transcerebellar measurements more or less correspond to gestational age until approximately
    A. 15 weeks
    B. 18 weeks
    C. 20 weeks
    D. 25 weeks
    E. 30 weeks

340. For hormone replacement therapy, progesterone is often given in addition to estrogen because it
    A. diminishes side effects
    B. decreases infection
    C. maintains a youthful appearance
    D. prevents menstruation
    E. decreases cancer

Questions 341 and 342

Refer to the sagittal transabdominal view of the pelvis below:

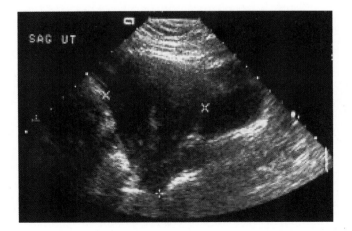

341. The uterus is
    A. anteverted and retroflexed
    B. anteverted
    C. retroverted and retroflexed
    D. normoverted
    E. normoverted and anteflexed

342. This patient is between
    A. 0 and 5 years of age
    B. 5 and 12 years of age
    C. 30 and 40 years of age
    D. 65 and 75 years of age
    E. 75 and 95 years of age

Question 343

Refer to the transabdominal sagittal (left image) and transverse (right image) views of the uterus below:

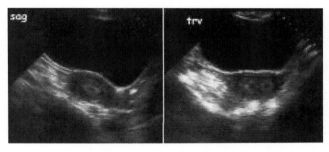

343. The sagittal view shows all of the information needed about this uterus. What does the transverse view show?
    A. Twin gestational sacs
    B. Blood in the endometrial cavity
    C. Rectus muscle artifact
    D. Bicornuate uterus
    E. Intracavitary fibroids

344. Which of the following structures is normally seen in the fetal thorax?
    A. Gallbladder
    B. Stomach
    C. Liver
    D. Spleen
    E. Heart

345. A biophysical profile examination is done at 32 weeks. Fetal breathing is seen, but there is no fetal movement. The amniotic fluid index is 10. A nonstress test was not performed. The biophysical profile score is
    A. 2
    B. 4
    C. 5
    D. 6
    E. 8

346. A cyst adjacent to the middle of the vagina is called a
    A. ureterocele
    B. paraovarian cyst
    C. Gartner's duct cyst
    D. nabothian cyst

347. After an initial sonogram at 18 weeks, which of the following placental positions is an indication for a follow-up sonogram later in pregnancy?
    A. Left lateral placenta with a full bladder
    B. Anterior, high placenta with an empty bladder
    C. Marginal placenta previa with an empty bladder
    D. Posterior, low placenta with a full bladder
    E. Partial placenta previa with a full bladder

348. During days 5–14 of the menstrual cycle, the endometrium is in the
    A. menstrual phase
    B. proliferative phase
    C. secretory phase
    D. follicular phase
    E. luteal phase

Questions 349 and 350

Refer to the midline transabdominal sagittal view of the pelvis below:

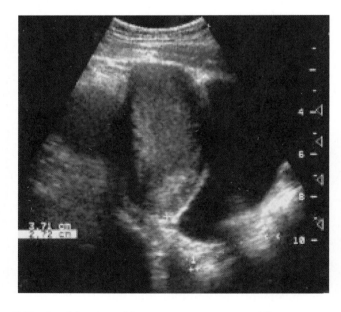

349. An 18-year-old woman presents with amenorrhea. Which of the following is the **MOST** likely cause of her absent periods?
    A. Imperforate hymen
    B. Transverse vaginal septum
    C. Absent cervix and vagina
    D. Absent uterus

350. Which of the following is the **MOST** likely explanation for the mass superior to the uterus?
    A. Dominant follicle
    B. Hematoma
    C. Ovarian cancer
    D. Corpus luteum cyst
    E. Dermoid

351. Which of the following fetal presentations is normally treated by cesarean section?
    A. Vertex presentation at 39 weeks
    B. Cephalic presentation at 36 weeks
    C. Breech presentation at 38 weeks
    D. Occiput presentation at 41 weeks
    E. Breech presentation at 22 weeks

352. Which of the following is **NOT** appropriately included in a satisfactory femoral length measurement?
    A. Femoral head
    B. Distal femoral epiphysis
    C. Lateral femoral shaft
    D. Medial femoral shaft

353. All of the following findings are suggestive of placenta accreta **EXCEPT**
    A. history of a previous cesarean section
    B. a thinned uterine wall
    C. vertically aligned intraplacental vessels
    D. history of intrauterine surgery
    E. an avascular area between the placenta and the uterine wall

Questions 354 and 355

Refer to the transverse transabdominal view taken low in the pelvis of a 45-year-old woman:

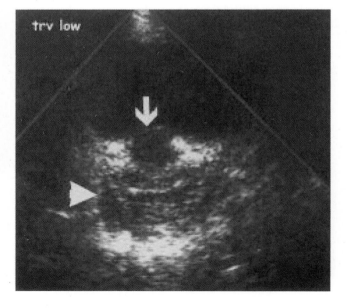

354. The arrow is pointing to
    A. a Gartner's duct cyst
    B. an intravaginal mass
    C. the urethra
    D. a urethral diverticulum
    E. a bladder wall mass

355. The arrowhead is pointing to
    A. the rectum
    B. the vagina
    C. a rectal neoplasm
    D. the cervix
    E. the piriformis muscle

356. Mirror artifacts can be seen
    A. with a dominant follicle
    B. beyond the sacrum
    C. with a full bladder
    D. with a large fibroid uterus

357. For a biophysical profile, which of the following is considered an indication of good fetal tone?
    A. Eye movement
    B. An erect penis
    C. Opening and closing the hand
    D. Yawning
    E. Gulping

358. All of the following findings make a head circumference measurement inaccurate **EXCEPT**
    A. asymmetrical hemispheres
    B. including the cerebellum
    C. including the orbits
    D. including the cavum septum pellucidum
    E. including the tentorium

359. On a transverse view of the fetal lumbosacral spine, the angle of the iliac wings in relation to the posterior elements should measure
    A. slightly less than 90°
    B. 45°
    C. 10°
    D. 180°
    E. 15°

360. A 17-year-old girl presents with secondary sexual characteristics without the onset of menses. Which of the following conditions is **MOST** likely present?
    A. Leiomyoma
    B. Hematocolpos
    C. Diethylstilbestrol exposure anomaly
    D. Unicornuate uterus
    E. Uterus didelphys

361. How is the amniotic fluid index measured?
    A. Measure the combined transverse dimension of the four largest fluid pockets
    B. Measure the transverse dimension and anteroposterior measurement of the largest fluid pocket only
    C. Measure the anteroposterior measurement of the largest fluid pocket only
    D. Measure the anteroposterior measurement of the largest fluid pocket in each quadrant
    E. Measure the transverse dimension of the largest fluid pocket in each quadrant

362. All of the following conditions may produce an abnormally thick placenta **EXCEPT**
    A. nonimmune hydrops
    B. maternal hypertension
    C. maternal diabetes
    D. triploidy
    E. syphilis

Questions 363 and 364

Refer to the sagittal view of the pelvis below:

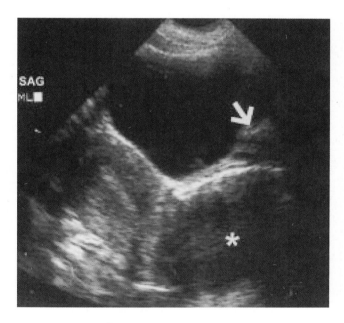

363. Which of the following is the **MOST** likely explanation for the area indicated by the asterisk?
    A. Intravaginal mass
    B. Rectal neoplasm
    C. Fecal material in the rectum
    D. Cervical fibroid
    E. Sacral mass

364. The arrow is pointing to
    A. a bladder wall mass
    B. a normal urethra
    C. a ureteral diverticulum
    D. a perineal neoplasm
    E. a Foley catheter

365. A patient is referred for her first obstetric sonogram in the third trimester. The sonogram confirmed the clinician's suspicion that she was small for gestational age. Which of the following conditions could NOT be responsible for causing the low fundal height on exam?
    A. Fetal renal anomaly
    B. Premature rupture of membranes
    C. Maternal hypertension
    D. Retroverted uterus
    E. Chromosomal anomaly

366. A procedure in which a catheter is guided sonographically into the edge of the gestational sac is
    A. chorionic villi sampling
    B. an amniocentesis
    C. a uterine biopsy
    D. percutaneous umbilical vein sampling
    E. a cordocentesis

367. A T-shaped uterus is the result of
    A. diethylstilbestrol exposure
    B. a career as a prostitute
    C. syphilis
    D. radiation therapy
    E. chemical poisoning

368. How is hydrops related to Rh incompatibility normally treated at 26 weeks?
    A. Amniocentesis
    B. Chorionic villi sampling
    C. Early delivery
    D. Exchange transfusion
    E. Pigtail catheter insertion

369. The **MOST** common cause of painless vaginal bleeding in the second and third trimesters is
    A. trauma
    B. ectopic pregnancy
    C. placenta previa
    D. placental abruption
    E. incompetent cervix

Questions 370 and 371

Refer to the sagittal transabdominal view of the pelvis of a 30-year-old woman below:

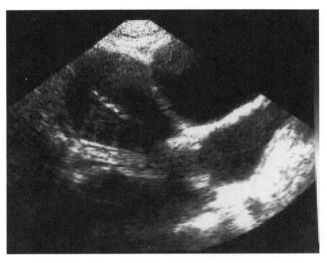

370. Which of the following can be seen in the uterus?
    A. Retained bony products of conception
    B. Dalkon shield intrauterine contraceptive device (IUCD)
    C. Lippes loop IUCD
    D. Endometrial neoplasm
    E. Arcuate artery calcification

371. What lies posterior to the bladder on this image?
    A. Rectal neoplasm
    B. Bladder wall mass
    C. Sacral mass
    D. Solid vaginal mass
    E. Fluid-filled vagina

372. Which of the following conditions is characterized by ectopic endometrial deposits in the myometrium of the uterus?
    A. Endometriosis
    B. Hypermenorrhea
    C. Adenomyosis
    D. Pelvic inflammatory disease

373. Endometrial thickening may be seen in all of the following **EXCEPT**
    A. an early pregnancy
    B. polyps
    C. a pedunculated fibroid
    D. the secretory phase of the menstrual cycle
    E. endometrial cancer

374. Which of the following approaches is **MOST** accurate for ruling out placenta previa?
    A. Transabdominal
    B. Translabial
    C. Transvaginal
    D. Transrectal
    E. Transperineal

375. Which of the following **MOST** accurately predicts fetal lung maturity?
    A. A grade 3 placenta
    B. The lecithin:sphingomyelin ratio from the amniotic fluid
    C. The presence of meconium in the fetal colon
    D. An increase in the echogenicity of the fetal lungs
    E. A proximal humeral epiphysis seen on the scan

Questions 376–381

Refer to the axial view of a fetal cranium below:

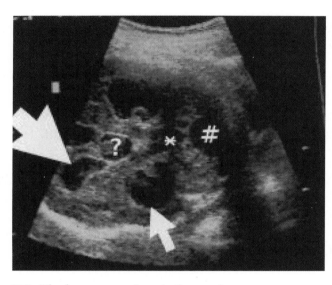

376. The large arrow is pointing to the
    A. temporal horn of the lateral ventricle
    B. anterior (frontal) horn of the lateral ventricle
    C. cavum septum pellucidum
    D. third ventricle
    E. fourth ventricle

377. The question mark indicates the
    A. cavum septum pellucidum
    B. anterior horn of the lateral ventricle
    C. cavum vergae
    D. third ventricle
    E. temporal horn of the lateral ventricle

378. The small arrow is pointing to the
    A. anterior horn of the lateral ventricle
    B. fourth ventricle
    C. third ventricle
    D. temporal horn of the lateral ventricle
    E. ambient cistern

379. The asterisk indicates the
    A. third ventricle
    B. fourth ventricle
    C. cisterna magna
    D. quadrigeminal cistern
    E. cavum vergae

380. The pound sign indicates the
    A. cisterna magna
    B. fourth ventricle
    C. third ventricle
    D. quadrigeminal cistern
    E. ambient cistern

381. What is the underlying cause of the ventricular enlargement?
    A. Aqueduct stenosis
    B. Arnold-Chiari malformation
    C. Dandy-Walker syndrome
    D. Unilateral ventriculomegaly
    E. Hydranencephalus

382. A biophysical profile is indicated in all of the following **EXCEPT**
    A. intrauterine growth restriction
    B. post-term gestation
    C. pregnancy-induced hypertension
    D. antiepileptic drug administration
    E. maternal diabetes

383. In the United States, which of the following is the **MOST** commonly inserted intrauterine contraceptive device?
    A. Dalkon shield
    B. Paragard
    C. Lippes loop
    D. Copper 7
    E. None of the above; they are all off of the market

384. The sperm unites with the ovum approximately
    A. 24 hours after ovulation
    B. 3 days after ovulation
    C. 7 days after ovulation
    D. 10 days after ovulation
    E. 14 days after ovulation

385. The dumbbell-shaped structure(s) inferior and posterior to the cerebrum is(are) the
    A. third ventricle
    B. sylvian fissure
    C. cavum septum pellucidum
    D. cerebellum
    E. lateral ventricles

Question 386

Refer to the transabdominal sagittal view of the pelvis of a 40-year-old woman below:

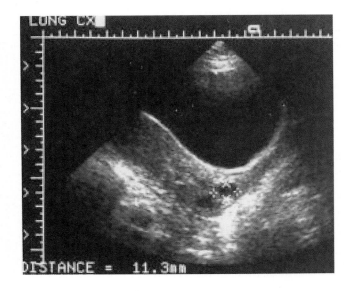

386. Which of the following entities is being measured on this image?
    A. Aborting gestational sac
    B. Cervical pregnancy
    C. Nabothian cyst
    D. Urine in the vagina
    E. Bladder neoplasm

387. All of the following are examples of fetal tone as used in biophysical profile **EXCEPT**
    A. opening and closing of the hand
    B. movement of the tongue
    C. flexion and extension of the spine
    D. flexion and extension of an upper extremity
    E. flexion and extension of a lower extremity

388. On an intracranial examination of the fetus, the cisterna magna should **NOT** measure more than
    A. 1 mm
    B. 10 mm
    C. 15 mm
    D. 20 mm
    E. 25 mm

389. All of the following are risk factors for endometrial cancer **EXCEPT**
    A. diabetes
    B. anorexia
    C. tamoxifen
    D. hypertension
    E. obesity

390. As a follicle grows, estrogen levels
    A. increase
    B. decrease abruptly
    C. taper off
    D. do not change
    E. plateau

391. An enlarged placenta in an otherwise healthy diabetic patient is **MOST** likely the result of
    A. a trisomy anomaly
    B. overeating
    C. obesity
    D. increased placental transfer of glucose
    E. VACTERL syndrome

392. A sonographic technique used to determine whether the fallopian tubes are patent is
    A. hysterography
    B. hysterosonography
    C. hysterectomy
    D. hysterosalpingography
    E. hysteroscopy

393. Female factors in infertility include all of the following **EXCEPT**
    A. obesity
    B. anorexia
    C. anxiety
    D. thyroid malfunction
    E. history of cesarean section

Questions 394–395

Refer to the endovaginal sagittal view of the uterus below:

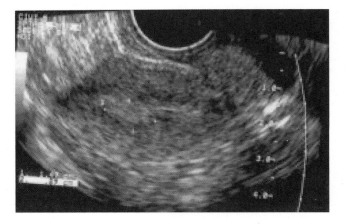

394. Which of the following findings is present on this image?
    A. Normal postmenopausal endometrial cavity
    B. Normal secretory phase appearances
    C. Normal proliferative phase appearances
    D. A small endometrial mass
    E. A small intrauterine contraceptive device

395. Which of the following procedures would be **MOST** helpful in the further assessment of this image?
    A. A transabdominal view with a full bladder
    B. Transrectal views
    C. A water enema
    D. A procedure in which saline is infused into the endometrial cavity
    E. A CT scan

396. In a postmenopausal patient taking hormone replacement therapy, what is the normal upper limit of size for the endometrial cavity?
    A. 3–4 mm
    B. 5–6 mm
    C. 8–10 mm
    D. 12–14 mm
    E. 16–20 mm

397. A female gynecologist was on her way to work when a heavy period began. She felt faint and called her office. She explained to her coworker that she would have to take the morning off because of
    A. metrorider syndrome
    B. dysmenorrhea
    C. menorrhagia
    D. menometrorrhagia
    E. mennonite syndrome

Appendices

LABORATORY VALUES

Laboratory Test	Pathology	Change
AFP	Neural crest abnormalities	Increased above about 2.1 MoM
	Abdominal wall defects	Increased
	Placental abnormalities	Mildly increased
	Intra-amniotic bleeding	Increased
HCG	Trophoblastic disease	Significantly increased
	Pregnancy	Increased
	Testicular tumor	Increased
	Ectopic pregnancy*	Increased
CA125	Ovarian cancer	Increased
	Early pregnancy	Mildly increased
	Benign ovarian cyst	Mildly increased
	Endometriosis	Mildly increased
	Pelvic inflammatory disease	Mildly increased
AST	Acute hepatitis	Increased
	Cirrhosis	Increased
	Hepatic necrosis	Increased
	Injury	Increased
	Metastases	Increased
	Fatty changes	Increased
	Biliary obstruction	Increased
ALT	Hepatitis	Moderately increased
	Obstructive jaundice	Moderately increased
	Hepatocellular disease	Moderately increased
	Shock	Increased
	Drug toxicity	Increased
Alkaline phosphatase	Bile duct dilation	Markedly increased
	Primary biliary cirrhosis	Markedly increased
	Primary sclerosing cholangitis	Markedly increased
	Abscess	Increased
	Carcinoma	Increased
	Cirrhosis	Increased
	Early biliary obstruction	Increased
	Bone metastases	Increased
LDH	Hepatitis	Mildly increased
	Cirrhosis	Mildly increased

Laboratory Test	Pathology	Change
	Hepatic congestion	Mildly increased
	Obstructive jaundice	Mildly increased
	Infectious mononucleosis	Moderately increased
	Myocardial infarction	Increased
	Pulmonary infarction	Increased
	Renal infarction	Increased
	Chronic renal disease	Increased
Albumin	Liver dysfunction	Decreased
	Malnutrition	Decreased
	Some renal diseases	Decreased
PT	Liver damage	Increased
	Clotting problems	Increased
γ-Globulin	Liver disease	Increased
SPEP	Liver disease	Increased
Bilirubin		
Serum bilirubin	Liver disease	Increased
	Hyperbilirubinemia	Increased
Indirect or unconjugated bilirubin	Hepatocellular disease	Increased
	Hemolytic anemia	Increased
Direct or conjugated bilirubin	Extrahepatic obstruction	Increased
Serum amylase	Acute pancreatitis	Increased
	Chronic pancreatitis	Increased or normal
Lipase	Pancreatitis	Increased
	Pancreatic duct obstruction	Increased
	Pancreatic cancer	Increased
	Cirrhosis	Increased
	Acute cholecystitis	Increased
WBC count	Leukemia	Increased
	Infection	Increased (rarely decreased)
	Infectious mononucleosis	Increased
	Splenic abscess	Increased
	Inflammation	Increased
	Hodgkin's lymphoma	Decreased
	Non-Hodgkin's lymphoma	Decreased
	Immune deficiency (AIDS)	Decreased
RBC count (hemoglobin, hematocrit)	Hemorrhage	Decreased
	Leukemia	Decreased
	Anemia	Decreased
BUN	Renal failure	Increased
	Renal parenchymal disease	Increased
	Obstructive uropathy	Increased
	Dehydration	Increased
	Hemorrhage	Increased
Creatinine	Renal failure	Increased
PSA[†]	Prostate cancer	Increased
	Acute prostatitis	Increased
	Chronic prostatitis	Mildly increased
	BPH	Mildly increased
	After a TURP procedure	Mildly increased
	After a digital rectal exam	Mildly increased
PAP	Prostate cancer	Increased
Urinalysis		
Specific gravity	Dehydration	Increased
RBCs	Hypernephroma	Increased

Laboratory Test	Pathology	Change
	Infarction	Increased
	Renal calculi	Increased
	Trauma	Increased
	Infection	Increased
WBCs (pyuria)	Infection	Increased
Proteinuria	Glomerulonephritis	Increased
	Nephrotic syndrome	Increased
	Renal vein thrombosis	Increased
Urine amylase	Pancreatitis	Increased
Amniotic fluid		
AFP	Neural crest abnormalities	Markedly increased
	Gastroschisis	Markedly increased
	Omphalocele	Increased
Acetylcholinesterase	Neural crest abnormalities	Increased
	Abdominal wall defects	Mildly increased

AFP = α-fetoprotein; ALT = alanine aminotransferase; AST = aspartate aminotransferase; BPH = benign prostatic hypertrophy; BUN = blood urea nitrogen; HCG = human chorionic gonadotropin; LDH = lactate dehydrogenase; MoM = multiples of the median; PAP = prostate acid phosphatase; PSA = prostate-specific antigen; PT = prothrombin time; RBC = red blood cell; SPEP = serum protein electrophoresis; TURP = transurethral resection of the prostate; WBC = white blood cell.

*Ectopic pregnancy can be diagnosed if there is no intrauterine pregnancy but the HCG level is above 1500 mIU/ml.

†PSA is considered abnormal if it is greater than 4 ng/ml.

WORD ORIGINS

Word	Origin	Meaning	Examples
abdomen	L	Belly	
allantois	GR	Sausage	
amnio-	GR	Lamb ("amnos")	Amnion
ampulla	L	Little jar	Ampulla of Vater
ante-	L	Before	Anteverted
anti-	GR	Against	Antiseptic
antrum	GR	Cave ("antron")	
	L	Cavity	
appendix	L	Hang to ("appendere")	
bio-	GR	Life ("bios")	Biology
-blast-	GR	Germ	Blastocyst
bruit	FR	Noise	
cancer	GR	Crab	
-cele-	GR	Hernia ("kele")	Ureterocele: prolapse of the ureter into the bladder
-centesis	GR	Puncture	Amniocentesis: removal of amniotic fluid by needle puncture
cephalo-	GR	Head	Cephalocele: protrusion of part of the brain through the skull (see -*cele*)
chole-	GR	Bile	Cholecystectomy
chorion	GR	Skin, leather	Outer membrane enclosing an embryo
chorion villus	L	Shaggy hair	
cirrhosis	GR	Yellow	See -*osis*
cisterna	L	A vessel	Cisterna magna: holds cerebrospinal fluid
coccus	GR	Berry ("kokkos")	Coccus: spherical or ovoid bacteria
contra-	L	Opposite	Contralateral
cotyledons	GR	Hollow of a cup	
decidua	L	To fall off	Decidualized: decidual tissue of the endometrium sheds at menstruation
decubitus	L	To lie down	
dia-	GR	Through	Dialysis: removing elements from blood or lymph by means of filtration through a membrane (see *lysis*)
duodenal	L	Measuring 12 finger breadths in length	
echino-	GR	Prickly husk	Echinococcosis: infestation by the larvae of the tapeworm (see *coccus*)
echo	GR	Sound	

Word	Origin	Meaning	Examples
ecto-	GR	Outside ("ektos")	Ectopic pregnancy: a pregnancy that is outside of the correct place (see *topo-*)
-ectomy	GR	To cut out	Sigmoidectomy: resection of the sigmoid portion of the colon
endo-	GR	Within	Endocarditis: inflammation within the heart
fenestra	L	Window	Fenestrated drape: a drape with an opening in the center
fetus	L	Bringing forth	
flexion	L	To bend	
gossy	L	Plant that provides cotton for fiber ("Gossypium")	Gossyphiboma: a "tumor" created by a retained surgical sponge
-gram	GR	Record ("gramma")	Gramophone, sonogram
gynecologic	GR	Of a woman	
hemo-	GR	Blood	
hepatic	GR	Liver	
hydro-	GR	Water	
-iasis	GR	State or condition of	Elephantiasis: condition resembling the state of an elephant
-infra-	L	Below	
-inter-	L	Between	
-intra-	L	Situated within	
ipsi-	L	Same	Ipsilateral: on the same side
-itis	GR	Inflammation	Pyelonephritis: inflammation of the kidney
lateral	L	Side	Ipsilateral: pertaining to the same side of the body (see *ipsi-*)
lipo-	GR	Fat ("lipos")	Lipoma: fatty tumor (see *-oma*)
litho-	GR	Stone ("lithos")	Cholelithiasis: stone in the gallbladder
-lysis	GR	Dissolution	Hemolysis: the breakdown of red blood cells and release of hemoglobin
morpho-	GR	Form	Morphology, ectomorph
morula	L	Mulberry	
mucin	L	Slime	
nephro-	GR	Kidneys	Nephrolithiasis: the condition of having stones in the kidney (see *litho-*)
obstetric	L	Midwife	
-ology	GR	Word, reason	Nephrology: study of the kidney
-oma	GR	Tumor	
oocyte	GR	Egg	
-osis	GR	Abnormal or diseased condition	Cirrhosis: condition of the liver that can cause jaundice
path-	GR	Disease, suffering ("pathos")	Pathology: the study of the nature and cause of disease; or, the condition produced by disease
peri-	GR	Surrounding	Pericardium
placenta	L	Flat cake	
previa	L	To come first	Placenta previa: condition in which the placenta lies in the lower uterine segment (i.e., before the fetus) [see *placenta*]
pus	L	Corrupt matter	
pyelo-	GR	Pelvis	
pylorus	GR	Gatekeeper	
pyo-	GR	Pus	
salpinx	GR	Tube	
scrotal	L	A bag	
sperm	GR	Seed	
stenosis	GR	A narrowing	Pyloric stenosis: narrowing of the opening between the stomach and duodenum due to hypertrophy
stomach	GR	Gullet	
sub-	L	Under, below	
supra-	L	Above, beyond, or on top of	
tera-	GR	Monster, a wonder	Teratogenesis: development of physical deformities in an embryo

Word	Origin	Meaning	Examples
thanato-	GR	Death ("thanatos")	Thanatophoric dwarfism: a fatal form of dwarfism
thrombo-	GR	Clot, a lump ("thrombos")	
thyroid	GR	Shield, form	
topo-	GR	Place or locale	See *ecto-*
tropho-	GR	Nutrition	Trophoblast (see *-blast*)
umbilicus	L	Navel	
uterus	L	Womb	
villus	L	Tuft of hair	Chorionic villi: tiny vascular projections of the chorionic surface
zygote	GR	Yoked, united	Sperm penetrates the ovum resulting in fertilization; the union of the sperm and ovum

This table was created using *Webster's New Universal Unabridged Dictionary,* published in 1996. Please note that word origins may vary from dictionary to dictionary.

FR = French; GR = Greek; L = Latin.

SUGGESTED READING LIST

Abbitt P: *Ultrasound: A Pattern Approach.* New York, McGraw-Hill, Inc., 1995.

Anderhub B: *General Sonography: A Clinical Guide.* St. Louis, Mosby, 1995.

Berman M, Cohen H: *Diagnostic Medical Sonography: Obstetrics and Gynecology,* 2nd ed. Philadelphia, Lippincott, 1997.

Callen P: *Ultrasonography in Obstetrics and Gynecological Sonography,* 4th ed. Philadelphia, WB Saunders, 2000.

Gill K: *Abdominal Ultrasound: A Practitioner's Guide.* Philadelphia, Saunders, 2001.

Hagen-Ansert S: *Textbook of Diagnostic Ultrasonography,* 5th ed. Philadelphia, Mosby, 2001.

Hagen-Ansert S: *Abdominal Ultrasound Study Guide and Exam Review.* St. Louis, Mosby, 1996.

Hickey J, Goldberg F: *Ultrasound Review of the Abdomen, Male Pelvis and Small Parts.* Philadelphia, Lippincott, 1998.

Hickey J, Goldberg F: *Ultrasound Review of Obstetrics and Gynecology.* Philadelphia, Lippincott, 1996.

Jaffee R, Pierson R, Abramowicz J: *Imaging in Infertility and Reproductive Endocrinology.* Philadelphia, Lippincott, 1995.

Kawamura D: *Diagnostic Medical Sonography: Abdomen and Superficial Structures,* 2nd ed. Philadelphia, Lippincott, 1997.

Kurtz A: *Ultrasound: The Requisites.* St. Louis, Mosby, 1996.

Nyberg D, Hill L, Bohm-Velez M, et al: *Transvaginal Ultrasound.* St. Louis, Mosby, 1992.

Rumack C: *Diagnostic Ultrasound,* vols 1 and 2, 2nd ed. St. Louis, Mosby, 1998.

Sanders R, Miner N (eds): *Clinical Sonography: A Practical Guide,* 3rd ed. Philadelphia, Lippincott, 1998.

Sanders R (ed): *Structural Fetal Abnormalities: The Total Picture.* St. Louis, Mosby, 1996.

Answers and Explanations

1. **E** [13,II]. **Linear array transducers** are also called sequential array transducers. *Curved linear transducers* are also sequential, but have a transducer surface in the shape of an arc. *Phased array transducers* are more or less square in shape and produce a pie-shaped image. A *mechanical sector transducer* is round; a soundbeam-deflecting mirror produces a sector-shaped image. *Intracavitary transducers* are small transducers that are sector or arc shaped and placed on the end of a catheter.

2. **A** [8,VI]. The retroperitoneum, particularly within the **psoas muscle,** is a likely site for a hematoma in a patient with a bleeding disorder such as hemophilia. Although the *spleen, liver, posterior cul-de-sac,* and *beneath the diaphragm* are also popular locations for fluid collections, the psoas muscle is the best answer given the patient's history.

3. **B** [8,II]. The **prone oblique decubitus** position is the best view to visualize the retroperitoneum around the kidneys while avoiding bowel gas that may obscure this area in a *supine* position.

4. **A** [8,IV]. The retroperitoneum is a common site for fluid collections that can be readily evaluated with ultrasound. The **spleen** is intraperitoneal, not retroperitoneal.

5. **C** [10,V]. Crohn's disease is an inflammatory bowel disease that most commonly affects the terminal ileum. The only finding listed that is not consistent with Crohn's disease is **lack of color flow Doppler signals.** Vascularity is typically increased in the presence of bowel inflammation.

6. **B** [6,V]. Benign prostatic hypertrophy is an enlargement of the prostate gland. It is not an infection; therefore, there is no **fever.** *Renal failure* and consequent *increased creatinine* levels may occur if the enlarged prostate causes urethral obstruction (thereby affecting the *urinary stream*) and subsequent hydronephrosis.

7. **E** [6,IV]. Seminal vesicles cysts are as a rule an incidental finding on a transrectal ultrasound study. *Prostatic calculi* are also readily seen with ultrasound. **Peyronie's disease** is a painful curvature of the penis when erect. Ultrasound findings include calcifications in the penis; these images are obtained with a small parts transducer.

8. **D** [11,IV]. **Abnormally low serum calcium levels** are not an indication for neck ultrasound. However, elevated serum calcium levels may be indicative of parathyroid disease, which is an acceptable indication for neck ultrasound.

9. **C** [11,I]. The normal size of a parathyroid gland is 5 mm, not **1 cm.**

10. **C** [11,II]. Thyroid masses, whether *malignant* or *benign,* are vascular. Color flow Doppler helps to delineate a mass that is isoechoic to the normal gland, consequently proving that it **is indeed a mass.**

11. **A** [11,VII]. This mass is most likely a **thyroglossal duct cyst,** which is an embryologic remnant developing in a midline location. *Branchial cleft cysts* and *lymph nodes* are more laterally placed. *Adenomas* are not typically cystic.

12. **E** [11,VIII]. Usually, an enlarged parathyroid gland is a cause of hypercalcemia. The **kidneys should be evaluated for renal calculi.** In addition, the remaining parathyroid glands should be examined because more than one gland may be enlarged in hyperparathyroidism.

13. **C** [11,II]. A high-frequency transducer (i.e., **7.5 MHz** or higher) is the best choice when imaging structures that lie close to the near field, such as the thyroid. If a lower frequency transducer has to be used, a standoff pad will help to place the area of interest further away from the probe, avoiding near field reverberation artifacts. A *sector scanner* may place important information out of the field of view because of its pie-shaped image.

14. **A** [11,VI]. **Thyroid adenomas** are benign masses that are usually multiple and typically have a halo appearance. *Hashimoto's disease* is a generalized disease of the entire thyroid gland. In *Graves' disease* (also referred to as diffuse hyperthyroidism) the thyroid gland appears hypoechoic and enlarged. *Thyroid cancer* is rare; typically the mass has irregular borders and no halo.

15. **D** [11,I]. **The common carotid artery lies lateral to the thyroid lobe; the internal jugular vein lies lateral to the common carotid artery.** The carotid artery does not divide into the *internal and external carotid arteries* until a level superior to the thyroid lobe.

16. **C** [11,II]. The isthmus is a very anterior structure; therefore, it may be obscured by near field reverberation artifacts. Both a *standoff pad* and a *higher frequency transducer* are helpful when imaging structures in the near field. *Color flow Doppler* may delineate a mass that blends in with surrounding normal tissue. *More acoustic gel* will ensure proper contact on the skin. However, even a **slight increase in pressure** may displace the structure under the transducer.

17. **A** [11,X]. The sonographer is most likely to find a **hypoechoic, homogeneous mass with an echogenic center lateral to the internal jugular vein.** This is a typical location for an enlarged *lymph node*, which fits with the patient's history.

18. **E** [11,III]. An <u>iodine deficiency</u> is responsible for endemic goiters, which typically appear as a diffusely enlarged thyroid gland on a sonogram. Thyroid function is measured by radioimmune assay of *triiodothyronine* (T_3) *and thyroxine* (T_4) levels, which would be decreased in iodine deficiency (endemic goiter) and increased in Graves' disease. In the United States, <u>multinodular</u> goiters are more common than endemic goiters. It is thought that the gland is damaged by a viral infection and responds by developing the nodules; **thyroid-stimulating hormone** can be mildly elevated to stimulate adequate function of thyroid hormone.

19. **D** [9,I]. The **renal arteries** are responsible for carrying 15%–30% of the total cardiac output. The *common carotid artery* supplies blood to the brain. The *superior mesenteric artery* supplies most of the small intestine and parts of the colon. The *common iliac arteries* branch off of the abdominal aorta at the level of bifurcation and supply the pelvic region.

20. **D** [8,I]. The **spleen** is an intraperitoneal structure, with the exception of a portion of the hilum.

21. **C** [1,I]. The **bare area,** in contact with the diaphragm, is the only portion of the liver that is not covered by visceral peritoneum.

22. **B** [1,I]. In the fetus, the right branch of the umbilical vein becomes the ductus venosus, which goes into the inferior vena cava. After birth, the ductus venosus becomes a fibrous cord called the **ligamentum venosum.** The *main lobar fissure* separates the right and left lobes of the liver. The *ligamentum teres* is the remnant of the left umbilical vein. The *hepatoduodenal ligament* surrounds the portal triad.

23. **A** [1,I]. The **main portal vein** and the *hepatic artery* are responsible for supplying the liver with oxygen and nutrients; however, the main portal vein is the larger contributor. The *common bile duct* drains waste products from the liver, and it is not a vessel.

The *celiac artery* (or axis) is the first branch off of the aorta it divides into the splenic artery, common hepatic artery, and often the left gastric artery. The *hepatic veins* drain the blood from the liver.

24. **B** [9,IX]. The waveforms of the *hepatic vein, jugular vein, femoral vein,* and *inferior vena cava* all vary with respiration. Only the **portal vein** waveform does not vary with respiration.

25. **B** [2,I]. **Cholecystokinin** allows the sphincter of Oddi to relax. Bile is released into the cystic duct, then into the common bile duct, and finally into the duodenum. *Bilirubin* is a product of the breakdown of old red blood cells that are converted into bile pigments. *Cholesterol* is a fat-soluble steroid alcohol found in animal food products. *Lecithin* is a phospholipid found in the liver and other structures and is responsible for metabolism of fats. *Renin* is an enzyme produced in the kidneys that affects blood pressure.

26. **B** [1,III]. **Alanine aminotransferase (ALT)** is also known as serum glutamic pyruvic transaminase (SGPT). It is the most specific laboratory test for liver function. ALT is an enzyme produced in the hepatocytes, and there are high concentrations of ALT in the liver. *Alkaline phosphatase* is an enzyme produced in the bile ducts, kidneys, bones, intestines, and placenta. *Serum protein* is any protein in blood serum. *α-Fetoprotein* (*AFP*) is present in the developing embryo and fetus; a high level in maternal serum or amniotic fluid is useful in the detection of spina bifida in the fetus. In adults, AFP is abnormal in liver disease and cancer, although it is not a specific marker.

27. **E** [1,III]. **Acid phosphatase** is not affected by normal liver functions; it is an enzyme elevated by some bone metastases. Alkaline phosphatase is elevated in some liver diseases.

28. **A** [1,III]. **Vitamin K** levels decrease in hepatocellular disease, resulting in a prolonged prothrombin time (PT). Prolonged PT carries a poor prognosis, but can revert to normal if the liver damage is reversed.

29. **D** [1,V]. Of the choices listed, only **intravenous antibiotics** are not a cause of fatty infiltration of the liver. Isolated fatty infiltration of the liver is a benign, reversible disorder that affects the hepatocytes and may interfere with liver function.

30. **E** [2,V]. The normal common bile duct increases in size by approximately 1 mm per decade, so an 8-mm duct is a *normal finding in an 80-year-old patient.* Duct size may normally increase *after cholecystectomy.* *Biliary obstruction* would be present in a 25-year-old patient with an 8-mm duct; **in an unobstructed duct, the width does not increase if food is eaten.** A poststenotic *hepatic artery* can

reach a size of 8 mm and may occasionally lie anterior to the duct; however, color flow Doppler will show it is a vessel.

31. **B** [9,IX]. In a normal patient, Doppler signals will change from **high resistance** to low resistance when the patient goes from a <u>fasting</u> to a postprandial state.

32. **E** [9,IX]. The renal arteries receive 15%–30% of the cardiac output and are a common site for aneurysm and *stenosis*. If vascular *hypertension* results, it is treatable. Color flow Doppler is useful in diagnosing renal artery vascular disease, which may be present in a patient with an *abdominal bruit, hypertension,* or a *small kidney*. **Renal calculi** are not an indication for renal artery Doppler imaging unless there are additional findings.

33. **D** [4,XIV]. Doppler findings are abnormal in *renal artery stenosis, renal vein thrombosis, rejection,* and *acute tubular necrosis*. Only a **urinoma** will result in normal findings on Doppler imaging.

34. **A** [4,XV]. **Schistosomiasis** is a common disease in semitropical areas (e.g., Egypt) that is caused by worms found in fresh water. Infection results when the worms puncture the skin and migrate to the bladder via the venous or lymphatic systems. *Ascaris* is a worm found in tropical regions that develops in the biliary system. *Hydatid disease* occasionally affects the kidneys, but not the bladder. *Malaria* is a tropical infection that causes anemia and splenomegaly. *Glycogen storage disease* is not an infection, and is unrelated to parasites.

35. **C** [1,VIII]. **Shepherds** are at risk for hydatid disease. The eggs of this parasite are excreted in the feces of infected animals, predominantly sheep, resulting in humans becoming hosts. The liver is the most common site for cyst development.

36. **A** [1,VI]. **Hepatoblastoma** causes liver enlargement and occurs in small children. *Rhabdomyosarcoma* affects the same age-group, but most often develops around the bladder. *Hepatocellular carcinoma* is typically seen in an older population. *Focal nodular hyperplasia* is a benign mass. A *hematoma* is a benign, blood-filled mass secondary to trauma.

37. **B** [2,V]. **Hydrops of the gallbladder** is caused by cystic duct obstruction and results in massive distention of the gallbladder. *Mirizzi syndrome* is a rare complication of untreated acute cholecystitis; a stone in the cystic duct compresses the common bile duct causing bile duct obstruction. Mirizzi syndrome is the only condition in which pathology involving the cystic duct obstructs the common bile duct. Because the gallbladder only acts as a biliary reservoir, blockage of the cystic duct does not cause *jaundice*.

38. **C** [2,VI]. A **Klatskin tumor** is an uncommon carcinoma of the bile ducts that originates at the junction of the right and left hepatic ducts. This poorly defined mass metastasizes late and can be confused with sclerosing cholangitis. *Budd-Chiari syndrome* results from hepatic vein thrombosis and spares the caudate lobe. *Arnold-Chiari malformation* is a cerebral ventricular problem related to spina bifida. *Intraductal metastases* are unlikely to involve this location. *Cystadenocarcinoma* is a tumor of the liver substance or ovaries rather than the bile ducts.

39. **A** [3,I]. Endocrine functions of the pancreas include secretion of glucagon and insulin. **Islet cells** secrete insulin and are found in the *islets of Langerhans,* the site from which endocrine tumors originate. *Acinar cells* secrete digestive enzymes. The production of *red blood cells* occurs in the bone marrow.

40. **D** [3,III]. Lipase is the key word that indicates that the pancreas, not the liver or gallbladder, is involved. The decreased hematocrit indicates that the **pancreatitis is hemorrhagic.** Although *cholelithiasis* can result in pain, nausea, vomiting, and possible distention of the abdomen, an increase in lipase levels and a decrease in hematocrit are not associated clinical findings.

41. **B** [3,VI]. **Adenocarcinomas** comprise almost all malignant tumors of the pancreas and are mostly located in exocrine cells. An *islet cell tumor* is an endocrine tumor of the pancreas. *Cystadenocarcinoma* of the pancreas is a malignant lesion typically located in the tail. *Pseudocysts* are benign masses that result from inflammatory disease, which leads to a walled-off collection of fluid from extravasated pancreatic secretions. *Phlegmon* is also of inflammatory origin and results in a focal edematous mass.

42. **A** [4,III]. **Serum creatinine** is the most sensitive laboratory test for determining renal function. Creatinine forms in the muscles, passes into the blood, and is excreted by the kidneys. *Blood urea nitrogen* is another determinate of renal function that measures the amount of urea nitrogen in the blood. Urea is an end product of protein metabolism. *Specific gravity* measures the kidneys' ability to concentrate urine. A *urinalysis* can detect hematuria and pyuria. A *24-hour urine collection* is typically used to measure the amount of protein in the urine.

43. **A** [4,VII]. A **parenchymal renal cyst** is located in the parenchyma of the kidney and displays the typical characteristics of a cyst. *Parapelvic cysts* do not communicate with the collecting system and are not true cysts, but are derived from the lymphatic system. *Pseudocysts* are usually associated with pancreatitis and are collections of digested material. A *biloma* is a collection of bile that has leaked from a bile duct. A *seroma* is a serum-filled fluid collection with no true walls.

44. **A** [4,VI]. **Transitional cell carcinoma** is a urothelial tumor that develops in the renal pelvis, ureter, or bladder and is the most likely diagnosis in this case. *Hypernephroma*, also referred to as *renal cell carcinoma*, is the most common solid renal mass in adults; however, it develops in the renal parenchyma. An *angiomyolipoma* is a common benign mass composed of fat, vessels, and muscle that develops in the renal parenchyma. *Adenomas* are small, echogenic, parenchymal tumors. *Renal lymphoma* is seen with more widespread disease. It is typically bilateral and presents with enlarged kidneys that contain multiple hypoechoic masses in all regions.

45. **C** [4,VI]. **Renal cell carcinoma,** *adenocarcinoma, Grawitz' tumor,* and *hypernephroma* are all names for the same malignant tumor. It is the only renal tumor that commonly calcifies and invades the renal vein. *Wilms' tumor* is the second most common solid tumor in children. It does not calcify, and it rarely invades the renal vein and inferior vena cava. *Multicystic dysplastic kidney disease* is a benign cystic process. The cysts first seen in infants gradually shrink and may eventually calcify. *Hemangioma* is a benign vascular tumor of the liver that occasionally occurs in the kidney. *Transitional cell carcinoma* is seen in the renal pelvis and is hypoechoic. It does not calcify or invade the renal vein.

46. **C** [4,VII]. **Autosomal dominant (adult) polycystic kidney disease** is a genetic disorder that results in multiple bilateral renal cysts, enlarged kidneys, and hypertension. Berry aneurysms in the circle of Willis may occur with this condition. *Autosomal recessive (infantile) polycystic kidney disease* is a genetic disorder associated with liver fibrosis. *Renal cell carcinoma, transitional cell carcinoma,* and *multicystic dysplastic kidney disease* are not associated with brain lesions.

47. **A** [4,XI]. A **calculus** is intrinsic, with a stone in either the kidney or ureter. *Uterine fibroids, trauma, pregnancy,* and *ovarian neoplasms* are all extrinsic causes of hydronephrosis that are not related to the kidneys, ureters, or bladder. However, when masses related to the adnexa enlarge or a sizable hematoma develops, impingement on the kidneys or ureters can result in hydronephrosis.

48. **B** [4,XI]. Overdistention of the urinary bladder can cause a temporary hydronephrosis that is usually relieved after voiding. Make sure you perform **previoid and postvoid views** if hydronephrosis is found but the bladder is large, particularly in children and transplant patients.

49. **E** [4,XIV]. **Cyclosporine toxicity** has no specific ultrasonic features. *Hydronephrosis, fluid collections, rejection,* and *kinked veins* are sonographically detectable complications of renal transplants.

50. **B** [4,XIV]. **Acute tubular necrosis** is a medical complication caused by ischemic damage to the kidney and is seen at approximately day 2 in most renal transplants. There are no distinctive sonographic features and, if uncomplicated, it is reversible. *Renal obstruction* after renal transplant is important, but not common. *Acute pyelonephritis* is an infectious process not typically associated with transplant failure. *Acute rejection* and *cyclosporine toxicity* usually do not occur within 2 days of a transplant.

51. **B** [4,XIV]. **Bladder distension** is not a feature of rejection. A *decrease in renal size* is associated with chronic rejection, and an increase in renal size is associated with acute rejection. A *high-resistance Doppler pattern* with low to absent end-diastolic flow or reversal of flow is typical of acute rejection. *Increased parenchymal echogenicity* is seen in chronic rejection.

52. **D** [4,IV]. **Benign prostatic hypertrophy** occurs only in older men. Most patients with myelomeningocele have a neurologic bladder. Typical urinary tract problems in children with a neurologic bladder due to myelomeningocele are a *large, trabeculated bladder; dilated ureters;* a *dilated renal pelvis* caused by obstruction or reflux; and infection with consequent *renal calculi.*

53. **B** [5,V]. **Torsion** causes complete infarction of the testicle when there is rotation or twisting of the spermatic cord with subsequent blood loss. *Cryptorchidism* is an undescended testicle and is not associated with pain. *Orchitis* is an inflammation of the testes that can be focal or diffuse. Unlike torsion, Doppler imaging will show increased vascularity in inflammation. *Epididymitis* is inflammation of the epididymis and can be either acute or chronic. A *spermatocele* is a cystic mass at the head of the epididymis or superior to the testicle, along the path of the vas deferens. It is filled with nonviable sperm, fat, cellular debris, and lymphocytes.

54. **A** [5,IV]. Cryptorchidism (i.e., undescended testicles) predisposes to cancer development. **Seminoma** is the most common germ cell tumor in the testicle. Undescended testicles are also associated with *infertility. Torsion, epididymitis, hydroceles,* and *spermatoceles* are not specifically associated with undescended testicles.

55. **D** [7,X]. Infarction is a loss of the blood supply that leads to a decrease in splenic size; a *thrombus in the splenic artery* would clearly accomplish this. *Bacterial endocarditis* can lead to splenic abscess and splenic infarction. *Sickle cell anemia* is a hematologic disorder that initially leads to splenomegaly; however, repeated infarctions often result in asplenia. A **splenic cyst** is not associated with infarction.

56. **A** [7,IX]. The thin-walled spleen is the most commonly ruptured internal organ; therefore, **splenic rupture** should be the primary concern when examining this patient. An *abscess* would be associated with elevation in temperature. *Renal artery aneurysms* are uncommon and are not usually of traumatic origin, unless caused by needle puncture. The *gallbladder* is located on the right side of the body and is not a typical site for rupture caused by trauma. The prostate is most unlikely to rupture unless there are pelvic factures, and *obstruction of the prostate* would not cause these symptoms.

57. **B** [12,V (BREAST)]. **Fibroadenomas** are the most common benign tumors in the breast. Slow growing and stimulated by estrogen, these solid tumors have homogeneous, low-level internal echoes and smooth borders. *Cysts* are anechoic, round, benign masses with good through transmission. *Galactoceles* are seen in lactating women and are typically anechoic. *Cystosarcoma phyllodes* is a large, well-defined, rapidly growing mass. *Ductal carcinoma* is irregularly shaped with acoustic shadowing.

58. **D** [12,V (BREAST)]. **Infiltrating ductal carcinoma** is by far the most common malignant breast tumor in the United States. *Medullary carcinoma* is less common. *Fibroadenoma* is a benign mass. *Lobular carcinoma* originates in the ductules of the lobules and is much less frequent than infiltrating ductal carcinoma. *Paget's disease* in the breast is a rare subvariant of ductal carcinoma that involves the skin.

59. **D** [9,VII]. An arteriovenous shunt, or fistula, is an abnormal communication between an artery and vein. It can be *congenital* or it can be caused by *trauma, surgery,* or an *aneurysm.* **Atherosclerosis** is the build up of cholesterol and lipids in the inner layers of the arterial walls. Gradual occlusion of the vessel occurs, but not arteriovenous fistula formation.

60. **E** [1,VII]. **Bilomas** are extrahepatic collections of bile resulting from trauma to the abdomen, biliary obstruction or surgery, or gallbladder disease. *Hematomas* are blood filled and result from blunt or penetrating trauma. *Choledochal cysts* are congenital dilations of the common bile duct. *Lymphoceles* usually result from surgery and are filled with lymph. *Urinomas* are extravasated urine from damage to the urinary tract.

61. **A** [10,I]. Although the *gallbladder* may border the lateral aspect of the C-loop of the duodenum, the **main lobar fissure** that connects the gallbladder to the portal vein is superior and lateral to the C-loop of the duodenum.

62. **B** [10,V]. The patient in this scenario presents with the typical history for **acute appendicitis.** *Gall-stones, pancreatitis, renal colic,* and *ulcerative colitis* do not typically cause this group of symptoms.

63. **D** [10,V]. **Polyps** are small, benign growths arising in many different organs. A *tubo-ovarian abscess,* a *torsed ovarian cyst,* a *ruptured ectopic pregnancy,* and *Crohn's disease* are all located in the pelvis and are good differential diagnoses for appendicitis. A good clinical history that includes patient gender, age, the date of the last normal menstrual period, and the presence or absence of fever and diarrhea helps to narrow the differential diagnosis.

64. **C** [11,V]. **Hashimoto's disease** is a form of autoimmune thyroiditis. It is a chronic, progressive inflammatory disease seen more frequently in women. It appears sonographically as a coarse lobular pattern to the thyroid. *Adenomas* are benign thyroid neoplasms that are usually multiple. *Multinodular and endemic goiters* are composed of multiple small masses and are not inflammatory in origin.

65. **B** [9,V]. Infective aneurysms are called **mycotic aneurysms.** *Pseudoaneurysms* have a wall composed of blood clot; the true wall of the blood vessel has burst. The terms *saccular* and *fusiform* refer to aneurysms of a particular shape. *Berry aneurysms* are found in the brain.

66. **B** [1,I]. The **hepatic veins** define the separation between the lobes and segments of the liver. The *umbilical vein* is no longer patent after birth. There is no *portal artery.* The portal vein and *hepatic arteries* supply the liver with oxygen and nutrients but do not separate the lobes. The *inferior vena cava* does not separate the lobes of the liver.

67. **A** [9,IX]. Because of their close proximity to the right atrium, **hepatic veins** exhibit a pulsatile, choppy flow. Normal *portal veins* have a nonpulsatile, even flow. The *hepatic arteries* have a low-resistance arterial pattern. In normal patients, the *superior mesenteric artery* Doppler signal changes from a high- to low-resistance arterial pattern when the patient goes from a fasting to postprandial state. The *iliac veins* do not normally pulsate, although the veins vary with respiration.

68. **D** [13,III]. **Picture-archiving systems (PACs)** are digital-archiving and image-storage devices that allow a true representation of the actual image seen on the monitor. Image quality does not deteriorate over time. There is some distortion of a *videotape* image, although very high quality videotape can largely compensate for this spatial resolution problem and long-term image-quality deterioration. There are several variations in *thermal paper* recording; some have better resolution than others, but most fade with time and exposure to light. *Polaroid film* was widely used in the 1970s, but because of cost, fading,

and storage problems it has been replaced by other recording methods. *Radiographic film* is still commonly used and allows for multiple images on a single sheet. This film requires the use of a darkroom and x-ray processor. Radiographic film can be subject to fog, and the chemicals used in processing may cause inconsistencies. When using radiographic film, the settings on the recording device must be carefully manipulated so that the image quality represents what is seen on the monitor.

69. **E** [2,VI]. **Gallbladder cancer** is a common biliary tract malignancy with increased frequency in Native Americans and workers in the automotive, rubber, textile, and fabric industries. It is associated with gallstones up to 90% of the time and with porcelain gallbladder. *Empyema* refers to pus in the gallbladder. *Cholecystitis* is an inflammatory process that leads to generalized, not localized, wall thickening. *Adenomyomatosis* is a benign condition leading to generalized thickening of the mucosa and cholesterol crystals in the Rokitansky-Aschoff sinuses, which exhibit bright reflectors with comet tail artifacts near the wall. *Hemobilia* refers to blood in the biliary system, and it does not cause wall thickening.

70. **C** [2,VIII]. By convention, the gallbladder wall is measured on the **anterior surface,** perpendicular to the gallbladder in the short axis and at right angles to the long axis. The anterior surface is usually where there is the best resolution.

71. **C** [2,V]. **Hydrops of the gallbladder** is caused by complete blockage of the cystic duct, leading to an increase in gallbladder size secondary to bile accumulation. A *biloma* is a bile collection. *Acalculous cholecystitis* refers to an inflammatory condition without gallstones. *Papilloma* and *megacystic* are not terms used in reference to the gallbladder.

72. **B** [4,XIII]. Renal sinus lipomatosis is the term used for increased fat deposition in the renal sinus resulting in **increased echogenicity and size of the renal pelvis.** It is a benign condition associated with <u>obesity</u>, chronic infection, or advanced age of the patient. Occasionally, areas of renal sinus lipomatosis can look hypoechoic and be mistaken for other pathology.

73. **B** [12,I (MUSCULOSKELETAL)]. The **diaphragm** refers to the muscle and tendon that separates the chest and abdominal cavities. The *internal oblique muscles* are fibers that run at 90° angles to the *external oblique muscles,* which are on the outer surface of the lower eight ribs and are the most superficial of the muscles. The *transversus abdominus muscles* are deep in relation to the internal oblique muscles and run horizontally. The paired *rectus abdominus muscles* run longitudinally from the front of the symphysis pubis and pubic crest.

74. **C** [8,I]. Also known as the cul-de-sac, the **pouch of Douglas** is a common site for fluid collections because of its dependent position posterior to the uterus. *Morison's pouch* is the potential space between the liver and right kidney. *Hartmann's pouch* is the proximal portion of the gallbladder. The *sacral and Chiari pouches* do not exist.

75. **E** [7,II]. In the **right lateral decubitus** position, the patient's left side is up. In a coronal view taken with the patient in this position, the spleen is relatively accessible when the patient takes a full inspiration. The spleen is difficult to see in the *prone* position because it is obscured by ribs. A *reverse Trendelenburg* position could further obscure the spleen by displacing it cranially. The *erect* position is a good fallback if the spleen cannot be found when the patient is lying down.

76. **D** [1,V]. A **lobular outline to the liver** is a feature of *cirrhosis,* not hepatitis. *Prominent portal vessels,* a *thickened gallbladder wall, splenomegaly,* and a *hypoechoic liver* are all seen in hepatitis. Prominent portal vessels, giving rise to the "starry night" appearance, are caused by edema of the liver.

77. **B** [9,V]. When **congestive heart failure** involves the right side of the heart, venous pressure rises and the hepatic veins and inferior vena cava dilate. In *portal hypertension,* the pressure increase is in the liver; collaterals form and shunt the blood via alternate routes other than the vena cava to the heart. *Uremia, hypertension,* and *mitral valve prolapse* do not affect the size of the inferior vena cava.

78. **D** [11,XI]. The *brachiocephalic trunk or artery* arises from the aorta and bifurcates into the right common carotid and subclavian arteries. The **right common carotid artery** does not normally arise from the aorta.

79. **A** [4,XII]. Renal vein thrombosis is uncommon; however, thrombosis with *low-level echoes* is occasionally seen in the main renal vein. A high-resistance arterial waveform in the renal artery with *no venous flow* detected on Doppler makes the diagnosis. There will not be **renal vein dilation distal to the thrombus** because of the lack of flow. The kidney will be *enlarged.*

80. **C** [4,XII]. This patient's symptoms are typical of those seen in **renal vein thrombosis.** *Renal cysts* and *multicystic kidneys* are typically asymptomatic, unless very large. *Pyonephrosis* causes fever. A *neuroblastoma* is a malignant adrenal tumor in children that would be unlikely to be associated with hematuria.

81. **E** [1,V]. Cirrhosis of the liver is a chronic, progressive disease caused by multiple factors that destroy

the liver. **Diabetes mellitus** is caused by faulty insulin production in the pancreas. If uncomplicated, diabetes mellitus does not affect the liver.

82. **B** [1,V]. Cirrhosis is a fibrotic process that causes the *liver to shrink*. An **enlarged liver** occurs in the early stages of alcohol-related liver disease when there is fatty infiltration or hepatitis. A *nodular outline, increased echogenicity,* and *hepatofugal flow of the portal veins* are all features of severe cirrhosis.

 When two choices are directly opposite to one another, one of them is almost certainly the correct answer.

---

83. **D** [1,III]. **Prothrombin time** is a measurement of one of the factors involved in blood clotting; it is affected by the amount of vitamin K. A prolonged prothrombin time is often an indicator of poor liver function. *Bilirubin* is a product of the breakdown of old red blood cells that are converted into bile pigments. *Aspartate aminotransferase (AST)* is associated with hepatitis, cirrhosis, necrosis, injury, metastasis, and fatty changes. *Alanine aminotransferase (ALT)* is more specific to liver disease. *Lactic acid dehydrogenase* is found in multiple organ systems and is typically used to detect myocardial and pulmonary infarction.

84. **A** [1,IX]. Because of its location, a subcapsular hematoma is **curvilinear** in shape. Blood, depending on its age, may be *anechoic,* **hypoechoic,** or echogenic.

85. **D** [2,I]. An **isthmus** is a band of tissue connecting two parts, as in the thyroid. No isthmus is present in the gallbladder. *Hartmann's pouch* is the name for the portion of the gallbladder between the neck of the gallbladder and the cystic duct.

86. **B** [2,IV]. **Melena** refers to black, tarry stool that contains digested blood, usually from an upper gastrointestinal tract bleeding disorder. *Nausea and vomiting, right upper quadrant pain, chest pain,* and *right shoulder pain* (referred from shared nerves) are all associated with gallbladder disease.

87. **C** [2,VII]. Gallstones are composed of either **cholesterol** or calcium bilirubinate; however, most are composed of cholesterol. *Sludge,* a precursor of gallstones, contains high levels of calcium bilirubinate and cholesterol crystals and is caused by stasis of bile. *Uric acid, cysteine,* and *xanthine* are all components of urinary tract calculi.

88. **D** [3,I]. The **pancreas** is an important endocrine and exocrine organ. The *gallbladder, appendix, uterus,* and *spleen* are all nonessential to life.

89. **A** [2,I]. Isolated **fatty infiltration of the liver** is not associated with gallbladder wall thickening. *Acute cholecystitis, AIDS, ascites,* and *hypoalbuminemia* all cause gallbladder wall thickening.

90. **C** [4,I]. The *formation,* storage, and *excretion* of urine, which removes waste products from the body, are the main functions of the urinary system. This in turn *regulates blood pressure* and *controls blood concentration.* The **regulation of body temperature** is controlled by the hypothalamus.

91. **B** [4,III]. **Red blood cells** (or erythrocytes) are found in the circulating blood and transport oxygen. Red blood cells are seen in urine only when a cause of bleeding is located in the urinary tract. *Water, carbon dioxide, nitrogenous waste,* and *protein* are normally excreted in urine.

92. **A** [4,XIII]. Ectopic refers to a structure that is out of place. An **ectopic kidney** is one that is normally formed but located in an unusual position, usually the pelvis. Most (i.e., 90%) of *crossed renal ectopic kidneys* are fused. *Pancake kidneys, horseshoe kidneys,* and *duplicated kidneys* are fusion anomalies.

93. **E** [4,XIII]. The prefix "a-" refers to an absence of something; **renal agenesis** is a condition in which a kidney is absent. The prefix "dys-" refers to pain; therefore, *renal dysgenesis* is a painful kidney. *Renal noesis, renal dysamyomenosis,* and *arenaluria* do not exist.

94. **B** [4,VIII]. Both history and description favor a gas-filled **abscess.** None of the other entities contain gas.

95. **C** [4,VIII]. The prefix "pyo-" refers to pus; therefore, **pyonephrosis** is the correct answer. *Acute and focal pyelonephritis* are infections that form in the renal parenchyma but do not form pus. *Lobar nephronia* is another name for focal pyelonephritis. A *renal abscess* is filled with pus but is located in the parenchyma, not the renal pelvis.

96. **B** [4,I]. The kidney is surrounded by **perirenal fat.** *Glisson's capsule* surrounds the liver, with the exception of the bare area. The *renal capsule* and *cortex* are both part of the kidney. The *tunica albuginea* surrounds the testicle.

97. **A** [6,I]. The prostate contains three zones. The **peripheral zone** is posterolateral and occupies most of the apex; 70% of cancers are detected in this zone. The *central zone* surrounds the ejaculatory ducts and houses 20% of glandular tissue and 10% of prostate cancers. The *transitional zone* is a bilobed area composed of glandular and stromal elements; benign prostatic hypertrophy originates in this zone.

98. **B** [6,III]. **Increased prostate-specific antigen (PSA)** is the most sensitive of the tests listed for detecting prostate cancer; however, it is not very specific. Many cancerous nodules cannot be palpated and many cannot be distinguished from the remainder of the prostate with ultrasound.

99. **D** [5,VII]. A cystic space around the testicle is most likely a hydrocele. Hydroceles can be *congenital*, idiopathic, or *acquired*. They can also develop after *trauma* or *infection*. Hydroceles do not occur with uncomplicated testicular **malignancy.**

100. **D** [4,III]. Blood urea nitrogen is a measure of renal function. It increases in renal failure, parenchymal disease, obstructive uropathy, **dehydration,** and hemorrhage. It decreases in *overhydration, pregnancy, liver failure,* and *decreased protein intake.*

101. **E** [4,III]. Leukocytosis is an abnormal increase in white blood cells typically accompanying a bacterial infection. **Pyelonephritis** is a bacterial infection associated with a rise in the white blood cell count. *Benign prostatic hypertrophy, AIDS, anemia,* and *goiter* do not cause an increase in white blood cells.

102. **B** [7,I]. *Accessory spleens* can match this description, but they are small, not "sizable." The prefix "poly-" means many or multiple; therefore, the best answer is **polysplenia.** *Ectopic and wandering spleens* are not located in the splenic fossa and are single.

103. **D** [7,X]. **Splenic infarcts** are commonly caused by homozygous sickle cell anemia and result in decreased spleen size. Splenomegaly, or enlargement of the spleen, occurs for a variety of reasons, including systemic disorders, portal hypertension (perhaps as a result of *portal vein thrombosis* or *cirrhosis*), infectious diseases (e.g., *mononucleosis*), hematologic disorders (e.g., *thalassemia*), lymphoma, leukemia, and AIDS.

104. **A** [9,V]. **Marfan's syndrome** is an autosomal dominant condition. Typically, patients with Marfan's syndrome are very tall with somewhat coarse features. In Marfan's syndrome, the fibers in the media of the aorta have a tendency to become fragmented, leading to an aneurysm. *Morison's pouch* is the potential space between the right kidney and the liver. *Atherosclerosis, dissecting aortic aneurysm,* and *aortic thrombosis* are all acquired, not congenital, diseases of the aorta.

105. **B** [1,VI]. **Hemangiomas** are benign, vascular tumors. *Hepatomas* are malignant. *Lymphomas* are malignant neoplasms of lymphoid tissue. *Hepatic adenomas* are glandular epithelial tumors. *Focal nodular hyperplasia* is benign, relatively rare, and can appear hypoechoic or hyperechoic. Neither hepatic adenoma nor focal nodular hyperplasia is highly vascular.

106. **B** [2,I]. **Rokitansky-Aschoff sinuses** are outpouchings of the gallbladder mucosa. These cavities may be filled with cholesterol crystals in adenomyomatosis. *Maxillary sinuses* are air-filled spaces in the bones of the face. The *pouch of Douglas* is a potential space in the pelvis posterior to the uterus. *Hartmann's pouch* is at the proximal part of the gallbladder. *Morison's pouch* is the potential space between the right kidney and the liver.

107. **D** [2,III]. **Presbyductia** is a term used to describe the normal enlargement of the common bile duct with age. Although hyperbilirubinemia is usually associated with *liver disease* or *biliary obstruction,* it can occur in the presence of *destruction of red blood cells,* as in hemolytic anemia.

108. **A** [2,V]. **Sclerosing cholangitis** is the result of inflammation and scarring of the bile ducts. Although the ducts may be obstructed, scarring prevents duct dilation. *Pneumobilia* is air in the biliary system from a surgical anastomosis between the bowel and biliary tree (e.g., sphincterectomy) or from gallstone ileus, in which a stone has perforated into the gut from the biliary tree. *Mirizzi syndrome* is a rare complication of untreated acute cholecystitis. An inflamed stone in the cystic duct is surrounded by so much edema that it compresses and obstructs the common bile duct. *Choledocholithiasis* is a stone in the bile ducts. *Klatskin tumor* is uncommon and is sometimes confused with sclerosing cholangitis. It is a cancer of the bile ducts that originates at the junction of the right and left hepatic ducts.

109. **B** [5,VI]. The majority of intratesticular tumors are **malignant.** The most common intratesticular tumors are seminomas, which are hypoechoic. Embryonal cell cancer, the second most common intratesticular tumor, has a more *complex* pattern. Teratomas are rare and may contain *cystic* or *echogenic* areas.

110. **A** [5,VI]. The majority of extratesticular masses are **benign.** Extratesticular masses include hydroceles, varicoceles, epididymal cysts, spermatoceles, and hernias. Most extratesticular masses are cystic.

111. **C** [5,VI]. **Choriocarcinoma** is an irregularly shaped tumor with cystic and calcified regions, which elevates the level of human chorionic gonadotropin. None of the other tumors mentioned are associated with abnormal laboratory values when confined to the testes.

112. **D** [5,VI]. **Seminomas,** germ cell tumors, account for 40%–50% of testicular tumors. Seminomas

usually occur between the third and fifth decades of life and have a good prognosis.

113. **B** [5,VII]. **Varicoceles,** seen in 40% of infertile men, can be associated with a low sperm count. Sonographically, there are tortuous veins situated superior and posterolateral to the testicles. *Epididymal cysts* can occur anywhere along the epididymis and are anechoic with posterior enhancement. *Spermatoceles,* although filled with sperm, are not associated with infertility.

114. **C** [5,VII]. Sonographically, the normal testicles can be differentiated from the hernia; however, the surrounding gut may look like a neoplasm. The presence of bowel **peristalsis** differentiates the gut from other processes.

115. **B** [8,V]. Because of its thick walls and high internal pressure, the **aorta** cannot be compressed by enlarged lymph nodes.

116. **E** [8,V]. Lymph nodes are small, oval structures that filter lymph and fight off infection. They are typically housed in areas such as the *groin,* axilla, neck, *para-aortic region, renal hilum,* and *porta hepatis.* Lymph nodes are not found **under the diaphragm.**

117. **C** [12,I (BREAST)]. As women age, **fatty tissue increases and glandular tissue regresses.**

118. **E** [12,II (BREAST)]. **Gynecomastia** is an abnormal increase in the size of one or both breasts in a man. It is usually a temporary, benign condition caused by hormonal imbalance. For a woman, a *family history of breast cancer* is pertinent. A *localized mass, nipple discharge,* and any *pain or tenderness* are all important clinical indications.

119. **D** [12,VI (BREAST)]. **Simple cysts have smooth walls, no internal echoes, and good through transmission.** *Fibroadenomas and medullary cell carcinomas have very similar sonographic appearances. Lactating breasts are difficult to examine* because of prominent glandular tissue. *Hematomas* are usually caused by trauma. *Breast malignancies are poorly circumscribed* and are associated with shadowing.

120. **C** [9,I]. The **celiac axis** is the first branch to leave the aorta that is easily visualized with ultrasound.

121. **A** [9,I]. The aorta bifurcates into the **iliac arteries.**

122. **D** [9,I]. The superior mesenteric vein and splenic vein join to form the **main portal vein** at the portal confluence, posterior to the pancreatic neck.

123. **D** [9,I]. The **left renal vein** passes between the aorta and the superior mesenteric artery.

124. **C** [9,I]. The only vessel normally seen posterior to the inferior vena cava is the **right renal artery.**

125. **A** [9,I]. The portal confluence is composed of the **superior mesenteric vein, splenic vein, and portal vein.** The portal confluence is where the splenic vein and superior mesenteric vein come together to form the main portal vein.

126. **B** [1,II]. A high **transverse view close to the diaphragm** best shows the three hepatic veins. The veins join the inferior vena cava just below the diaphragm. *Longtudinal views* only show a single vein.

127. **A** [1,I]. The **sphincter of Oddi** is at the entrance of the common bile duct and pancreatic duct into the duodenum; it does not lie in the porta hepatis. *Glisson's capsule* refers to the fibrous tissue surrounding the portal veins, bile ducts, and hepatic arteries as they travel together in the liver. Glisson's capsule also surrounds the liver. The common hepatic duct becomes the *common bile duct* at the point where it is joined by the cystic duct, which is in the porta hepatis.

128. **C** [3,I]. The **gastroduodenal artery** is a landmark for the anterior aspect of the pancreatic head.

129. **B** [1,I]. Hepatic veins do not have **echogenic walls.**

130. **A** [9,I]. The gastroduodenal artery is a branch of the **common hepatic artery.**

131. **B** [9,I]. The **hepatic artery** normally runs between the common bile duct and the portal vein. It may have a tortuous course and usually bifurcates proximal to the bifurcation of the common hepatic duct.

132. **E** [3,I]. The **inferior vena cava** lies posterior to the head of the pancreas.

133. **C** [9,I]. The **intima, media, and adventitia** are the three layers that compose an arterial wall.

134. **A** [1,II]. Budd-Chiari syndrome is characterized by thrombosis of the **hepatic veins** and may be associated with ascites and liver failure.

135. **B** [1,I]. The **common bile duct is not always anterior to the hepatic artery;** occasionally, the hepatic artery runs anterior to the common bile duct as a normal variant.

 Watch out for words such as "always" and "never;" there are few absolutes in human anatomy.

136. **C** [9,I]. The normal **inferior vena cava does not lie to the left of the aorta.**

137. **D** [1,V]. Portal hypertension refers to an increase in pressure in the portal venous system, usually caused by liver disease or possibly portal vein thrombosis. **Hepatic artery thrombosis** is not a typical result of portal hypertension; however, the portal vein often becomes thrombosed in portal hypertension. *Collaterals* and *splenomegaly* result from the pressure being reversed or forced to create new paths.

138. **A** [1,V]. **Common bile duct obstruction** is not associated with hepatofugal flow. Hepatofugal flow occurs when the pressure in the portal system of the liver is increased and blood cannot flow through the portal vein. A reversal of the normal direction of flow is detected with Doppler imaging; however, a *poor Doppler angle* may create *false direction of flow.*

139. **A** [1,V]. Blood in the normal portal vein and the hepatic artery is *detectable with Doppler.* In both vessels, the **blood flows in the same direction—hepatopetal flow** (i.e., toward the liver). *Turbulence* is not a characteristic of the flow in either vessel.

140. **C** [9,IX]. The normal portal vein flows continuously into the liver, which makes it a **monophasic waveform.** *Triphasic* describes a waveform seen particularly in the leg arteries and hepatic veins.

141. **C** [9,IX]. **High flow velocity** in the portal vein will evoke a detectable portal vein flow. The presence of a *clot* in the portal vein may obstruct blood flow. From a technical standpoint, a Doppler shift may not be detected with either *low flow velocity* or a *perpendicular transducer angle.*

142. **A** [3,I]. The **splenic artery** normally runs along the posterosuperior aspect of the pancreas.

143. **B** [9,IX]. **Acceleration time** is the most sensitive indication of renal artery stenosis. The *resistive and pulsatility indices* are altered when the process is more severe.

144. **B** [4,VI]. Wilms' tumor is a malignant tumor that occurs in the 1- to 6-year-old age-group and is usually unilateral. However, it is *bilateral* in 10% of cases. Because it is malignant, careful attention must be paid to the *great vessels* for tumor involvement and to the *liver* for metastases. There is no reason to suspect involvement of the **pancreas.**

145. **D** [4,XI]. **Ureteroceles** cause hydronephrosis, usually in the superior component of a duplex kidney. A *rhabdomyosarcoma*, typically found in the bladder or the heart, is a solid sarcomatous mus-cle tumor. It is unlikely that a *bladder diverticulum* would cause hydronephrosis. A *pelvic kidney* is a normal kidney in an ectopic location, but not in the bladder. An *ovarian cyst* would not be found in the bladder.

146. **C** [4,XI]. Because the pelvis is dilated but the ureter is not, the most likely diagnosis is **ureteropelvic junction obstruction.** The level of an obstruction in the urinary system determines the location of the dilation. Typically, everything above the level of the obstruction dilates.

147. **D** [8,VIII]. **Neuroblastomas** usually occur in the adrenal glands and are common in infants. *Wilms' tumor* occurs in the kidney but is rarely seen in infants. A *teratoma* is a benign tumor that usually develops in the sacrococcygeal region. *Infantile polycystic kidney* and *adrenal hemorrhage* are not tumors.

148. **A** [4,VII]. Multicystic dysplastic kidney disease is usually unilateral (not **bilateral**) and is predominately characterized by *cysts of variable sizes.* The condition is *fatal if it is bilateral,* unless there are spared areas. Only a small amount of echogenic parenchyma is present. The parenchyma is not evenly echogenic.

149. **A** [4,I]. Because the renal cortices in infants are more echogenic than in adults, the **renal pyramids appear more prominent.** Be careful not to mistake prominent renal pyramids for renal cysts.

150. **B** [4,XIII]. **Renal agenesis** refers to absent kidneys. If bilateral, renal agenesis is incompatible with life. *Hydronephrosis*, an *enlarged bladder,* a *dilated posterior urethra,* and *hydroureter* are all characteristics of prune-belly syndrome.

151. **B** [4,XI]. *Posterior urethral valves* is the correct answer—a membranous valve usually located in the posterior urethra partially obstructs the urethra. Because the obstruction is located in the urethra it causes dilation of the bladder, ureters, and renal pelves. *Vesicoureteral reflux* is the retrograde flow of urine from the bladder to the ureters and renal pelves and usually presents in female children. It may also present with enlarged ureters, renal pelves, and bladder. *Cryptorchidism* refers to undescended testicles. *Ureteropelvic junction obstruction* is a high ureteral obstruction that is not gender specific.

152. **C** [4,XI]. Because the ureter and kidney lie proximal to the vesicoureteral junction, **hydronephrosis and hydroureter** will be seen.

153. **A** [4,I]. In the normal adult kidney, the echogenic central sinus echoes are mainly composed of **fat** surrounded by the less echogenic *renal pyramids* (*medulla*) and *renal cortex.* The *renal capsule* is a

well-defined, echogenic line around the kidney. In the pediatric patient, the capsule and the central sinus echoes may be difficult to see because of the absence of perinephric and renal sinus fat.

154. **C** [4,II]. Because of the location of the right kidney, the **liver affords the best acoustic window.** The *prone, posterior approach* is sometimes helpful in a pediatric patient with bones that are not calcified enough to cause obstructing acoustic shadows.

155. **E** [4,I]. The correct order from least to greatest echogenicity is the **pyramids, cortex, and sinus fat.** In a normal individual of any age the sinus echoes, and to a lesser extent the cortex, are more echogenic than the pyramids.

156. **E** [4,XIII]. The **echogenicity of the renal parenchyma is normally less than that of the liver, not greater.** A *dromedary hump,* a normal variant, refers to a bulge in the lateral border of the left kidney. A *column of Bertin* is a normal variant of enlarged cortex between groups of calyces.

157. **A** [4,VII]. **Bilateral, enlarged, echogenic kidneys** are seen in autosomal recessive (infantile) polycystic kidney disease. Although *multiple small cysts* are present in infantile polycystic kidneys, they are too small to be resolved with ultrasound and are seen as interfaces.

158. **A** [4,VII]. **Small, shrunken kidneys** are not a feature of adult polycystic kidney disease; in fact, the kidneys become very large. *Renal failure* in adult polycystic kidney disease usually occurs at 40–50 years of age. The cysts may *distort the central sinus echoes* in the kidney. Associated *liver cysts* occur in 40% of cases.

159. **C** [4,II]. An accurate comparison of the renal cortex with the liver requires a consistent standard. The liver texture and echogenicity change in the presence of a parenchymal liver disease, such as **cirrhosis.** This condition would render a comparison invalid.

160. **C** [4,XI]. A **renal vein stent** would not relieve obstruction in the urinary system (i.e., bladder, ureters, kidneys) because it dilates a vascular structure. Apparent hydronephrosis may be caused by overdistension of the bladder, particularly in children and patients with renal transplants. *Voiding* will cause the apparent hydronephrosis to disappear. A *nephrostomy tube, bladder catheterization,* and *prostatectomy* are all techniques that may be used to relieve urinary tract obstruction.

161. **A** [4,VII]. An **angiomyolipoma** is a benign, highly echogenic, vascular tumor; however, the blood flow is usually too slow to be picked up with Doppler. A *staghorn calculus* will appear echogenic with acoustic shadowing. A *renal lymphoma* will appear hypoechoic and is not vascular. *Wilms' tumors* are only moderately echogenic, and *adenomas* are so small they are difficult to see at all.

162. **E** [4,XIII]. A horseshoe kidney has **two collecting systems,** one from each kidney, that are **fused together by an isthmus of tissue.** S̲upernumerary kidney̲ occurs when there are *two normal kidneys and a pelvic kidney. Malrotated kidneys* lie in an unusual axis but are otherwise normal. *Crossed renal ectopia* is a condition in which the *two kidneys are on the same side of the body.*

163. **D** [4,X]. **Nephrocalcinosis** is the term used for the accumulation of small stones in the renal pyramids. *Cystitis* is inflammation of the bladder wall. *Pyelonephritis* refers to an infection in the kidney, and *pyonephrosis* is pus in the collecting system. *Staghorn calculi* are large calculi located in the renal pelves.

164. **B** [4,II]. The urinary bladder is examined transabdominally when it is **distended.** If the patient is unable to fill his bladder, a *catheter* may be placed. A transvaginal approach with an empty bladder may also be helpful in female patients.

165. **E** [4,IV]. **Renal sinus lipomatosis** is a condition found in elderly patients. It causes excessive fatty infiltration in the renal pelvis, but not gross hematuria. *Bladder calculi, benign prostatic hypertrophy, renal stones,* and *bladder tumors* all cause hematuria.

166. **B** [4,VIII]. Low-level echoes in the renal pelvis are suggestive of **pyonephrosis;** another unmentioned possibility is blood in the renal pelvis. If the gain is turned up too high a structure may be artifactually filled with low-level echoes, mimicking pathology. If the *gain is too low,* low-level echoes will be obliterated. *Peripelvic cysts* are not part of the collecting system and will likely be echo-free. *Medullary nephrocalcinosis* does not cause hydronephrosis. A *staghorn calculus* would cause high-level echoes with shadowing rather than low-level echoes.

167. **C** [3,I]. The **uncinate process** extends between the superior mesenteric vein and the aorta. It may also extend posterior to the superior mesenteric artery.

168. **C** [3,I]. Wirsung's duct is the **main pancreatic duct.** There is also an accessory pancreatic duct in the head of the pancreas called Santorini's duct.

169. **D** [3,III]. The **urinary amylase** level is typically *elevated* in acute pancreatitis, especially early in the course of the disease. As with other organs, such as

the prostate, disease may be present but not seen with ultrasound. However, the pancreas is usually hypoechoic and edematous in acute pancreatitis.

170. **A** [3,V]. A shrunken, echogenic pancreas is a feature of **chronic pancreatitis.** Elderly patients and patients with cystic fibrosis also commonly have a small, echogenic pancreas, so the clinical history is important. Edema and enlargement of the pancreas are common in *acute pancreatitis.* A small, echogenic liver characterizes *cirrhosis. Pseudocysts* are associated with acute pancreatitis and appear as cystic or complex fluid collections.

171. **B** [10,I]. The **duodenum** normally encircles the pancreatic head. Watching for peristalsis or filling the duodenum with water by having the patient drink will help differentiate it from a pancreatic mass. The *stomach,* which may also be confused with a mass, lies anterior to the pancreas. A *pancreatic pseudocyst* is not a normal finding. The *gastroduodenal artery* is easily distinguished because it has flow on color flow Doppler.

172. **C** [3,II]. **Gas in the abdomen** will prevent sound transmission. Therefore, ask the patient to avoid ingesting air when drinking the water.

173. **D** [3,VI]. The features described (i.e., dilated common bile duct, ill-defined pancreatic head mass with poor through transmission) are the typical features of **pancreatic cancer.** *Gallstone pancreatitis* and *common bile duct calcification* do not cause this type of mass. *Pseudocysts* should have good through transmission because they are fluid filled. A *hepatoma* is a malignant tumor found in the liver.

174. **E** [3,III]. In acute pancreatitis, **serum amylase** is elevated during the first 24 hours, after which it decreases.

175. **A** [3,II]. The pancreas lies posterior to the inferior portion of the liver, so an **intercostal approach** here would be high and would place the beam at the wrong angle. The *left lobe of the liver* lies anterior to the pancreas (usually) and is a valuable acoustic window. The *spleen* is a fairly useful window to image the pancreatic tail. The *fluid-filled stomach and duodenum* provide windows to the head and body of the pancreas.

176. **C** [3,V]. Calculi associated with pancreatic duct dilation are characteristic of **chronic pancreatitis.** *Gallstones* are found in the gallbladder. When they pass into the biliary tree and impact at the sphincter of Oddi they may be a cause of pancreatitis. A *pseudocyst* is a fluid-filled mass associated with pancreatitis. *Cancer* presents with an irregular mass in the pancreas. Simple cysts in the gland

may indicate *polycystic disease;* one should then carefully scan the kidneys and liver.

177. **A** [2,II]. All of the options listed will work as acoustic windows. However, considering the anatomy of the very distal common bile duct as it curves laterally through the head of the pancreas to enter the ampulla of Vater, the best access is through the **head of the pancreas.** The beam is often angled from medial to lateral to visualize that portion of the duct. The *duodenum, gallbladder,* and *liver* are all windows that lie lateral to the duct. Furthermore, they are variable in size and location whereas the relationship between the pancreatic head and common bile duct is constant. In the case of the duodenum, air pockets will occur.

 If all answers are true, look for the one that is always correct.

178. **B** [3,I]. The order from right to left is the gallbladder, duodenum, and pancreas. Therefore, the gallbladder and duodenum can be found **to the right** of the pancreas.

179. **B** [3,II]. The **spleen and left kidney** provide a reasonably good window to the tail of the pancreas.

180. **B** [3,VII]. Only a **pancreatic pseudocyst** explains an elevated serum amylase level. The trauma to the abdomen is responsible for an acute pancreatitis that leaked enzymes to form a pseudocyst.

181. **C** [3,II]. Giving the patient **fluid by mouth** will distinguish the duodenum from the pancreatic head. Giving the patient *cholecystokinin* will make the gallbladder contract but will not help to identify the pancreatic head. A pancreatic head mass is not always accompanied by *dilation of the bile duct.* Placing the patient in the *Trendelenburg position* will push the pancreas toward the chest and make the examination more difficult. *Firm pressure to the midabdominal region* would not help because this is not the usual location of the pancreas. Increased epigastric pressure may push gas away from the pancreas, but is not often of use.

182. **E** [3,I]. The **entrance of the common bile duct and pancreatic duct into the duodenum** is called the ampulla of Vater.

183. **A** [3,IV]. **Hypertension** is not a cause of acute pancreatitis. *Alcoholism, pancreatic duct calculus, blunt trauma,* and *gallstones* are all causes of acute pancreatitis.

184. **D** [3,IV]. **Dysuria** (i.e., painful urination) suggests a urinary tract problem rather than pancreatic disease. *Weight loss, chronic severe abdominal pain,*

and an *epigastric mass* are suggestive of pancreatic cancer. *Vomiting* is common in pancreatitis.

185. **B** [2,V]. Jaundice, no visible dilated ducts, and usually an absent gallbladder characterize **biliary atresia.** A *choledochal cyst* is a focal dilation of the biliary tree. *Intussusception* is a telescoping of the bowel and is characterized by a donut or target sign on a sonogram. *Budd-Chiari syndrome* is a condition in which there is obstruction of the hepatic veins. *Cirrhosis* is advanced liver disease characterized by a small, fibrotic, echogenic liver.

186. **E** [10,VII]. The **pyloric length** will be abnormally *long* rather than short in the presence of pyloric stenosis. A *thickened pyloric wall, projectile vomiting,* an *epigastric mass,* and a *persistently fluid-filled stomach* are all features of pyloric stenosis.

187. **A** [10,VII]. In **intussusception,** a proximal portion of bowel invaginates into more distal bowel and causes gut obstruction.

188. **D** [11,I]. The small arrow is pointing to the **isthmus** of the thyroid, which is the connection between the two lobes of the thyroid. The *strap muscles* can be seen in the area in front of the arrow. *Reverberation artifact* from air in the trachea can be seen behind the arrow. The *piriform extension* is superior to the isthmus and is not seen on this transverse view.

189. **D** [11,I]. The question mark appears in the **carotid artery.** The *jugular vein* is not visible in this patient and is more ovoid in shape. It is not a *thyroid cyst* because it is outside of the thyroid. It is unlikely to be a *parathyroid adenoma* because it is a cystic structure, and it is too anterior for the usual parathyroid location. It is too posterior and lateral to be a *strap muscle.*

190. **A** [11,I]. The large arrow represents the **longus colli muscle.** The area marked by the large arrow is too far posterior to be the *jugular vein* or an *adenoma of the thyroid.* No calcification is seen in this location, so it is not *reverberation artifact.*

191. **E** [11,VII]. A **thyroid cyst** showing through transmission is present in the right lobe of the thyroid.

192. **A** [6,I]. The area delineated by the white arrow is the **peripheral zone.**

193. **C** [6,I]. The black arrow is in the central zone, which is an unusual site for *cancer* and *prostatitis.* The area is not cystic, so it is not a *utricle* or a *prostatic cyst.* The arrow most likely indicates an area of **benign prostatic hypertrophy.**

194. **A** [6,VI]. The hypoechoic area seen in the left peripheral zone is typical of **prostate cancer.** Al-

though *prostatitis* can cause hypoechoic areas, the findings are more diffuse and the usual appearance is an echogenic area. Although the area is hypoechoic, it is not cystic (i.e., there is no through transmission). Therefore, a *prostatic cyst* and *transurethral resection of the prostate (TURP) defect* are both incorrect.

195. **B** [12,III (NONCARDIAC CHEST)]. A solid mass is seen on the image. Of the options listed, only a **pulmonary sequestration** usually appears as a solid mass. Pulmonary sequestration is a congenital pulmonary malformation in which part of the bronchopulmonary mass is not connected to the normal bronchial system. *Pleural effusion, left-sided diaphragmatic hernia, mediastinal teratoma,* and *bronchogenic cysts* all contain avascular cystic areas.

196. **D** [12,II (NONCARDIAC CHEST)]. A single, large, aberrant vessel arising from the distal aorta is usually visible supplying a sequestration; therefore, **color flow Doppler** is the most helpful modality.

197. **D** [9,IX]. The vessels being sampled are the **portal vein and hepatic artery.** The *hepatic veins,* which lie at the superior aspect of the liver, cannot be sampled at the same time as the vessels in the porta hepatis (i.e., the hepatic artery and portal vein). Because there is no flow in the *common bile duct,* it cannot be a correct answer.

198. **D** [1,V]. Both the portal vein and the hepatic artery need to be sampled so that the direction of flow in the portal vein can be assessed. A consequence of chronic liver disease is the development of portal hypertension. Flow in the portal vein is normally in the direction of the liver (i.e., *hepatopetal flow*), but with worsening cirrhosis and liver fibrosis it reverses direction and flows away from the liver (**hepatofugal flow**). Consequently, flow in the hepatic artery and portal vein is in opposite directions, whereas normally it is in the same direction.

199. **D** [1,VII]. Many small cystic areas are seen in the region posterior to the liver. In view of the patient's history, the most likely explanation is multiple small **varices.** *Budd-Chiari syndrome* refers to occluded vessels in the liver. *Pseudocysts* do not present as multiple tiny cysts. A *multicystic kidney remnant* could have this appearance, but not this location.

200. **C** [3,VII]. The varices lie within the **pancreas,** which is a common location.

201. **E** [3,II]. The **hepatic veins** are not affected by portal hypertension, but all the remaining suggestions are worth trying to make the diagnosis more specific.

202. **C** [4,XV]. Given the history of the biopsy, a **blood clot** would be the most likely diagnosis, although a *tumor* could have the same appearance. Because there is no shadowing, *calculi* can be excluded. No discrete fluid level is seen, so *sediment* can be excluded. *Fungal balls* do not grow to this size and are typically seen in the renal pelvis.

203. **A** [4,II]. When the patient's position is changed, blood clots often move to a dependent position because of gravity; therefore, taking **decubitus views** will help to confirm the diagnosis. Bladder tumors do not change position because they are fixed to the bladder wall.

204. **E** [2,V]. The sonogram shows massive **common bile duct dilation,** with the bile duct much larger than the portal vein. *Choledocholithiasis* refers to a stone in the common bile duct—none is seen. *Cholangitis* (i.e., inflammation of the bile ducts) does not cause an enlarged common bile duct. *Cholesterolosis* is a disease affecting the wall of the gallbladder, which is not shown.

205. **B** [2,I]. The arrow is pointing to the **hepatic artery**. The hepatic artery can sometimes look like a small stone in the common bile duct because of its proximity to the duct.

206. **D** [2,VII]. The image indicates that this patient has **choledocholithiasis with a dilated common bile duct.** The massively dilated common bile duct is seen on the transverse view of the head of the pancreas, and a small stone in the duct is causing shadowing. The *pancreatic duct* would run transversely. Most *duodenal diverticula* contain food and gas rather than fluid, and the gas would be seen in the anterior aspect of the diverticula. *Pancreatic pseudocysts* can form in this location but would not contain calcification. The cystic area is too far posterior to be the *gastroduodenal artery.*

207. **E** [9,I]. This image nicely shows the *aorta, left renal vein, superior mesenteric artery, superior mesenteric vein,* and *common bile duct.* It does not show the **splenic artery.**

208. **E** [2,VI]. A **comet tail artifact** is not seen on this image. This artifact occurs when small cholesterol stones form in Aschoff-Rokitansky sinuses. Reverberations in these small calculi form a strong linear echo posterior to the small stone. *Gallstones, gallbladder wall thickening, gallbladder distention,* and *perigallbladder fluid* are visible on this image.

209. **C** [2,VIII]. This patient has **acute cholecystitis.** The findings of gallstones, gallbladder distention, a gallbladder wall greater than 3–5 mm thick, pericholecystic fluid, and a positive sonographic Mur-

phy's sign all support the diagnosis. *Acalculous and chronic cholecystitis* might show wall thickening, but not the other findings.

210. **D** [8,V]. The sonogram shows a **retroperitoneal mass.** The mass is posterior to the liver with the retroperitoneal fat line running anterior to it; therefore, it is not *intraperitoneal.* The mass is not *subcapsular* or *intrarenal* because it is not deforming the renal outline.

211. **C** [8,VII]. **Lung cancer metastases to the adrenal glands** are common in older patients. In addition, this patient has been exposed to second-hand smoke in his bar, further confirming the diagnosis. *Metastases from the kidneys* to the adrenal glands are very rare. *Pheochromocytoma,* unless malignant, is not as large as the mass seen on this sonogram. *Neuroblastoma* does not occur in 60-year-old individuals. *Myelolipoma* is densely echogenic with good through transmission because it is filled with fat.

212. **C** [4,XI]. Generalized dilation of the complete collecting system is present; therefore, the correct answer is **hydronephrosis.** *Pyonephrosis* is unlikely in view of the history and absence of internal echoes in the dilated renal pelvis. A dilated ureter (*hydroureter*) is not shown. A *duplex collecting system* is not present.

213. **D** [4,X]. The echogenicity in the region of the pyramids represents **milk of calcium,** presumably related to papillary necrosis. No *tumor* can be seen on the sonogram. The calcification does not have a double-line (tram-line) appearance as is seen with *arcuate artery calcification.*

214. **B** [13,II]. **Increasing the frequency of the transducer** will improve the resolution and enhance the shadowing from the renal calculi.

215. **E** [4,X]. This patient has kidney stones (i.e., **nephrolithiasis**). Shadowing is seen from portions of the extensive intrapelvic stone. *Air in the collecting system* would shadow along its entire length. *Renal cell carcinoma, angiomyolipoma,* and *papillary necrosis* all occur in the parenchyma, not in the renal pelvis.

216. **A** [11,VIII]. The patient's history of repeated attacks of abdominal pain suggests that he often produces renal calculi. The clinician might ask for his **parathyroid glands** to be examined because parathyroid adenoma induces hypercalcemia and, secondarily, renal calculi.

217. **B** [5,I]. The arrow is pointing to the **appendix epididymis** alongside the testicle. This is a normal structure, not a *mass, calculus,* or *blood clot.*

218. **A** [5,VII]. There is a large **hydrocele** surrounding the testicle. *Spermatoceles* and *epididymal cysts* are both cysts that occur in the epididymis. *Varicoceles* are large, dilated veins that lie alongside the epididymis and superior to the testicle. The majority of *hematoceles* (i.e., blood collections) contain internal echoes.

219. **C** [5,VII]. The hydrocele is located **between the two layers of the tunica vaginalis.**

220. **C** [4,VIII]. This patient's right kidney is enlarged (7–12 cm is normal in a 12-year-old girl) with a hypoechoic parenchymal area toward the lower pole. These findings suggest **acute pyelonephritis.** Because her other kidney is normal, *hemihypertrophy* and *Beckwith-Wiedemann syndrome* can be excluded. The kidney shrinks rather than enlarges in *chronic glomerulonephritis,* and the process is bilateral. In *pyonephrosis,* the renal pelvis would be distended, most likely with echogenic pus.

221. **D** [4,VIII]. This patient has a **renal abscess,** which appears as a thick-walled, hypoechoic, complex mass. The contents may show through transmission, internal debris, or gas. *Hepatic cysts, simple cysts,* and *parapelvic cysts* are not appropriate diagnoses because of the internal debris seen on the sonogram. A cystic *renal cell carcinoma* of this size would be very unusual.

222. **D** [4,XV]. Based on the patient's history and the thick-walled bladder on the sonogram, **pus** is the most likely diagnosis. *Hematoma* is less likely because there is no history of hematuria or trauma. A *bladder wall tumor* can be ruled out because the mass does not appear to arise from the bladder wall and it has a fluid–fluid level. If the findings were reverberation or mirror *artifacts,* the echoes would not be so well formed and would be adjacent to the anterior bladder wall.

223. **E** [4,XV]. A **bladder calculus** can be seen posteriorly in a dependent position in the bladder with acoustic shadowing. Bladder stones are most often associated with infection.

224. **C** [1,VI]. **Air in the biliary system** is almost never seen as a single focus and causes dirty shadowing rather than the clean shadowing seen on this image. The shadowing seen on this image is from the *tip of a biopsy needle;* however, *calcified granulomas* and *calcified hematomas* also cause this type of well-defined shadowing.

225. **C** [4,V]. Markedly **narrowed renal parenchyma** is seen on this patient's sonogram. The renal hypertension is a result of renal artery stenosis or chronic pyelonephritis. The renal pelvis appears large because of the parenchymal loss. No *tumors* or *calculi* are seen on this sonogram.

226. **D** [12,II (NONCARDIAC CHEST)]. The spleen is enlarged (i.e., **splenomegaly**) for a small child and there is a **pleural effusion** above the diaphragm. No *adrenal mass* is visible, and the intrathoracic fluid can be seen above the diaphragm rather than around the heart.

 It is difficult to think of wrong answers; if you see options repeated, then doubled up like this, heads up! The right answer is answer is probably the one that includes both.

---

227. **C** [9,I]. The letter **C** identifies the right adrenal gland. *E* is the common bile duct, *D* is the main portal vein, *A* is the right renal artery, and *B* is the hepatic artery.

228. **B** [3,VII]. A **pancreatic pseudocyst** is the most likely explanation for the multicystic, complex mass seen on this sonogram. The internal echoes in the cystic structure are not dependent, as they would be in a *dilated stomach. Mucinous cystadenoma* is a tumor of the ovary. *Cystic fibrosis* causes chronic pancreatitis appearances. A small portion of a normal-appearing pancreas is seen, so the findings are not the result of *acute pancreatitis.*

229. **D** [7,VIII]. **Granulomas** are seen on this sonogram. They are focal, bright, echogenic lesions with or without shadowing. *Infarcts, metastases, hemangiomas,* and *hematomas* are not typically calcified.

230. **E** [7,VIII]. In the United States, the most common cause of multiple, calcified, splenic granulomas is **histoplasmosis;** however, in many other countries *tuberculosis* is more common.

231. **C** [7,I]. The mass medial to the spleen is a fluid-filled **stomach,** which nestles in the hilum of the spleen. The thick wall and location are almost specific to the stomach. *Pseudocysts* can form in almost any location, but do not have such a thick wall. The thick wall and internal echoes are also not seen in any of the cysts mentioned.

232. **A** [7,II]. **Filling the stomach with water** usually improves visualization of the left upper quadrant; however, in this case, the stomach is already fluid filled. Having the patient drink would initially fill the stomach with air bubbles. All of the other options would result in better definition of the area of dropout

233. **E** [4,I]. The sonogram shows a collection in the **perinephric space.** Although the kidney is com-

pressed, the parenchyma is not thinned. If the collection were in the *subcapsular space,* the shape of the kidney would be distorted in the area of the collection. The *subphrenic space, subdiaphragmatic space,* and *submarine space* do not relate to the kidney.

234. **A** [4,IV]. The collection seen on the sonogram is suggestive of a *hematoma* around the kidney; therefore, a recent history of trauma (e.g., **recent kick in the side during a fight**) is likely. Infection (resulting in *fever and abdominal pain*) is less likely, but possible. The location is not a likely site for metastases, so a history of *loss of weight and appetite* is unlikely.

235. **C** [7,VIII]. Although **splenic abscesses** can resemble *splenic cysts,* they are typically complex collections containing debris such as that seen on this sonogram. *Pancreatic pseudocysts* occasionally extend into this area and can have a similar appearance; however, the amount and shape of the debris on this sonogram is not typical of pseudocysts. Both *splenic infarcts* and *splenic metastases* are solid rather than cystic masses.

236. **B** [2,I]. After choledochojejunostomy (i.e., a surgical connection between the biliary tree and the jejunum), **air in the biliary tree** is common. *Bile duct stones* are unlikely because of the absence of well-defined shadowing and the linear pattern of the echogenic areas. No dilated ducts, as would be seen with *biliary obstruction,* are visible. *Granulomas* form as scattered echogenic foci, not in a tubular configuration.

237. **E** [4,XI]. The ureter can be traced below the level of the renal pelvis; therefore, the obstruction is in the **ureter.** The obstruction is not in the *calyx* or *infundibulum,* and it is below the level of the *ureteropelvic junction.* An obstruction at the *glomerular level* cannot be seen with ultrasound.

238. **C** [4,II]. The **distal ureter,** bladder, and urethra should be examined **transabdominally** with a **full bladder** to find the cause of the obstruction.

239. **C** [1,V]. Tumors occur frequently in AIDS patients; therefore, Kaposi's sarcoma is more common in patients with **AIDS.**

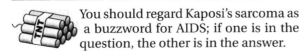 You should regard Kaposi's sarcoma as a buzzword for AIDS; if one is in the question, the other is in the answer.

240. **E** [2,VIII]. Massive **gallbladder wall thickening** is present on this sonogram. *Ascaris lumbricoides* is a worm seen in tropical countries. It enters the biliary tract and may appear in the gallbladder as a curvilinear mass that may be moving. The sonogram does not show a *gallbladder tumor* or a *cystic tumor in the liver.*

241. **E** [2,VIII]. Severe thickening of the gallbladder wall may be caused by *acute cholecystitis, hepatitis A, ascites,* and *AIDS.* **Chronic cholecystitis** does not result in a massively thickened gallbaldder wall.

242. **B** [5,VIII]. Greatly increased flow is seen in an enlarged epididymis; therefore, this patient most likely has **acute epididymitis.** Inflammation increases flow to most organs initially. Flow is not increased in the testicle, so *orchitis* (i.e., testicular inflammation) is not present. No mass is seen in the normal-appearing testicle, so *seminoma* and *torsion* are not present.

243. **B** [7,IX]. Keep in mind that this patient was struck by a car, and the spleen is one of the organs most vulnerable to **trauma.** A splenic contusion, not a splenic fracture, often results in inhomogeneous, hypoechoic areas. *Splenic torsion* only occurs if the spleen is not anchored, as in a wandering spleen. *Splenic hemangiomas* and *granulomas* would be echogenic rather than echopenic.

244. **A** [12,II (NONCARDIAC CHEST)]. The arrow is pointing to a **pleural effusion,** a common finding with splenic contusion. The fluid is above the diaphragm, so it is not a *fluid-filled stomach,* a *perirenal collection,* or a *perisplenic hematoma.* It has the typical wedge shape of a pleural effusion; a *pericardial effusion,* which has a circular border, would not be seen unless the heart was so large that it came in contact with the left diaphragm.

245. **C** [12,II (NONCARDIAC CHEST)]. The asterisk is placed over a **lung,** which is outlined by the pleural effusion. The sharp angulation is the normal shape of the inferolateral margin of the lung. A *lung mass* has a rounder shape and is more echogenic. The *heart* has a rounded outline and is fluid filled. The suspect area is well above the *diaphragm,* which is well outlined by fluid.

246. **C** [7,IX]. The echo-free area posterior to the spleen is a **perisplenic hematoma.** Bleeding is likely in a patient with a history of trauma, and hematomas form around injured organs. The collection does not lie in the kidney or adrenal gland and it is within the splenic outline, eliminating the other possibilities.

247. **A** [7,I]. The arrow is pointing to the **left hemidiaphragm.** It is outlined on either side by fluid alongside the spleen in a subphrenic location and by a pleural effusion. *Blood clots* rarely appear as a single line and are not as smooth. The *stomach* lies medial to the spleen. The *splenic capsule* is thin and

is usually not seen sonographically. The *phrenico-colic ligament* is rarely seen and, compared with the diaphragm, is not such a well-seen interface.

248. **C** [2,V]. The **parallel channel sign** is present on this sonogram. A dilated duct can be seen running anterior to the smaller portal vein, which indicates biliary obstruction. The *light bulb sign* is seen when a cyst is compared with neighboring structures (rather obsolete). The *comet effect* is an artifact seen when sound interacts with metallic or calcified structures. A *mirror artifact* is present when sound is refracted from a curved surface before it returns to the transducer. *Dirty shadowing* is the type of acoustic shadowing caused by gas. In comparison with shadowing from calculi, the borders are fuzzy and the shadowed area contains a few echoes. No artifacts are present in this case.

249. **E** [1,IX]. The lesion seen on the sonogram is distorting the portal vein by pushing it anteriorly. Simple *liver cysts* do not displace liver vessels and have sharply defined walls, so a traumatic hematoma related to **domestic violence** is the most likely diagnosis. Hematomas may vary from cystic to solid in appearance. The lesion is fluid filled (note the subtle through transmission); therefore, *metastasis*, *hemangioma*, and *renal tumor* are unlikely. In addition, the lesion is anterior to the inferior vena cava and is therefore intrahepatic.

250. **C** [9,VI]. **Portal vein thrombosis** is present because an echogenic thrombus can be seen filling the lumen of the portal vein. No flow is seen in the portal vein whereas the hepatic artery is patent and seen with color flow Doppler. *Budd-Chiari syndrome* involves the hepatic veins, not the portal vein. No *cavernous transformation* has occurred as yet because there are no collaterals alongside the thrombosed vein. Neither a *portal vein aneurysm* nor an *enlarged, patent portal vein* is seen.

251. **C** [10,IX]. All of the conditions listed can cause ascites. Because there is no internal echogenic material in the ascites, *peritonitis* and *malignancy* are unlikely. The liver shape is abnormal with border nodularity, which is indicative of **cirrhosis.** In addition, the portal vessels are difficult to see because the overall echogenicity of the liver is increased.

252. **C** [5,II]. The lesion looks like a cyst, but the through transmission is questionable. **Increasing the transducer frequency** will make it easier to see through transmission and confirm that it is a cyst. *Decreasing the transducer frequency* will make the image worse. *Surgery* is not the standard treatment for cysts; they are a common incidental finding. The lesion does not look vascular because there is no supplying vessel, so *color flow Doppler* will not solve the problem. *Percutaneous biopsy* of

testicular lesions is currently not performed because it is thought to encourage metastases if the lesion is malignant.

253. **E** [4,XIV]. A **renal stent** is present in the transplant; note the smooth double-line (tram-line) appearance typical of a man-made tube. Renal stents are placed between the bladder and the kidney in patients with transient or inoperable obstruction, typically after recent surgery when there is ureteral edema. The arrow points to the renal stent. Incidentally, another portion of the stent can be seen coiled in the posterior aspect of the bladder. Therefore, a *calcified ureter* and *arterial calcifications* are not viable options. *Bladder calculi* would fall to a dependent location.

254. **D** [5,V]. The testicle has the typical appearance of a recent **infarct;** note the pie-shaped echopenic area. In *cystic dysplasia* and *rete testis*, small cysts would be visible in the echopenic area. A *testicular abscess* would have a complex but basically cystic appearance. *Lymphoma* in the testicle would be echopenic with rounded borders.

255. **B** [5,II]. Because the lesion is avascular, no flow will be seen in the infarct; however, **color flow Doppler** should show flow in the remaining tissue of the testicle. Reexamination with *Valsalva maneuver*, a *standoff pad, needle aspiration*, or a *different patient position* would not be helpful in this case.

256. **E** [11,V]. No **calcification** is seen on this sonogram. The fine-needle aspiration biopsy that was performed after the sonogram showed a multinodular goiter. These three masses show most of the features of multinodular goiters—*multiple lesions*, the *halo effect*, and *cystic and echogenic areas*.

257. **C** [9,VI]. The internal echoes in the inferior vena cava represent an **inferior vena cava thrombus.** An *inferior vena cava filter* is an echogenic, intracaval metallic structure often associated with a distal vena cava clot. There is no *extrinsic compression of the inferior vena cava.*

258. **B** [9,II]. The inferior vena cava thrombus may have originated in the renal vein; therefore, the **kidneys** should also be examined. Approximately 5% of hypernephromas extend into the renal vein and eventually into the inferior vena cava. The *parathyroid glands, pancreas, testicles*, and *spleen* are not associated with vena cava thrombi.

259. **C** [4,XIV]. In diastole, the flow is below the line, which indicates reversal of flow. **Reversed diastolic flow** in a renal transplant is most likely caused by renal vein thrombosis, although rejection can give the same kind of signal. With a *normal flow* pattern there is some flow in diastole (i.e., a *low-resistance flow* pattern). *Triphasic flow*, seen in the iliac artery,

shows brief reversal of flow after systole and then a bounce back with flow in diastole.

260. **D** [1,VI]. Multiple hypoechoic lesions typical of **lymphoma** are seen. The lesions are not *cystic* because there is no increased through transmission. A *liver laceration* is unlikely to lead to numerous, separate damaged areas. A *hepatoma* may be multifocal, but it would be unusual to have five separate foci. The pattern is not typical of a *hemangioma*, which is usually echogenic.

261. **D** [4,XIII]. The sonogram shows a **horseshoe kidney.** The isthmus that connects the two kidneys can be seen anterior to the spine. *Column of Bertin, duplicated collecting system, crossed renal ectopia,* and *fetal lobulation* would be better visualized on a longitudinal view because they affect individual kidneys.

262. **D** [5,VI]. An echopenic, multilobular mass is seen without good through transmission; therefore, it is not a *testicular cyst.* This appearance is most consistent with a **malignant testicular mass,** such as a seminoma, which is usually seen in young adults. The epididymis is not seen, so *epididymitis* cannot be diagnosed. The testicle is in its usual location, so an *undescended testicle* is not a possibility. *Partial torsion* would not give rise to a focal, hypoechoic lesion.

263. **E** [8,VII]. The mass on the image represents a **metastatic lesion in the right adrenal gland,** which is found in 30% of lung cancer patients. Note that it is separate from the kidney, unlike a primary *renal cell carcinoma.* The recurrent urinary tract infections have no clinical significance; they were the reason for the renal sonogram. The mass was an incidental finding. *Pyelonephritis* is an infection in the kidney that may cause narrowing of renal parenchyma as a result of scarring. *Adrenal hemorrhages* are usually found in infants. A *pheochromocytoma* is a benign tumor of the adrenal gland that causes an increase in blood pressure.

264. **C** [5,I]. Multiple small cysts are seen in the hilum of the testicle, which is a finding consistent with **rete testis.** In this normal variant, multiple small tubules are seen as small cysts. No *solid mass* is seen, and the cysts are too small to be considered *benign testicular cysts.*

265. **D** [5,VII]. The multiple anechoic and hypoechoic areas in and superior to the epididymis indicate a **varicocele.** *Spermatoceles* are typically seen in the epididymis, especially the head, and are usually single or few in number. They also tend to be larger than varicoceles. A *hydrocele* would surround the testicle with fluid. *Epididymitis* and *epididymal masses* are not "cystic."

266. **D** [5,II]. To confirm a varicocele, have the patient perform a *Valsalva maneuver* and look for veins with *color flow Doppler.* When you have located a large vein, place a *pulsed Doppler* tracing over the vein. Have the patient perform and then release a Valsalva maneuver. If a varicocele is present, flow will reverse because of incompetent venous valves. Having the *patient stand upright* during the procedure will make the veins become engorged; a **Trendelenburg position** will make the veins less visible.

267. **D** [5,V]. **Microlithiasis** is present on this image. Multiple small calcifications are seen in the testicle, which may or may not shadow because they are small. *Scrotal pearls* are small calcifications outside of the testicle, usually in a hydrocele. *Fungal balls* rarely occur in the testicle. *Tuberculosis* and *chronic infarcts* give rise to hypoechoic areas in the testicle.

268. **C** [5,VI]. Microlithiasis is an asymptomatic condition; however, it is associated with an **increased risk of malignancy.** Serial sonograms every 6 months to 1 year are recommended.

269. **B** [5,I]. The linear echogenic area is the **mediastinum testis,** which is a normal variant that marks the hilum of the testicle where the tubules enter the testicle from the epididymis. *Calcification, arterial* or otherwise, is not present because there is no shadowing or evidence of flow in the echogenic area. *Infarcts* of the testicle form hypoechoic areas. *Gangrenous infection* would produce areas of gas with acoustic shadowing.

270. **E** [4,I]. The **left renal vein** courses between a cross-sectional aorta and superior mesenteric artery and enters the inferior vena cava. The superior mesenteric artery is surrounded by fat, which appears as an echogenic ring around the artery.

271. **A** [3,I]. The **gastroduodenal artery** may be seen outlining the lateral border of the pancreatic head just anterior to the common bile duct.

272. **C** [9,I]. The **inferior vena cava** is seen transversely, posterior to the head of the pancreas. Posterior and adjacent to the body of the pancreas is the portal confluence (i.e., the junction of the splenic vein, superior mesenteric vein, and portal vein).

273. **D** [9,I]. The **common bile duct** is seen entering the posterolateral pancreatic head.

274. **E** [2,I]. The **gallbladder** typically lies lateral to the duodenum, which encircles the pancreatic head.

275. **B** [3,I]. The pancreas can be seen on this transverse view. The cystic structure is tubular and located in the center of the pancreas. Its location

and tubular shape make it most likely to be a dilated **pancreatic duct.**

276. **D** [3,VI]. The pertinent finding on this image is a complex, irregular **mass in the head of the pancreas,** which represents pancreatic cancer. *Gallstones* and *hepatomas* are located in the gallbladder and liver rather than in the pancreas. *Lymphoma* is possible, although it is much less common in the pancreas than cancer.

277. **E** [3,VI]. The *biliary system,* both intrahepatic and extrahepatic, should be examined for dilation and obstruction. The *liver* should be examined for possible metastases, and all the sites where abdominal adenopathy can occur should be visualized. The **ligamentum teres** need not be examined closely because recanalization occurs as the result of portal hypertension, not pancreatic cancer.

278. **C** [3,IV]. Patients with cancer of the pancreas usually present with weight loss (not *weight gain*), **chronic epigastric pain,** and possibly a midepigastric mass. The prognosis is usually poor because of spread to the liver and lymphatic system, which often occurs by the time of the diagnosis.

279. **C** [5,VIII]. The image shows thickening of the scrotal wall, a small hydrocele, and a swollen echopenic epididymis, which causes **acute tenderness in the groin.** These are the features of *acute epididymitis.*

280. **D** [5,VII]. The cyst seen on this sonogram lies in the **epididymis,** which is found posterosuperior to the proximal end of the testicle.

281. **B** [5,VII]. The cystic structure seen on this scrotal sonogram represents a spermatocele (i.e., a collection of **sperm**).

282. **E** [5,IV]. Spermatoceles have no clinical significance and are discovered as an incidental **scrotal lump.**

283. **A** [5,VII]. Spermatoceles are of little pathologic significance; therefore, **no management** is required.

284. **D** [4,V]. This renal sonogram demonstrates small, shrunken kidneys with multiple cysts, which is consistent with chronic medical renal disease (e.g., **end-stage renal failure**). Prolonged dialysis is the usual cause for small, cystic kidneys. End-stage renal failure is not likely to cause *hematuria, flank pain,* or *fever. Adult polycystic kidney disease* is characterized by very large kidneys; in this case, the kidneys are only 7.5 cm in length.

285. **A** [4,V]. In end-stage renal failure, it is not unusual for the renal pelvis to be **distorted by cysts.**

286. **B** [4,II]. The structure identified by the thin arrow is a dilated renal pelvis. With careful technique, the many causes of hydronephrosis can be significantly narrowed down. If the cause is reflux, the apparent hydronephrosis will disappear when the *patient stands* and will change with *voiding.* The use of *color flow Doppler* and an attempt to connect the structure to the inferior vena cava will differentiate the dilated pelvis from a vascular structure. **Changing the gain** will not help because it will not provide an explanation for the mild dilation of the collecting system.

287. **D** [4,XI]. Once hydronephrosis is confirmed, an attempt must be made to determine the cause. The *degree and location of ureteral dilation* may determine the level of the obstruction. *Calculi* in the urinary tract or a mass may be obstructing the system; therefore, the *ureterovesical junction* must be interrogated to rule out a ureterocele. The **blood urea nitrogen and creatinine** levels will indicate renal failure, but will not be helpful in determining the cause of the hydronephrosis.

288. **B** [4,VIII]. Given the patient's history of recurrent fevers and infections and the low-level echoes seen in the dilated system, the most likely cause of dilation is **pyonephrosis** (i.e., pus in the collecting system). An *angiomyolipoma* would not be the cause of the obstruction because it is a cortical lesion. In the absence of infection, *diabetic nephropathy* does not dilate the collecting system. A *lower pole calculus* is not seen and would not cause pelvic dilation. A *ureterocele* would not cause echoes in the collecting system unless there was superimposed infection.

289. **C** [4,VI]. The echogenic focus in the lower pole of the kidney is an incidental **angiomyolipoma,** which is a benign, fatty, vascular tumor. A *renal calculus* of this size would cause acoustic shadowing. None of the other possibilities cause an echogenic mass.

290. **E** [4,I]. The renal sonogram shows hydronephrosis and hydroureter. The arrow points to a dilated **calyx,** which is the area located adjacent to the renal *pyramid* where urine collects. The *infundibulum* connects the renal pelvis to the calyx. The *hilum* refers to the concavity on the medial edge of the kidney. The *medulla* is the portion of the renal parenchyma between the pyramids.

291. **D** [4,X]. The image on the right is a dilated **ureter** that contains a **calculus,** which is causing the obstruction in the kidney. *Milk of calcium* would appear as a nonshadowing, echogenic focus in the region of the calyx.

292. **B** [4,IV]. Symptoms of calculi in the urinary system include flank pain and **hematuria.** *Anuria* means

no urine production, *oliguria* means too little urine production, and *polyuria* means too frequent urination, none of which occur with an obstructing renal calculus in only one ureter. *Pyuria* may occur with calculi if the cause of the stone is infection, but this is not as consistently present as hematuria.

293. **A** [3,I]. The large arrow is pointing to **Wirsung's duct** (i.e., the pancreatic duct), which contains a calcification. The duct is clearly dilated in this patient (2 mm is normal) as a result of obstruction of the duct by the stone. Be sure to identify pancreatic tissue on either side of Wirsung's duct so as not to confuse it with the *splenic artery, stomach, lesser sac,* or *cystic duct.*

294. **C** [3,II]. The small arrow is pointing to the spine, which is very posterior and has strong acoustic shadowing. Because it is not vessel, flow will be **absent.**

295. **E** [3,V]. The **echogenicity of the pancreatic tissue is normal** (i.e., hyperechoic to the liver). This is an accurate comparison, as long as it is known that the liver is normal.

296. **C** [3,II]. Image A is a *transverse section* through the midabdomen. Image B is a **longitudinal section** through the pancreatic head area. If *water* had been given by mouth, which is sometimes helpful in imaging the pancreas, we would most likely see a fluid-filled stomach or duodenum on the image. A *fatty meal* causes the gallbladder to contract, but would have no effect on this image of the pancreas.

297. **D** [9,V]. This image demonstrates a **false aneurysm** (i.e., pseudoaneurysm) that is seen as a collection adjacent to the femoral artery. The false aneurysm is secondary to trauma (i.e., the catheterization).

298. **C** [9,V]. The wall of the false aneurysm is formed by clot, which appears as a **defect in the wall of the femoral artery.** The color flow Doppler shows swirling blood flow in the mass, which has a typical mushroom-like appearance with its stem arising from the vessel. Flow in the normal femoral artery is shown, but the vein is not demonstrated.

299. **E** [9,V]. The arrowhead points to the **thrombus,** which forms the wall of the false aneurysm.

300. **A** [10,II]. The patient's clinical history is classic for pyloric stenosis, which occurs mostly in male infants and is caused by a thickening of the outlet portion of the stomach wall. Therefore, the sonographer should focus on the **stomach.**

301. **E** [10,I]. The arrow is pointing to the **fluid in the distended stomach.**

302. **D** [10,VII]. The thickness of the **pyloric wall** is being measured on image B. In a transverse view, which is demonstrated on image B, the thickness of the pyloric wall should not exceed 4–6 mm. The pyloric length should not be more than 14–16 mm, when normal.

303. **B** [10,VII]. The appearances are typical of pyloric stenosis, which causes a **stomach outlet obstruction** and is treated by **pediatric surgery.**

304. **C** [1,VIII]. **Abscess formation** is indicated by the sonogram and the patient's history; in fact, the patient's history of fever, tenderness, and an increased leukocyte count almost negates the necessity of looking at the image. *Pneumobilia,* or air in the biliary tree, results in "soft" or "dirty" shadowing that is arranged in a horizontal linear fashion and follows the pattern of the biliary tree. The lesion indicated by the arrow is not the normal size or position for a *porcelain gallbladder.* Calcification of any kind (e.g., *staghorn calculus*) is a poor choice because there would be dramatic acoustic shadowing.

305. **D** [1,VIII]. If the patient stays **supine and the transducer is moved to a right coronal approach,** the beam can often come in under the air and define the walls of the abscess.

306. **B** [1,VIII]. The bright echoes are caused by **gas** sitting in the top of a hepatic abscess, producing a "dirty" shadow. This "dirty" shadowing is most compatible with gas, letting some sound through but obliterating the detail posterior to it.

307. **E** [4,XI]. This image of the bladder is **normal.** A *Foley catheter with an inflated balloon* is in place and must not be mistaken for a mass (e.g., *transitional cell tumor*) or a *ureterocele,* which would be positioned more posteriorly, where the ureter inserts into the base of the bladder. It is not a ureterocele, which has a similar appearance, because it is located on the anterior aspect of the base of the bladder. None of the other options are cystic.

308. **B** [4,I]. The arrow is pointing to the **vagina** as it is seen through a distended bladder.

309. **A** [6,III]. The image shows benign prostatic hypertrophy. **Prostate-specific antigen (PSA)** is typically elevated in this condition.

310. **E** [6,II]. The structure being measured on the image is an enlarged prostate with hypertrophy. A **transrectal ultrasound** is a more accurate method of measuring prostate size; it aids in the evaluation of cancer and biopsy performance.

311. **C** [4,XI]. These images demonstrate a ureterocele or an expansion of the **distal ureter** (indicated by

the arrow on image A) as it inserts into the bladder. Note that on the longitudinal image (B), the tortuous dilated ureter is seen posterior to the bladder. The membrane is within the bladder outline; therefore, it is not the *bladder wall.* The membrane encloses a tubular structure that does not have the shape or the location of a *Foley catheter,* which is round and more anterior. A *mirror image artifact* would be an apparent cyst located posterior to the bladder. The *proximal urethra* is seen inferior to the bladder as a solid mass.

312. **E** [4,XIII]. In most cases of ureterocele, a **duplicated collecting system** is present and the dilated ureter connects the upper half of the kidney to the ureterocele. In this case, unilateral hydronephrosis, either segmental or involving the entire kidney, can be assumed to be present. Large ureteroceles may cause bilateral hydronephrosis, but without images of the kidneys we cannot be certain in this particular patient. The appearance is not compatible with a diverticulum of the bladder, which often occurs in *benign prostatic hypertrophy.* A diverticulum protrudes outside the bladder wall and has a narrow neck. None of the other three entities are associated with ureteroceles.

313. **B** [4,VII]. The correct diagnosis in this case is a **multicystic, dysplastic kidney,** which is thought to be caused by urinary obstruction during kidney formation. Multicystic dysplastic kidney disease is not a *genetic syndrome* when it is an isolated finding. In *Meckel-Gruber syndrome,* small renal cysts that are uniform in size are scattered throughout the kidney. In *infantile polycystic kidney disease,* the kidneys are greatly enlarged without visible cysts. *Trisomy 13 syndrome* kidneys are enlarged and echogenic with occasional small cysts.

314. **D** [4,VII]. **Bilateral multicystic, dysplastic kidneys are incompatible with life** without a renal transplant. If multicystic kidney disease is unilateral, *it will resolve over time.*

315. **E** [4,I]. This image is typical of medullary nephrocalcinosis. The *pyramids,* or **medulla** (indicated by the white arrow), are filled with tiny, nonshadowing calcifications.

316. **A** [4,III]. Nephrocalcinosis is often found in patients with increased serum calcium, resulting in **hypercalciuria.** A *serum creatinine value of 0.4* is normal. None of the other options have associations with hypercalciuria.

317. **E** [4,X]. Nephrocalcinosis can be caused by *long-term furosemide (Lasix) administration, renal tubular acidosis, hypervitaminosis D,* and *hypercalcemia.* **Milk of calcium,** which refers to an echogenic focus in a calyceal diverticulum, is not a cause of nephrocalcinosis.

318. **D** [8,I]. The structure identified by the black arrow is the **psoas muscle,** which lies posterior to the kidneys and alongside the spine.

319. **D** [1,II]. The echogenicity of the kidney can only be accurately compared to a liver with normal echotexture. In this case, **an accurate comparison cannot be made because the liver is abnormal.**

320. **A** [4,VII]. This image demonstrates infantile polycystic kidney disease, which is characterized by bilaterally enlarged, echogenic kidneys (note the 12-cm length). Therefore, the contralateral kidney will have the **same appearance as the kidney on the sonogram.**

321. **B** [1,III]. The **hepatic fibrosis** seen on this image is associated with infantile polycystic kidney disease in the older child. Although most commonly diagnosed in infants, this disease can present later in childhood. All patients with infantile polycystic kidney disease will have fibrotic changes in the liver, although the changes may not be visible sonographically. *Forty percent* of patients with autosomal dominant adult polycystic kidney disease will have cysts in the liver.

322. **A** [4,VII]. Infantile polycystic kidney disease is an *autosomal recessive disorder.* Parents with the condition have a **25% chance** of having another child with the same condition.

323. **D** [13,IV]. This image demonstrates a simple renal cyst. The arrowheads are pointing to **acoustic enhancement** or through transmission, which is one of the sonographic features of a cyst. Because kidney texture can be seen distal to the cyst, the area indicated by the arrowheads is not an *area of dropout* or *acoustic shadowing. Slice thickness artifacts* are seen in fluid-filled structures only. *Reverberation artifacts* are seen deep to strong acoustic interfaces and represent secondary echoes sent back and forth from the transducer surface to the strong interface.

324. **E** [4,VII]. The **size of the entity** is irrelevant because renal cysts may be very small or extremely large. All of the other features are typical findings in cysts.

325. **D** [2,I]. A **phrygian cap** is seen on this sonogram. Phrygian caps at the fundus are separated from the body of the gallbladder by an incomplete septum, with fenestration [see Appendix B]. *Fundal fenestration* is an invented term. *Hartmann's pouch* is formed by the neck of the gallbladder folding back over the region of the cystic duct en-

trance. *Septal defect* implies a cardiac anomaly. The *colonic bulb* refers to the cecum of the colon.

326. **B** [1,VI]. This image shows "*bull's eye*" *metastases* of the liver; therefore, it would be logical to choose **primary breast cancer** as an indication for scanning as opposed to *alcohol abuse*. Both of the laboratory values, *carcinoembryonic antigen* (*CEA*) and α-*fetoprotein* (*AFP*), should be increased in the presence of metastases, not decreased. While many forms of cancer metastasize to the brain, *primary brain cancer* does not metastasize outside of the central nervous system.

327. **E** [2,VI]. The crystals seen on this sonogram set off a particular *reverberation artifact* called a **comet tail artifact.** *Shadowing* is seen from an incidental gallstone on the posterior wall of the gallbladder but is *not diffuse*. Because the area of interest is on the anterior wall of the gallbladder and is not dependant, it is not *debris*.

A bold word in a question (e.g., **BEST**) usually means that at least two answers will work. Go for the more specific answer (e.g., comet tail artifact, which is a subset of reverberation artifact).

---

328. **B** [2,VI]. The crystals seen on this sonogram are **cholesterol crystals in the Rokitansky-Aschoff sinuses.** *Air* would cause areas of shadowing rather than a linear echo. *Sludge* accumulates on the dependant wall and does not cause the shadowing or comet tail appearances seen here. Although a single gallstone may be adherent to the gallbladder wall, most *gallstones* fall into a dependant position and are associated with shadowing.

329. **C** [2,VI]. This sonogram shows the most common form of **adenomyomatosis,** a condition in which cholesterol crystals form in the Rokitansky-Aschoff sinuses. The sinuses form as a result of hypertrophied gallbladder mucosa. Other forms of adenomyomatosis are multiple septa and multiple small polyps on the gallbladder wall (cholesterosis). *Staghorn calculus* does not occur in the gallbladder, but only in the kidney. *Adenomyosis* is a disease of the uterus. *A porcelain gallbladder* is a rare condition in which the walls of the gallbladder become calcified.

When a question has two answers that are very similar (e.g., adenomyosis and adenomyomatosis), one of them is probably right. We just want to see if you really know the answer.

---

330. **A** [2,VII]. The arrow is pointing to **shadowing from an incidental gallstone.** Shadowing is created by large differences in acoustic impedance created by dense material, such as calculi or gas. *Fat* and *polyps* are similar in composition to the gallbladder wall and fluid in the gallbladder and do not create shadowing.

331. **A** [2,V]. In a patient with a normal common bile duct and no jaundice, one would expect a normal bilirubin level, not an **increased bilirubin** level. However, this image does show focally dilated peripheral bile ducts showing a typical *parallel channel sign*. Something in the left biliary duct is causing the obstruction. The history gives every indication that the patient could have a lung mass, so a metastasis to the liver is the likely culprit. It *does not show* on this image, however. If a malignancy is present or even suspected, one should always look for *ascites* and *lymphadenopathy*.

332. **E** [1,I]. The section must be taken close to the diaphragm because all three hepatic veins are visible. The mass lies posterior to the right hepatic vein; therefore, it must be in the **superior portion of the right posterior lobe of the liver.**

333. **A** [1,VI]. **Metastases** are the most common cause of malignant solid liver masses in the United States. If the patient lived in Asia, where there is a high incidence of hepatitis B infection, *hepatocellular carcinoma* might be the most likely diagnosis. In the United States, hepatocellular carcinoma is more often associated with chronic cirrhosis, and this patient does not drink excessively. *Kaposi's sarcoma* would not be the first differential unless it was indicated by the patient's history. Most *hemangiomas* are echogenic, and *hepatocellular disease* causes diffuse changes, not a focal lesion.

334. **D** [2,I]. The arrows are pointing to the **right and left bile ducts,** which are flowing into the common hepatic duct.

335. **D** [2,V]. The key to this image is in the orientation. The pathology is clearly **biliary duct obstruction** when you realize that it is a right oblique sagittal view; therefore, the arrows are pointing to the dilated right and left bile ducts. Your nervous brain, however, might jump to the erroneous conclusion that it is seeing a transverse image of a large splenic vein anterior to the superior mesenteric artery. It is not a *Klatskin tumor;* if the cause of the obstruction were a mass, the common hepatic duct distal to that region would not be dilated. The portal vein is clear and is not dilated, ruling out *portal vein thrombosis*.

Be certain of the orientation of your image. Pathology can create very deceptive appearances. And if you did not fall for that one, it is to be hoped that you did not call it a Klatskin tumor just because you were shown a dilated left/right biliary junction. Remember, if the obstruction was caused by a mass there, the common hepatic duct distal to that region would not be dilated.

336. **E** [2,VIII]. Correct! **Testicular torsion** does not cause thickening of the gallbladder wall. The problem is that there are many conditions that do, including nonbiliary conditions like *portal hypertension* (due to venous congestion) and *ascites*. *Hepatitis,* although it can be responsible for a contracted gallbladder, often causes a marked thickening of the wall. Patients with *AIDS* often show effects throughout the biliary tree, with irregularly thickened walls in the ducts as well as gallbladder walls that measure over 3 mm.

337. **C** [7,IX]. In a patient with mononucleosis, the spleen is at high risk for rupture or fracture, even with no more provocation than letting a pitbull take you for a walk. The hypoechoic line in the image represents a **splenic fracture.** *Scarring* would appear echogenic, not hypoechoic. A *dilated venous structure* would show flow on color Doppler. A *normal variant* would be unlikely, and would have been seen on the initial scan. The spleen, unlike the liver, is not made up of *multiple lobes.*

338. **B** [7,IX]. A fracture logically leads to a bleed that pools below the diaphragm or beneath the splenic capsule. It is difficult to tell from this image which is happening; either way, the anechoic space represents a **hematoma.** Abscesses and hematomas can irritate the diaphragm, causing left shoulder pain; however, an *abscess* would most likely be accompanied by fever and focal pain. Abscesses also tend to have internal echoes and irregular borders. The echo-free nature of this collection points to a 2-day-old collection of blood. On the initial scan, the fresh clot was echogenic and could not be differentiated from the splenic texture. After 2 days of organization, the blood was homogeneous enough to be echo-free, both in the fracture and the hematoma. *Ascites* is also echo-free, but unlikely to loculate in that isolated spot. An *infarct* is unlikely given the patient's history. The collection could not be a *pleural effusion* because it is below the diaphragm.

339. **A** [7,VIII]. *Acoustic enhancement, debris in an irregularly shaped collection, fever,* and a *high leukocyte count* all describe the classic sonographic and clinical appearance of an intra-abdominal abscess.

Knowing the *location* relative to the spleen is helpful should drainage be planned. Abscesses can vary greatly in **size,** so this feature is not helpful in making the diagnosis.

340. **C** [7,VIII]. On ultrasound studies, there are similarities between the appearance of an abscess and an organizing hematoma; both can contain low-level echoes or a debris-fluid level. **Inserting a needle under ultrasound control** is the only option that would allow a distinction to be made between an abscess and an organizing hematoma.

341. **D** [7,I]. The image demonstrates the classic appearance of a **splenule** (i.e., accessory spleen), which is isoechoic to the spleen and ovoid or round in shape. At a glance, the round area may be considered a *renal mass,* but the interface of Gerota's fascia and perinephric fat clearly separates the splenule from the kidney.

342. **B** [7,I]. Splenules receive their vascular supply from **branches of the splenic artery.**

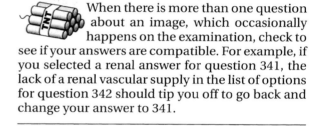
When there is more than one question about an image, which occasionally happens on the examination, check to see if your answers are compatible. For example, if you selected a renal answer for question 341, the lack of a renal vascular supply in the list of options for question 342 should tip you off to go back and change your answer to 341.

343. **C** [1,V]. *Splenic vein varices* are seen on this sonogram. These varices are usually secondary to **portal vein hypertension.** Although the image does look as though it could be a grossly dilated renal collecting system, it was stated that no kidney is on the image, which rules out secondary hyronephrosis due to a *large pelvic mass.* The varices do not resemble anything *metastatic, aneurysmal,* or *lymphatic.*

344. **C** [7,II]. A **decubitus view of the gallbladder** is unlikely to be useful in evaluating splenic vein varices; however, it is necessary to include the gallbladder for a complete examination. The varices do not resemble anything metastatic, aneurysmal, or lymphatic, which would be ruled out immediately if *color flow Doppler* were turned on. Even without a color image, direction of flow can be demonstrated with *pulsed Doppler* flow patterns. The reversal of flow away from the liver seen in portal hypertension causes recanalization of the fetal paraumbilical vein, which lies in the region of the *ligamentum teres.* Complex cystic masses in the left upper quadrant can be confusing, and it is conceivable that *water in the stomach* could clarify the issue.

345. **D** [1,V]. You would not expect to see **hepatopetal flow** in severe portal hypertension because the resistance to flow causes a reversal of flow away from the liver (i.e., *hepatofugal flow*). This reversal often causes recanalization of the fetal paraumbilical vein. *Splenomegaly, ascites,* and *echogenic liver texture* are all features of severe portal hypertension due to liver disease.

346. **A** [7,VI]. The lesions seen on this image were determined to be metastases based on all the mentioned criteria except the **cystic contents of the lesions** (note the *absence of through transmission*). The *lack of air in the lesions* supports the diagnosis; lesions that contain air are most likely abscesses. *Patient history* was very helpful, however, because this patient had melanoma, the malignancy most likely to metastasize to the spleen.

347. **E** [7,VI]. This patient had **melanoma,** which is the tumor most likely to metastasize to the spleen. Note: this is a tricky question because the other tumors mentioned are more common, and therefore more likely to be seen in the spleen. That, however, does not answer the question—be careful.

348. **C** [9,I]. The structure labeled C is the **C-loop** (i.e., second portion) of the duodenum that lies between the gallbladder and the *head of the pancreas.*

349. **D** [9,I]. The **right portal vein** is seen here posterior to the *bile ducts* and the *hepatic artery.*

350. **A** [9,I]. The **ampulla of Vater** is the opening in the second portion of the duodenum where the distal common bile duct enters.

351. **D** [9,I]. The **gastric artery** comes off of the aorta superior to the celiac axis; it is small and often not seen with ultrasound.

352. **A** [9,I]. The point at which A is labeled is just past the junction of the right and left bile ducts. Because the cystic duct has not entered the duct before this point, it cannot be the *common bile duct* yet; it is still the **common hepatic duct.**

353. **C** [9,I]. The **superior mesenteric artery** arises from the aorta.

354. **D** [2,V]. The image demonstrates the classic appearance of **peripheral duct dilation.** The *common bile duct* is not seen and *no cysts in the liver* are visible.

355. **B** [2,V]. Traditionally, the more anterior segment of the parallel channels is the **biliary radicle,** but there is such variation in anatomy that this is not always the case. A *recanalized paraumbilical vein* would be surrounded by the echogenic walls of the ligamentum teres. *Hepatic veins* do not travel in pairs, and *Kupffer tubule* is simply a creative invention.

356. **A** [2,II]. **Color flow Doppler** is the most efficient method to use when deciding which vessels are biliary and which are vascular. *Guessing* is admittedly the quickest method, but hardly the most efficient.

357. **E** [1,V]. Given the patient's history of alcoholism and the echogenic regions caused by hepatocellular destruction seen on the image, the most likely diagnosis is **chronic cirrhosis.** *Hepatitis* does not usually show much sonographically, except occasional prominence of the Glisson's capsule surrounding the portal veins that is thought to be caused by hypoechogenicity of the surrounding parenchyma. *Hepatic infarcts* often have a wedge shape and range from hypoechoic (new) to echogenic (chronic).

358. **A** [1,V]. The asterisk marks the area of a regenerating nodule, or what is essentially **normal parenchyma.** However, the round shape of the nodule could cause it to be confused with a *metastatic* lesion or *hepatoma.* The textural changes are not related to *acoustic enhancement from ascites,* because the texture is variable posterior to the fluid.

359. **C** [1,V]. In end-stage cirrhosis, it is often difficult to discern the portal vasculature; therefore, **prominent borders to portal vasculature** is the only sonographic sign mentioned that does not fit the scenario. The *nodular* outline of the liver (arrow), *ascites,* and *portal hypertension* are all regular components of chronic cirrhosis.

360. **D** [1,VI]. This image demonstrates a typical **hemangioma.** Hemangiomas are typically echogenic; however, it is possible that the lesion could undergo necrosis or thrombosis and develop an inhomogeneous, more hypoechoic appearance. *Adenomas* and *hepatomas* are typically less echogenic and more inhomogeneous in appearance. Fat-spared areas related to *fatty infiltration* are hypoechoic rather than echogenic.

361. **A** [1,VI]. Hemangiomas are the most common *solitary lesion* in the liver; most are *isolated,* but 10%–20% are multifocal. They are *more common in women,* and are generally asymptomatic; the right upper quadrant pain this patient is experiencing can be explained by her gallstones. Although hemangiomas are vascular lesions, the flow is generally **too slow to be visible on conventional color flow Doppler.** If arterial flow is seen, a malignancy should be considered.

362. **E** [1,VI]. The hemangioma seen on this image is less than 3 cm in size, which will most likely remain **unchanged** on subsequent scans.

363. **C** [9,II]. The sonogram demonstrates an abdominal aortic aneurysm. It is important for the surgical management of this condition to evaluate the major arterial vessels (i.e., *renal arteries, celiac axis, superior mesenteric artery, iliac bifurcation*) for involvement. It is not necessary to evaluate the **inferior vena cava.**

364. **E** [9,VI]. The low-level echoes seen in the aorta represent a **thrombus** or clot. Although a *reverberation artifact* may be mistaken for pathology, the artifact appears as parallel linear echoes, which are not evident on this image. The *intima* can be seen as a line along the border of a vessel, particularly in the carotid artery, which is examined with a higher frequency transducer; it cannot be seen here. *Slow blood flow* is occasionally visible in the inferior vena cava, but in the aorta the flow is always fast.

365. **C** [9,II]. **Color flow Doppler** may be helpful in evaluating thrombus in the aneurysm. Be careful not to alter the *gain settings* and prevent visualization of the thrombus in the vessel. None of the other options would help in showing clot.

366. **C** [1,IX]. If the image were not available, the history of trauma with symptoms of shock and hypovolemia alone would make a **hematoma** the most likely diagnosis. *Bilomas* and *hepatic abscesses* do not produce symptoms within minutes of a provoking incident. *Hepatic infarcts* are rare, especially in young children, because the liver has a dual blood supply from the hepatic artery and portal vein.

367. **D** [1,IX]. Based on the ultrasound findings alone, with no history, **any of the entities** listed (i.e., hepatic abscess, hemorrhagic cyst, degenerating hepatoblastoma) would have been possible. However, none of these diagnoses would have been correct.

> Do not just look at the image and try to find your diagnosis in the answer choices, no matter how much time you have left. History matters, so you always have to read the entire question.

368. **D** [1,IX]. If the hematoma had been scanned when fresh, it would have appeared **more hypoechoic** and looked different than it does in its organizing state.

369. **E** [2,VII]. This patient has the classic "4 Fs" that put her at risk for **cholelithiasis** (i.e., female, fertile, forty, fat). Given her colicky right upper quadrant pain, her clinician would expect the sonogram to show gallstones. *Sclerosing cholangitis* occurs commonly in young men and in the presence of cirrhosis. *Biliary atresia* is diagnosed in infants. *Acalculous cholecystitis* occurs most often in postoperative patients and is not related to age, size, or gender. The location of the pain is not good for *renal colic*

370. **E** [2,VII]. Although it is not clear on image A, image B shows a mass that is attached to the wall of the gallbladder, not floating. A **floating gallstone** is the only diagnosis that can be ruled out. A *cholesterol polyp* is the most logical choice, but you could not rule out *cholesterolosis*, an *adherent gallstone*, or *gallbladder cancer.*

> In addition to the history, always look at pathology in two planes, because an isolated image can be very deceptive. You will see some questions on the exam that refer to only a single image, which will be sure to contain all of the information you will need.

371. **E** [2,VII]. If you looked only at image A, a **floating gallstone** would seem to be the correct diagnosis.

372. **A** [2,II]. Trying to prove that a polyp is a polyp requires moving the patient around. It is necessary to scan the gallbladder with the patient in various positions (e.g., *erect, prone, decubitus*) while looking to see if the polyps move, because they seldom become dependent. If the patient has had an *oral cholecystographic agent*, the density of the bile will be increased, which can cause gallstones to float. A **lower frequency transducer** would not help to distinguish between a floating gallstone and a polyp; it would just diminish detail.

373. **C** [5,III]. An elevated human chorionic gonadotropin (HCG) level in a male patient raises concern for testicular malignancy; therefore, the **scrotum** should be scanned.

374. **B** [6,I]. The largest proportion of peripheral zone tissue lies at the **apex** (i.e., the inferior portion) of the prostate.

375. **C** [13,III]. An increase in **power** could theoretically cause harmful effects (e.g., thermal effects) to biologic tissue. Power is the amount of energy transmitted. Current ultrasound equipment power output is preset at the factory, and can be varied. The other controls mentioned do not change heat production.

376. **E** [10,VII]. The "olive" sign refers to the palpable epigastric mass found in infants with pyloric stenosis. It can be identified on a targeted **sonogram of the stomach.** The pyloric mass can be seen connected to the stomach, which is often enlarged and fluid filled after feeding.

377. **D** [13,III]. As sound travels (in depth and time) it loses amplitude and intensity through absorption,

scattering, and reflection. The time gain compensation (TGC), depth gain compensation (DGC), or swept gain compensates for this **attenuation** by decreasing the near field received signals.

378. **D** [13,I]. Hyperechoic (or echogenic) is the term used for a structure containing **many reflectors.** Hypoechoic (or echopenic) describes a structure with few reflectors. If a structure is anechoic (or echo-free), there are *no reflectors.*

379. **A** [13,V]. **Quality assurance must be performed routinely** on all ultrasound equipment to assure accuracy in the recording devices, measurement devices, and image quality. This is typically done through routinely scheduled preventive maintenance programs, which examine tissue-mimicking phantoms and check the accuracy of measurements. *A variable aneurysm* does not exist. *Transducer* frequency, *patient position,* and *fasting versus nonfasting* would not effect the size or measurement of the aorta.

380. **C** [1,V]. In Budd-Chiari syndrome, the hepatic veins are partially or completely thrombosed. The **caudate lobe** is not affected because it is the only lobe that has vessels draining directly into the inferior vena cava, not into the hepatic veins.

381. **A** [13,I]. The liver is so close to the lung that the pleural cavity can be brought into the needle path at the time of a pleural effusion aspiration or mass biopsy simply by varying the amount of inspiration; **pneumothorax** is always a risk. Although *bowel perforation* can be a complication of liver biopsy, the term "intercostal" places the needle between the ribs. Intercostal needles almost always traverse the pleura, if not the lung. A *retroperitoneal bleed* is a possible but unlikely complication of an intercostal biopsy. An intraperitoneal or intrahepatic bleed is much more likely. A *liver abscess* complicating an intrahepatic bleed is possible, but rare. The *pancreas* is too remote from an intercostal site to be traumatized by an intracostal liver biopsy.

382. **C** [12,II (NONCARDIAC CHEST)]. The collection described is a pleural effusion, which is best punctured with the patient in a **sitting position.** If the fluid had been below the diaphragm, it would have extended only as far medially as the bare area, where the peritoneum attaches to the abdominal wall.

383. **D** [12,II (NONCARDIAC CHEST)]. A **posteroanterior chest x-ray taken on expiration** is recommended after pleurocentesis. With less air in the lungs, any air that lies outside of the lungs is more obvious.

384. **B** [8,V]. **Flukes** are a form of parasite, and may be one of the few disease processes that cannot be directly attributable to AIDS, at least in the United States.

385. **C** [8,VI]. The fever and drop in hematocrit point to a *hematoma,* which can occur after cesarean deliveries. There are three types of hematomas: superficial, subfascial, and bladder-flap hematomas. Superficial hematomas can be found *anterior to the rectus muscles.* Subfascial hematomas occur *posterior to the rectus muscles,* extending anterior to the bladder into the space of Retzius. Bladder-flap hematomas begin at the incision in the uterus behind the bladder and lie between the bladder and the lower segment of the uterus. A postcesarean hematoma would not develop **posterior to the sacrum.**

386. **D** [10,V]. A **gossyphiboma,** or retained sponge, has a distinctive appearance on CT and ultrasound scans (see Appendix B if you are not familiar with the term). *Calculus* is improbable in this location, and a *hematoma* is unlikely with a normal hematocrit and no recent trauma. A *lymphocele* would appear more cystic. Besides, the midline in the pelvis is not a logical place for the lymphatic chain to get nicked.

387. **C** [2,V]. **AIDS cholangitis,** caused by the cytomegalovirus or *Cryptosporidium* organisms, causes thickened biliary duct mucosa and duct dilation. The mucosal thickening can appear as an irregular beading or a smooth wall thickening. *Primary biliary cirrhosis, choledochal cysts, biliary atresia* do not cause a thickened duct wall and *Heister's biliary hypertrophy* is a test-writer's invention.

388. **B** [9,V]. A surgeon planning **abdominal aortic aneurysm** surgery would be interested in learning whether or not the arteries coming off of the aorta are involved, as well as the length and extent of the aortic aneurysm. *Glomerulonephritis* and *osteoporosis* are not treated with surgery. If the surgeon were operating for *hydronephrosis,* the sonographer would be tracing the urinary tract for the nature of the obstruction.

389. **C** [1,VIII]. This patient has right shoulder pain because the shoulder and diaphragm share the same nerves, and there is referred pain from a **subphrenic abscess.** The suction created by the diaphragm can draw the pus from the ruptured appendix upward to form an abscess in this location. No respectable sonographer would stop with just an examination of the pelvis if an abscess was in question, even if one was found there.

The shoulder pain is an unexpected history for an appendix wound, and you are informed that it is relevant. The folks at the Registry are trying to test your knowledge, not trick you; so if they tell you that something is relevant, heads up. (They may not, however, be so blatant as to point out that the information is relevant.)

---

390. **A** [8,VI]. The patient's history leads to the correct answer—the patient has back pain when he walks or bends his legs at the hip, which requires use of the **iliopsoas muscles.** A **hematoma** causes a focal bulge in the normal linear muscle pattern seen on ultrasound, and can be confirmed, if unilateral, by demonstrating the same muscle on the other side. A *renal fracture* would probably create hematuria. A *retroperitoneal abscess* would result in an abnormal white blood cell count. A *ruptured spleen* would be much more likely to cause pain on the patient's left side.

391. **B** [2,VI]. A 5-cm mass in the region of the porta hepatis would impinge on the common bile duct, obstructing the flow of bile and causing **jaundice.**

392. **D** [1,V]. Jaundice brings to mind obstruction from *choledocholithiasis,* but with an absence of gallstones or shadowing throughout the liver a nonobstructive cause should be considered. A subtle increase in echogenicity of the portal triads is one of the few sonographic indications of **hepatitis;** however, this finding is not always present. It is possible that the increase in periportal echogenicity is caused by the decreased parenchymal echogenicity sometimes seen in hepatitis. *Pneumobilia* would cause linear echogenicity with dirty shadowing. *Choledocholithiasis* would be seen as one or more echogenic densities with acoustic shadowing.

393. **A** [1,II]. A history of alcohol abuse may suggest acute pancreatitis, but this diagnosis is not backed up by the patient's laboratory or sonographic data. Even the normal echogenicity of an 82-year-old pancreas should be great, so a liver that is more echogenic than the pancreas clearly has another manifestation of alchohol—fatty infiltration. Only a low-frequency transducer (e.g., **2 MHz**) would give a clear view of the right diaphragm in such a patient.

394. **D** [1,I]. The **middle and left hepatic veins** border the medial segment of the left lobe of the liver. The *ligamentum teres* separates the lateral and medial segments of the left lobe at a more inferior level. A mass that touches the *gallbladder* would have to be in the right anterior lobe. The *main portal vein and hepatic duct* are down by the porta hepatis.

The *left portal vein* lies exclusively in the lateral segment of the left lobe, not the medial segment.

395. **A** [1,I]. The **falciform ligament** itself is seldom visualized on ultrasound unless there is ascites, when the ligament can be seen at the dome of the liver connecting it to the anterior abdominal wall. The folds of the falciform ligament enclose the *ligamentum teres,* which can be seen on ultrasound and is a useful landmark for separating the lateral and medial segments of the left lobe of the liver. All the other structures delineate the separation between the right and left lobes of the liver.

396. **B** [9,VII]. Hepatofugal portal flow occurs in advanced portal hypertension, a common sequel to chronic cirrhosis. When sinusoidal resistance to flow is so great that the direction of flow reverses, portosystemic collaterals open up; the easiest to detect is the recanalized paraumbilical vein that travels in the **ligamentum teres.** To locate the paraumbilical vein, find the ascending portion of the left portal vein and follow the umbilical portion of it inferiorly between the medial and lateral segments of the left lobe of the liver. Color flow Doppler will demonstrate flow and that the vein is indeed recanalized.

397. **B** [1,I]. A Riedel's lobe is a long, thin extension of the right lobe of the liver that can put the liver edge well below the lower pole of the right kidney. Sonologists using this criterion to make a diagnosis of **hepatomegaly** will be guilty of not seeing the forest for the trees—the entire liver must be taken into account. The left lobe is often small in patients with a Riedel's lobe, and patients with a small anteroposterior diameter have livers that extend more inferiorly to compensate. A Reidels lobe is unlikely to be mistaken for any of the other options.

398. **C** [9,I]. A vessel coming from the superior mesenteric artery and supplying the liver is a **replaced hepatic artery,** present as a variant in approximately 20% of the population. A *portosystemic collateral* is a venous rather than arterial structure. The *gastroduodenal artery* supplies the head of the pancreas and is a branch of the hepatic artery. The *gastric artery* supplies the stomach and is a branch of the celiac trunk. The *coronary arteries* supply the heart and are in the chest.

399. **D** [2,II]. A gallbladder full of stones contains no bile to define its borders, but the main lobar fissure acts as a road map from the right portal vein to the gallbladder fossa. In the *decubitus* position, the gallbladder can fall into a variety of places depending on many factors (e.g., the patient's body habitus, the size and position of the gallbladder). The *duodenum* is too medial, and the *right portal vein*

is too lateral to show the gallbladder and main lobar fissure. A *sagittal view through liver and kidney* may reveal the gallbladder; however, only a longitudinal view that includes the right portal vein and main lobar fissure will definitely be successful.

400. **C** [1,III]. **Alkaline phosphatase** is an enzyme produced in the liver, bone, and placenta that is released into the blood in the event of liver injury or bile duct obstruction. *Hematocrit* quantifies the red blood cells. *Creatinine* is a measure of renal function. *Amylase* is elevated in pancreatitis.

401. **A** [1,III]. All of the enzymes listed are made in the liver. *Aspartate aminotransferase* (*AST*), *gamma-glutamyltransferase* (*GGT*), and *alanine aminotransferase* (*ALT*) are elevated in both biliary obstruction and intrinsic liver disease. **Acetylcholinesterase** is detected in amniotic fluid when a neural crest anomaly is present. If looking at a list of laboratory values sends you into a mild panic, review Appendix A.

402. **D** [2,II]. While all of the structures listed should be visualized on an abdominal sonogram, it is possible to miss choledocholithiasis by looking only at the biliary tree within the liver. Intrahepatic ducts could all be normal despite a stone in the distal **common bile duct in the head of the pancreas,** which may or may not be dilated.

403. **D** [1,I]. To answer this question, think of the classic sagittal view of the right portal vein, right hepatic artery, and common duct. Picture the bifurcation of the common hepatic duct just superior to that image and it is clear that it occurs **anterior and superior to the right hepatic artery.**

404. **B** [2,IV]. The administration of fat *increases the release of cholecystokinin,* thereby increasing the bile flow. A common duct that is large but otherwise unobstructed and normal should decrease in size after a fatty meal; an increase in size is not a *normal response* to the ingestion of fat. There will be an increase in the size of the common duct if there is an obstruction, such as a **stone.** In this patient, the stone must be in the extrahepatic duct. If the duct was large in size because a *gallstone was recently passed* and the duct was now unobstructed, fat would not change its size.

405. **C** [2,I]. A **7-mm duct is usually normal in an 80-year-old patient.** Asymptomatic gallstones are common, so *surgery* on this elderly woman is not necessary. If she *recently passed a stone* or had an aneurysm so large it was *obstructing her biliary system,* she would not be asymptomatic. *Murphy's sign* is local tenderness when the gallbladder region is palpated or examined sonographically; we are told the patient is asymptomatic, so this cannot be correct.

406. **A** [2,V]. This question describes pneumobilia, or air in the biliary tree. **Surgical clips from a cholecystectomy** would not be scattered throughout the liver, but would be clustered in the gallbladder fossa and cause "clean" or clear-cut shadowing. A surgical clip may cause a ring down artifact, but so can air, which fits the description better. Any procedure that opens the biliary system to an outside source of air (e.g., endoscopic retrograde cholangiopancreatography, surgical connection to bowel such as *choledochojejunostomy* or *sphincterotomy*) can cause pneumobilia. Pneumobilia may also result from *gallbladder ileus.*

407. **A** [2,VIII]. **Mirizzi syndrome** is a rare condition in which the obstructing stone is located in either Hartmann's pouch or the cystic duct. Only the ducts proximal to the stone are dilated, often including the common hepatic duct. This is a tricky diagnosis because a low-inserting cystic duct often runs in a common sheath with the common duct in this condition. The surgeon also finds this condition a challenge and appreciates forewarning. *Ascaris lumbricoides* are roundworms that live in the intestines. *Caroli's disease* is a disease of the biliary system in which the intrahepatic ducts have outpouchings that can resemble cystic lesions. *Sclerosing cholangitis* is fibrotic thickening of the bile ducts that sometimes causes dilation from the strictures. *Klatskin tumor* is a cholangiocarcinoma that occurs at the bifurcation of the common hepatic duct and involves the right and left biliary ducts.

408. **B** [1,VI]. If a mass and ascites are discovered, it is necessary to search carefully for metastases and enlarged lymph nodes, treating the lesion as a possible malignancy. However, in their absence, this woman's history—especially the *oral contraceptive use*—is appropriate for hepatic adenoma. Hepatic adenomas are benign, so **metastatic lesions ("bull's eye" or otherwise)** would not be present. The free fluid in her abdomen is from the *bleeding* going on in her mass, which has ruptured through the *capsule* into the peritoneum, irritating it and causing her diffuse pain.

409. **E** [1,VI]. *In the United States,* the **most common cause of hepatocellular carcinoma is advanced cirrhosis.** In Asia, hepatitis B is the most common cause of hepatocellular carcinoma. Of course, there are solid *liver tumors that are benign.* Even if a malignant tumor is vascular, it may not light up on *color flow Doppler.*

In question 409, although answer B is true, it does not answer the question. Be careful of nonsequiturs in the answer choices, and read all of the answers. An early answer may be true, but a later answer may be, well, more true.

Watch out for words like "always" and "never." There are few absolutes in medicine (or life), and these terms should raise a red flag if they are present in the answer or the question.

410. **E** [1,VI]. The first four answers are absolute statements: *melanomas* frequently *metastasize to the gallbladder; colon metastases are sometimes "bull's eye" lesions; color flow Doppler* may *show vascular flow;* and *lymphomatous lesions in the liver are* usually *hypoechoic,* but not always. Actually, this was a trick question to ask after the cautionary tip about "never" being in the answer. However, in this case "never" means "not always," so it is stopping you from making an absolute statement.

Absolute statements seldom work in ultrasound or in test answers. Read carefully for the answer that is invariably true.

411. **C** [1,II]. There will be **no Doppler signal** in a bile duct. A Doppler study is a good way to settle any vascular versus biliary questions.

412. **B** [1,VII]. Cysts from *autosomal dominant polycystic disease* do occur in the liver, but the key here is that these "cysts" are connected. **Caroli's disease** exhibits saccular dilations of the intrahepatic (not extrahepatic) bile ducts, which can look like cysts if the connecting, unaffected portions of the duct are not demonstrated. While Caroli's disease is a form of localized *biliary dilation,* the cyst-like nature of the ducts is what makes the sonographic diagnosis. Caroli's disease is strongly associated with hepatic fibrosis and medullary sponge kidney. *Autosomal recessive polycystic disease* is associated with hepatic fibrosis rather than cysts. *Meckel-Gruber* syndrome is a lethal congenital disease that causes cysts in the kidneys but does not affect the liver.

1. **E** [28,III]. **Atrophy of the endometrium,** a common entity after menopause, results in a reduced endometrial width. Endometrial thickening is symmetrical with *estrogen therapy* and *benign endometrial hyperplasia* and irregular with *polyps* and *cancer.*

2. **E** [14,VII]. Ectopic pregnancy does not result in **broad ligament hypertrophy.** The *adnexal ring sign* is a term used for a gestational sac–like appearance in the adnexa, which is commonly seen with ectopic pregnancy. *Fluid in the cul-de-sac* is a dangerous finding with ectopic pregnancy. It usually indicates tubal rupture and is often an indication for emergency surgery. *Decidual thickening,* sometimes with the formation of a decidual cast, is usually seen with ectopic pregnancy. An *adnexal mass* is a common finding that is usually caused by a hematoma accompanying the ectopic pregnancy.

3. **E** [18,III A]. The incidence of fetuses with neural tube defects increases **ten times** in diabetic mothers.

4. **C** [22,III]. The arrow is pointing to the border of a **cystic hygroma.** Note the septa in the hygroma. *Amniotic bands* are not as thick, symmetrical, or smooth. A *membrane between twin sacs,* an *amniotic sheet,* and the *borders of a bleed* do not attach to the fetus.

5. **A** [22,III]. This image was obtained at the level of the **neck,** which is the typical location of cystic hygromas. Because no ribs or iliac wings are visible relative to the spine, the view was not taken at the level of the *sacrum* or *chest.*

6. **C** [29,II]. An anterior fundal **fibroid** is present on this image. The pathology could ostensibly be *choriocarcinoma,* but it does not have the mixture of echogenic and cystic areas typical of that entity. A *partial mole* would present with a fetus and amniotic fluid. *Uterine cancer* is much less common than fibroids. This mass displaces rather than emerges from the endometrium, ruling out an *endometrial mass.*

7. **A** [29,II]. The fibroid is *intramural* because it is in the uterine wall. However, more importantly, it abuts on the endometrial cavity, so it is characterized as partially **submucosal.** Submucosal fibroids are more likely to induce vaginal bleeding.

 It is tricky when there are two correct options, but sometimes that is the reality in medicine. Pick the answer that is the most clinically significant.

---

8. **C** [29,II]. Fibroids often present with frequent and excessive vaginal bleeding (i.e., **menorrhagia**). Submucosal fibroids do not often cause pain (e.g., *pain on intercourse, leg pain*).

9. **D** [18,II]. A fetus with grossly thickened skin is anterior and a smaller, normal fetus is posterior and to the right. The intersac membrane is visible posterior to the abnormal head. This severe skin thickening is virtually specific for **acardiac twins.** It is too severe for the hydrops sometimes seen in *twin-to-twin transfusion syndrome* and *stuck twin syndrome.* Skin thickening is not seen in the other types of twins mentioned.

 Studying at the image before you skim the options can waste time. For example, in question #9 the options tell you that twins are present, putting you on the right track and preventing you from thinking of incorrect possibilities.

---

10. **C** [22,I]. **Severe ventriculomegaly** is seen in the brain of the more anterior twin. Some brain tissue is visible around both lateral ventricles. In *alobar holoprosencephaly,* only one large ventricle would be seen. The fourth ventricle is not dilated, so *Dandy-Walker syndrome* is not present. In *hydranencephaly,* both cerebral hemispheres would be absent.

11. **A** [18,II]. Although the image does not show any cystic areas, the majority of acardiac fetuses have large **cystic hygromas** in the neck associated with the severe skin thickening. Despite the absence of a heart, there is *leg movement. Omphalocele, poly-*

dactyly, and *pleural effusion* are not features of an acardiac fetus.

12. **B** [18,II]. Because the normal "pump" twin is supplying blood to the acardiac twin, heart failure with secondary **hydrops** often develops. Although *fetal death* is common, it is not inevitable. Normal growth of the pump twin is the usual finding with, if anything, polyhydramnios rather than *oligohydramnios.*

13. **C** [24,V]. The **rectus abdominis muscle** extends from the xiphoid process of the sternum to the pelvis in the midline.

14. **C** [18,II]. In a **singleton pregnancy** there is one amniotic sac and one chorionic sac. *Ectopic pregnancy* refers to a gestation implanted outside of the uterus. *Fraternal twins* are dizygotic dichorionic diamniotic twins. *Stuck twins* and *identical twins in two sacs* are monochorionic diamniotic twins. Identical twins in one sac are monozygotic monochorionic monoamniotic twins; however, this was not one of the answer choices.

15. **D** [17,X]. The lecithin:sphingomyelin ratio is measured in an amniotic fluid sample to assess **fetal lung maturity.**

16. **E** [27,II]. Although dilation of a fallopian tube is usually caused by previous *pelvic inflammatory disease,* it can also result from bleeding into the tube or obstruction of the tube. Of the conditions listed, only an **endometrial polyp** does not cause bleeding into the tube or obstruction.

17. **D** [29,III]. A **complex mass** that is partially solid and partially cystic is seen on the left. The shadowing from the solid component is too distinct (or "clean") to be the result of air in a *loop of bowel.* Regardless of how great the resolution is, it is not possible to make a histologic diagnosis on ultrasound, so *ovarian cancer* is not a correct choice.

18. **A** [29,III]. An echogenic area with shadowing in addition to a cystic area, the "tip of the iceberg" sign, is strongly suggestive of a **dermoid cyst** (i.e., benign cystic teratoma). *Dominant follicles* are cystic. *Ovarian cancers, ovarian cystadenomas,* and *corpora lutea* do not contain internal structures with much shadowing.

19. **B** [29,III]. A **CT scan** will show fat in the dermoid, confirming that it is a benign lesion. A *percutaneous biopsy* would be unnecessarily invasive and hazardous. A *liver scan* and a *white blood cell count* would remain unaffected by this benign mass. *Dilation and evacuation* would not be helpful because this mass is in the adnexa, not the endometrium.

20. **D** [29,III]. Approximately 15% of dermoids are bilateral; therefore, the **other ovary** would be the most likely place to find additional pathology. Because it is a benign process, one would not have to look for fluid in the *cul-de-sac,* enlarged *para-aortic nodes,* or *liver* metastases.

21. **A** [22,VI]. A bilateral **pleural effusion** is present. The lung is surrounded by fluid, and the heart is poorly seen. A *pericardial effusion* would surround the heart but not displace it, as does fluid in the pleural cavity.

22. **A** [20,III]. There is an association between pleural effusion and chromosomal anomalies, particularly Down syndrome. Therefore, an **amniocentesis** would be the most appropriate next step in the management of this fetus. The combination of α-fetoprotein, estriol, and human chorionic gonadotropin assay, known as the *triple screen blood test,* only indicates if the patient is at risk for trisomy 21 and trisomy 18, and the pleural effusion has already established a significant level of risk. *Drainage* is not recommended for small pleural effusions because most of them resolve spontaneously.

23. **C** [15,II E]. Of the choices provided, only the **spleen** can be seen, posterior to the stomach.

24. **E** [15,II E]. The white arrow is pointing to the **gallbladder,** which is to the right of the *umbilical vein.* The *stomach* is posterior and to the left. The area that the arrow is pointing to is too far anterior to be the *right portal vein* or the *right renal pelvis.* Note that this is not an ideal abdominal circumference view.

25. **C** [17,V]. This is an **oblique view** because ribs are seen on the right but not on the left. The fetal trunk is also mildly flattened by transducer pressure. For a satisfactory abdominal circumference measurement, the sonographer obtains a right-angle view of the fetal trunk at the level of the umbilical vein, stomach, adrenal gland, and liver, which does not show the kidneys or lungs. The *heart, lungs,* and *kidneys* are not seen on this image.

26. **C** [25,I]. The endometrium is in the **secretory phase** of the cycle after ovulation. It coincides with the *luteal phase* of the ovarian cycle.

27. **C** [21,II]. **Spalding's sign** is the term given to the overlapping of the skull bones after a fetal demise. It is an indication that the death was not recent. The *lemon sign* is the shape seen in Arnold-Chiari II malformation, along with a banana-shaped cerebellum. Although a pregnant woman may have a locally tender gallbladder, *Murphy's sign* will not occur *in utero.*

28. **C** [14,I]. An early **intrauterine pregnancy** is the most likely cause of this appearance. Note the thick trophoblastic reaction. An *interstitial pregnancy* would not be centrally located. A *choriocarcinoma* would be more irregular in shape with several cystic areas. A *fibroid* would be most unlikely to be echogenic with a cystic center. *Intracavitary blood,* even if it were echogenic, would be most unlikely to have a cystic center.

29. **B** [14,I]. A **pregnancy at 4.5 weeks' gestation** is most likely because no yolk sac or crown-rump length can be seen. At *3 weeks' gestation* no gestational sac is visible. A *pregnancy at 8 weeks' gestation* or a *missed abortion* would show all or part of a remaining fetus. If a *12-week blighted ovum* were present, the sac would be larger and not as well formed.

30. **E** [31,III]. The supine hypotensive syndrome is a common event in the third trimester. Because the weight of the fetus is compressing the maternal inferior vena cava, venous return to the heart is impaired. **Turning the patient on her side** usually immediately relieves the symptoms. If symptoms are very severe, perform the examination with the patient in a sitting position. The examination does not need to be *discontinued.* It is not uncommon for the syndrome to return at a second examination, so having the *patient come back another day* will not help. Putting the patient in the *Trendelenburg position* will worsen the syndrome.

31. **C** [29,III]. The bilateral, multicystic masses are thecalutein cysts associated with a **hydatidiform mole.** Multiple large cysts are present in both ovaries in approximately 40% of hydatidiform moles.

32. **E** [25,III]. Thecalutein cysts are associated with high levels of **human chorionic gonadotropin.** The *erythrocyte sedimentation rate* is a blood test that is elevated in infections and connective tissue disease. The *CA125 test* is used to detect ovarian cancer. The *white blood cell count* is used to detect infections. *α-Fetoprotein* is principally used to detect neural crest anomalies or as a component of the triple screen test for Down syndrome. None of these tests would help with mole detection.

33. **E** [22,VII]. The sonogram shows several noncommunicating cysts, which is a typical finding with a **multicystic, dysplastic kidney.** Because the cysts extend posteriorly along the spine, they are of renal origin, not gastrointestinal origin (i.e., unless there is renal agenesis). Because the cysts do not communicate, they are not in the configuration typical of *ureteropelvic junction obstruction.*

34. **D** [22,VII]. Both **ureteropelvic junction obstruction** and *reflux* are common in the kidney opposite from a multicystic, dysplastic kidney. In most instances, renal pelvic dilation related to *posterior urethral valves* is symmetrical.

35. **D** [24,V]. The **levator ani muscle** lines the floor of the pelvis.

36. **D** [27,IV]. Hyperstimulation is due to excess human chorionic gonadotropin administration and results in *enlarged ovaries* filled with theca-lutein cysts. These cysts can obstruct the ureters, causing *hydronephrosis* and water retention with subsequent *ascites* and *pleural effusion.* Hyperstimulation does not affect the **cervical canal,** although it may cause endometrial cavity thickening.

37. **B** [18,VI]. Postpartum hemorrhage from **placenta percreta** would be immediate, not delayed. *Retained products of conception* (i.e., *retained placenta*) and a *cesarean section hematoma* cause bleeding that continues for many days if untreated.

38. **B** [17,III]. The biparietal diameter can be accurately measured starting at **12 weeks** gestational age. The crown-rump length, which is routinely measured in the first trimester, becomes inaccurate after about 12 weeks.

39. **E** [28,III]. The endometrium has undergone *localized thickening* with a possible *intracavitary mass.* A *poly*p may be present, but it is too poorly seen for a definitive diagnosis. The endometrium is thickened in the *secretory phase* and thin in the **proliferative phase** of the menstrual cycle.

40. **A** [28,III]. A **hysterosonogram** saline infusion study was performed; note the fluid (saline) in the endometrium. The other procedures (*dilation and curettage, cone biopsy, percutaneous biopsy,* and *voiding cystogram*) do not involve the injection of saline into the endometrium.

41. **C** [28,III]. As a consequence of the procedure, there is **air trapped in front of a mass.** Normally, gas bubbles float to the fundus. Incidentally, a subtle endometrial wall *polyp* without a stalk is present. During hysterosonography, a soft catheter is introduced through a speculum; no *metallic instrument* enters the endometrium.

42. **D** [29,II]. **Nabothian cysts** are located in the cervix, not the vagina.

43. **A** [17,III]. The only landmark seen on this image that is essential for a biparietal diameter or head circumference measurement is the **cavum septum pellucidum.** Because the *cerebellar vermis* is visible, this view is angled improperly toward the posterior fossa and cannot be used to measure head circumference. Because the *cerebral peduncles* are present instead of the *thalamus,* this view is clearly

at too inferior a level for proper measurement of biparietal diameter or head circumference.

44. **E** [17,IX]. This skull is **normal.** It is not *brachycephalic* (i.e., short and fat) or *dolichocephalic* (i.e., long and thin). No *skull fracture* is present; however, some gaps in the skull outline are visible. The gap at the anterior aspect of the skull is related to dropout because at that point the skull is at a 90° angle to the beam. The occipital posterior gap is related to a suture. *Frontal bossing* would not be seen because this is not a profile view.

45. **C** [22,IX]. This is a view of the **distal arm.** The structures of the hand are poorly visualized.

46. **C** [22,IX]. The long bones are broken into small fragments, which is indicative of **osteogenesis imperfecta.** In *thanatophoric dwarfism, achondrogenesis, achondroplasia,* and *diastrophic dwarfism* the bones are short but not fractured.

47. **C** [16,VI]. Classic placental abruption is almost always associated with **pain and bleeding,** usually in the **third trimester.** Marginal bleeds, which are sometimes classified as a form of abruption, are often asymptomatic.

48. **E** [14,VII]. Common features of an ectopic pregnancy include *fluid in the cul-de-sac,* a *decidual reaction, local tenderness over the mass,* and a *pseudogestational sac.* A ruptured ectopic pregnancy with internal bleeding would result in a decreased hematocrit level, not an **increased hematocrit level.**

49. **A** [31,II]. Some patients are offended by the use of their **first name** on an initial meeting. Once you have an established relationship with a patient, this may be acceptable.

50. **C** [25,I]. This image shows the three-line phase, which is when **ovulation** normally takes place (day 14, or in the middle of the cycle). The three-line phase is the beginning of the secretory phase.

51. **A** [29,III]. A **dominant follicle is present** because this is the time of ovulation. If ovulation recently occurred, an early corpus luteum (not a *calcified corpus luteum*) may be present.

52. **D** [19,IV,V]. The image shows **significantly more** amniotic fluid than normal (severe polyhydramnios), with a fluid distance greater than 8 cm anterior to the fetus.

53. **B** [22,II]. This profile view shows severe **micrognathia,** demonstrating a very small jaw. Micrognathia can cause severe polyhydramnios, as in this case, because it interferes with swallowing.

54. **D** [18,I]. A nonstress test measures fetal heart rate accelerations, which normally follow fetal movement. **Two or more fetal heart rate accelerations in 20 minutes** earn the fetus 2 points on a biophysical profile. *Sustained fetal breathing* is also a biophysical profile parameter, but is unrelated to the nonstress test. None of the other choices are part of a nonstress test.

55. **C** [24,II]. The arrow is pointing to the **vagina.** The image shows an anteverted uterus with an almost empty bladder.

56. **C** [29,IV]. An **endometrioma** is the most likely explanation for the area indicated by the question mark. The mass is full of fluid judging by the through transmission, which excludes the possibility of a *fibroid.* The mass also contains many internal echoes, which rules out a *simple cyst.*

57. **E** [29,VII]. **Changing the transducer frequency** is unlikely to improve the image, which is of adequate quality. A higher frequency transducer would have less penetration, which is necessary to visualize this dense mass. An endometrioma is avascular and consists of old blood, so *color flow* would be helpful in showing lack of vascularity in the lesion. *Endovaginal* and transrectal *probes* might help to better define the relationship of the mass to the uterus. If the mass is fluid filled, the contents will show movement when shaken. Therefore, *observing the contents of the mass for movement* would be helpful.

58. **C** [22,II]. The orbits are too close together, which is a finding consistent with **hypotelorism** rather than *hypertelorism* when the orbits are too far apart. Only the orbits are visible, so *micrognathia* and *cleft lip* cannot be assessed on this view. No *proboscis,* which would extend from the forehead, is seen.

 When there are opposite choices (e.g., hypertelorism and hypotelorism), one of them is usually the correct answer. The incorrect choice is included to see if you really understand the concept.

59. **A** [17,VIII]. The **interocular distance** is a measurement of the distance between the eyes, which is necessary to diagnose hypotelorism or hypertelorism. *Ocular measurement* implies that one is measuring the width of the orbit itself. The *binocular distance* is the distance from the outer edge of one eye to the outer edge of the other eye.

60. **C** [22,I]. There is a strong association between hypotelorism and holoprosencephaly, which is a **brain** disorder. There are three types of holoprosencephaly: alobar, lobar, and semilobar.

61. **B** [18,I]. **Asymmetrical intrauterine growth retardation (IUGR)** is the most common type. It allows for the normal growth of the head and brain while the abdomen lags behind. *Symmetrical IUGR* is a lag in growth of the head and body. *Femur-sparing IUGR* is a term used by some when the femur is the only parameter not affected by growth retardation.

 "None of the above: is never used as a correct option in the current examination, so you can eliminate this option.

62. **C** [29,I]. The terms aplasia and agenesis refer to the absence of a structure. Because the uterus and kidney are both derived from the genitourinary system, they both may be affected by agenesis of the genitourinary system. Therefore, bilateral partial agenesis of the genitourinary system is likely to cause **uterine aplasia.** Complete bilateral renal agenesis would be fatal. A *septate uterus, uterus didelphys,* a *bicornuate uterus,* and a *T-shaped uterus* are all congenital uterine anomalies.

63. **B** [14,I]. The blastocyst has an outer layer of trophoblastic cells called the **chorionic villi** that surround a fluid-filled inner cell mass. After the blastocyst attaches to the endometrium, it begins to produce human chorionic gonadotropin along with the corpus luteum. The *decidua* refers to the endometrial changes. The *decidua capsularis* surrounds the blastocyst. The decidua vera or parietalis lines the remainder of the endometrial cavity. *Mesoderm* and *ectoderm* refer to the thickening line of germ cells that will become the embryo.

64. **B** [15,II E]. **Male genitalia,** large testicles and a small penis, are seen on the left side of the image.

65. **C** [18,II]. In this example of **cord entanglement** with monoamniotic twins, two cords originate from the placenta at C1 and C2 and wind around each other. A portion of the second fetus is visible. Fetal death *in utero* in monoamniotic twins is a common finding with cord entanglement; therefore, twins of this type need to be followed closely. *Cord knots* can look similar to cord entanglement if only one fetus is present. *Vasa previa* refers to the insertion of the cord at the margin of the placenta, so the cord insertion lies adjacent to the internal os and may impede delivery.

66. **B** [30,II]. As with most other neoplasms, ovarian cancer usually metastasizes to the **liver.**

67. **D** [19,V]. No fluid can be seen around the fetus; therefore, this image shows **anhydramnios.** The *placenta, cervix,* and *cord* are not visible. No *second twin* is present.

68. **E** [22,VII]. This image shows renal agenesis with *absence of the kidneys.* The **adrenal glands (A) are laterally displaced** as a consequence of the renal agenesis. Because there is renal agenesis, no amniotic fluid is present.

69. **D** [24,V]. The two symmetrical masses on either side of the pelvis posterior to the uterus and adnexa represent the **piriformis muscle.** A *hydrosalpinx* would contain fluid. A *rectal neoplasm* would have an echogenic center. The *sacrum* is bone, so it would create shadowing. The *left ovary* is more anterior.

70. **D** [24,V]. The only muscle that cannot be seen with ultrasound is the **levator ani muscle,** which is too thin to visualize.

71. **D** [16,V]. The white arrow is pointing to the **umbilical artery.** This is the ideal view to show the two umbilical arteries alongside the bladder. This image proves that there is a three-vessel cord.

72. **D** [15,II]. The black arrow is pointing to the left **iliac crest.** A view that shows the bladder and the umbilical arteries will not show the *lumbar spine.* The bony structure is the wrong shape and location for the *femoral head.* The *pubic symphysis* is not located laterally and is poorly ossified *in utero. Osteochondroses* are small bony fragments in a joint; these have not been reported *in utero.*

73. **C** [22,IX]. The scenario should lead the sonographer to suspect dwarfism. The **renal length** is not altered in skeletal abnormalities.

74. **A** [17,XI]. The lateral ventricular width is measured in the region of the atrium of the lateral ventricle (i.e., **posterior to the bulkiest part of the choroid plexus**). It is measured on an **axial view** of the fetal head because the measurement standards are based on that view.

75. **D** [22,I]. This is an image of alobar holoprosencephaly, showing a single, horseshoe-shaped *lateral ventricle.* As is usually the case in holoprosencephaly, the **thalamus is fused** and no *third ventricle* is visible. No *cavum septum pellucidum* is seen; this structure is also absent in holoprosencephaly.

 When two choices are similar (e.g., normal thalamus and fused thalamus), one of them is often the correct answer.

76. **A** [22,I,V]. Holoprosencephaly has a 50% association with trisomy 13, and **omphaloceles** are associated with trisomies 13, 18, and 21. Therefore, an omphalocele should be carefully sought if holo-

prosencephaly is found. *Gastrochisis, cataracts,* and *ureteropelvic junction obstruction* are not associated with chromosomal anomalies or holoprosencephaly. A *short femur* is associated with trisomy 21 rather than trisomy 13 and holoprosencephaly.

77. **E** [27,IV]. In GIFT procedures, the fertilized egg is placed into the **fallopian tube,** allowing fertilization (conception) to occur at the usual site.

78. **D** [15,II A]. This axial view taken low in the skull shows two normal structures: the bony **petrous and sphenoid ridges.** Moving the transducer level approximately 3 mm superior, up to the level of the biparietal diameter, would eliminate these normal structures from the image.

79. **D** [22,V]. A large **omphalocele** is present on this image. The umbilical vein is seen passing through the center of the liver that lies within the omphalocele. In *gastroschisis,* the liver is never seen outside of the abdomen and the umbilical vein inserts separately in the normal location to the left of the abdominal defect. In *bladder extrophy, limb/body wall complex,* and *pentalogy of Cantrell,* additional organs would be seen outside of the trunk.

80. **D** [22,V]. This omphalocele contains **liver and ascites.** Ascitic fluid is often seen in omphaloceles.

81. **B** [22,V]. Liver-containing omphaloceles have a relatively low association with chromosomal anomalies (i.e., **20%**). Gut-containing omphaloceles have a much stronger association with chromosomal anomalies (i.e., *80%*).

82. **C** [22,V]. There is a 50% association of **cardiac** anomalies with omphaloceles, even in the absence of chromosomal abnormalities.

83. **D** [29,IX]. The prefix "para-" refers to "beside." **Paraovarian cysts** are commonly seen in the region of the broad ligament. *Follicular cysts, corpus lutein cysts,* and *serous cystadenomas* all lie within the ovary, and *nabothian cysts* are located in the cervix.

84. **C** [18,II]. There are not **four membranes in the intersac septum;** in fact, there is no intersac membrane in a monochorionic monoamniotic pregnancy.

85. **D** [24,VI]. The **anterior cul-de-sac** is located between the posterior bladder wall and the fundus of the uterus. The *pouch of Douglas,* also called the *posterior cul-de-sac,* is located between the posterior uterine wall and the rectum. The *fornix* is the region of the vagina around the cervix. The *space of Retzius* is between the anterior bladder wall and the symphysis pubis.

86. **B** [17,III]. Dolichocephaly refers to the flattening of the fetal head due to molding; therefore, the **biparietal diameter** would be too short. *Cephalic index, head circumference, intraocular distance,* or *transcerebellar diameter* would provide a better assessment of gestational age in a dolichocephalic head.

87. **A** [18,I]. If **amniotic fluid volume** is low, this indicates a condition that has taken hours or days to develop. *Fetal heart rate, breathing, movement,* and *tone* respond to the hypoxia within minutes.

88. **C** [28,III]. The appearances on this image are typical of **benign endometrial hyperplasia.** The endometrial cavity echoes can be traced through the center of the thickened endometrium, making it unlikely that an intracavitary mass (e.g., *intracavitary polyp, intracavitary fibroid*) is present. The patient is 60 years of age, so this is not the endometrium of a *normal secretory phase of the menstrual cycle,* which can be this thick; however, if that were the case, the endometrial cavity line would probably not be visible.

89. **D** [29,II]. The most likely diagnosis is a **degenerating fibroid** that is undergoing cystic changes. Note that the echo-free area intrudes into the uterine configuration in an irregular fashion, indicating that it is likely of uterine origin. The location of the black area is not appropriate for *uterine cancer,* which arises from the endometrium. The area does not outline bowel in a fashion that suggests *ascites.*

90. **A** [31,VI]. **Trying to go between the mass and the uterus with the endovaginal probe** would not be helpful because the fibroid is inaccessible to the endovaginal approach (i.e., it is on the opposite side of the uterus to the vaginal probe). All of the other techniques listed (*color flow, transrectal probe, MRI,* and *manually pushing the abdomen*) might help with this diagnostic dilemma.

91. **D** [29,I]. The two endometrial cavities appear to join in the middle of the uterus, which is a finding consistent with a **subseptate uterus.** A *uterus didelphys* presents with two separate uterine bodies. A *bicornuate uterus* can be ruled out because although two endometrial cavity echoes can be seen, each entering a cornu, the outline of the uterus is normally shaped.

92. **C** [29,I]. The small cavities of the two abnormal uterine horns do not easily support a normal pregnancy, so the typical history with this type of patient is of **repeated miscarriages.**

93. **D** [29,I]. There is a strong association between uterine anomalies and **kidney** anomalies (e.g., renal agenesis, renal malposition), so be sure to look at the kidneys if you find such a case.

94. **D** [30,I]. Posterior to the uterus is an irregular cystic area consistent with **fluid in the cul-de-sac.**

95. **E** [27,II]. The sonogram shows adhesions; note that the space in the cul-de-sac is oddly shaped due to the fixed pelvic structures. Both ovaries lie posteriorly in the cul-de-sac close to the uterus. Adhesions do not cause **metromenorrhagia,** which means frequent, lengthy periods. However, patients with adhesions may have any or all of the other symptoms listed (i.e., *infertility, chronic lower abdominal pain, pain on intercourse, constipation*).

96. **D** [28,III]. Most gynecologic neoplasms occur **after menopause.**

97. **B** [16,V]. Unless the cord is straight with the arteries uncoiled, the best technique for determining that a two-vessel cord is present is a **transverse oblique color flow view** that shows the **bladder and only one umbilical artery** alongside. No other technique is as reliable, and some feel it should be routine.

98. **A** [25,I]. The Doppler pattern shows low-resistance flow typical of the **secretory phase** once the corpus luteum has developed. The *follicular phase* of the ovary and *proliferative phase* of the endometrium both refer to the first half of the cycle, before ovulation, when the resistance is high.

99. **D** [25,I]. Note that the cystic area has a thick, echogenic wall around it; therefore, it is most likely a **corpus luteum,** which the Doppler study supports. *Cancer* usually has a more complex pattern. Unfortunately, the pulsed Doppler pattern with ovarian cancer and a corpus luteum is often similar.

100. **C** [22,VI]. This image shows a massive **cystic adenomatoid malformation of the lung.** A *teratoma of the lung* would have a more mixed pattern. A *hemothorax* would have the appearance of a pleural effusion. The *heart* is not seen on this low view (note that almost no ribs are shown).

101. **C** [22,VI]. **Hydrops** is a complication of cystic adenomatoid malformation. The development of hydrops with cystic adenomatoid malformation results in fetal death unless *in utero* surgery is performed. Polyhydramnios rather than *oligohydramnios* may develop with large cystic adenomatoid malformations. If at all affected, the placenta will be swollen in association with hydrops rather than showing *placental atrophy*. *Vein of Galen malformation* does not cause an echogenic mass in the lung, and cystic adenomatoid malformation of the lung is not associated with *nuchal thickening*.

102. **D** [27,I]. Intrauterine contraceptive devices (IUCDs) are best located **at the fundus of the uterus.** If located lower in the uterus, IUCDs may fall out. IUCDs that extend *into the myometrium* are difficult to remove and less effective.

103. **D** [17,IX]. Dolichocephaly (i.e., a long, thin head) is present on this sonogram, and can only be revealed by determining the **cephalic index.** The cephalic index is the ratio of the occipitofrontal distance to the biparietal diameter. However, this measurement is usually unnecessary because the cranial shape is obviously long and flattened. In dolichocephaly the *head circumference* remains normal and the *biparietal diameter* appears abnormally small. *Ventricular width* and *intraorbital distance* generally remain unaffected.

104. **C** [15,II A]. Dolichocephaly is seen most often with **breech presentations.** It may also be found with oligohydramnios, not *polyhydramnios*. On rare occasions, it is a feature of craniosynostosis or skull deformity by compression with a fibroid. *Lethal dwarfism* syndromes are associated with brachycephaly or clover-leaf skull deformity rather than dolichocephaly. When the cranium is affected by *osteogenesis imperfecta*, the skull shape is normal. *Undue transducer pressure* can cause a dolichocephalic appearance in osteogenesis imperfecta because the skull is so malleable.

105. **D** [23,I]. A small **fibroid** is seen anterior to the fetal head. Note the discrete rounded shape with normal myometrium on either side ruling out *myometrial contraction*. The mass is not a *cesarean section incision scar* because it is at too high a level on the uterus and does not have the normal echogenic appearance of a scar.

106. **E** [23,I]. Fibroids do not cause **early placental maturation.** The two most significant problems associated with fibroids during pregnancy are *pain if "red" degeneration occurs* and *obstruction of delivery by a large fibroid*. However, fibroids may also result in *prolonged labor* and *difficulty clinically dating the pregnancy*.

107. **C** [14,VII]. Little or no myometrium surrounds this 8-week pregnancy with the uterus adjacent, which is a finding consistent with an **interstitial pregnancy.** Note the endometrial cavity echoes in the uterus far from the pregnancy. A *normal pregnancy* would be located in the endometrium and has myometrial tissue around it. An *intrasac bleed* would show a small fluid-filled, crescent-shaped area adjacent to the sac. A *bicornuate uterus* would show two uterine cavities with a pregnancy in one and a decidualized endometrium in the other.

108. **E** [14,VII]. **Free fluid with internal echoes (i.e., blood) in the cul-de-sac** means that the ectopic pregnancy has or is in the process of rupturing. This is a dangerous sign that requires the patient to undergo immediate treatment. *High diastolic flow on Doppler* can be a nonspecific finding seen in ectopic pregnancies and corpus luteum cysts.

An *extrauterine adnexal mass* and *adnexal ring sign* are other findings seen in ectopic pregnancy but do not indicate imminent rupture. β-*Human chorionic gonadotropin levels* are usually low in ectopic pregnancy and do not correlate with the likelihood of rupture.

109. **E** [20,IV]. **Fetal breathing** does not occur before 23 weeks, and chorionic villi sampling is performed at approximately 10 weeks. Ultrasound is necessary before chorionic villi sampling because no one would consider an invasive procedure without first ensuring that everything is in order. Chorionic villi sampling is normally performed at about 10 weeks—dating confirms that the fetus is not too young or too old. Because a large number of early pregnancies result in spontaneous abortion, a quick scan to verify that *there is fetal heart motion* is necessary before starting the procedure. The *position of the placenta* needs to be assessed to determine whether a transvaginal or transabdominal approach is to be used and to determine the curvature of the catheter. The presence of a multiple pregnancy might change the procedure if the fetuses are fraternal.

110. **C** [18,VI C]. *Hematomas* and *infections* are common after cesarean sections. Uncomplicated maternal **jaundice** does not cause fever and is not associated with delivery.

111. **E** [29,III]. Adhesions, which limit mobility, may result from *metastases, pelvic inflammatory disease, endometriosis,* and *pelvic surgery.* Of the conditions listed, only unruptured **dermoids** do not cause adhesions.

112. **D** [29,V]. The appearances on this image are consistent with **polycystic ovary syndrome.** Note the enlarged ovary with a length of 5.5 cm, the multiple peripherally placed cysts, and the increased stromal tissue at the center of the ovary.

113. **C** [29,V]. **Infrequent, light periods;** infertility; and obesity with excessive hair are the clinical findings associated with polycystic ovary syndrome. Note that the ovarian changes can occur in asymptomatic women.

114. **C** [18,II]. In most cases, the onset of stuck twin syndrome is before 26 weeks' gestation, so *early delivery* is not practical. Repeated therapeutic amniocenteses (i.e., **removing fluid from the amniotic sac around the second twin**) have decreased the high mortality associated with this condition. *Prolonged bed rest* and a *left-side-down position* would not have any effect on the pregnancy. These are used in conditions such as preeclampsia, bleeding, and severe intrauterine growth restriction. A *high-protein diet* would not selectively help the stuck twin, which is the only way to resolve this syndrome.

115. **E** [28,III]. Because there is a complex mass pushing the uterus forward, a neoplasm is a strong possibility in this elderly woman. The **gallbladder** is not a site for ovarian cancer metastases. However, ovarian metastases often go to the *liver, para-aortic nodes,* and *peritoneum.* The *kidneys* are often hydronephrotic if local spread involves the ureters.

116. **C** [28,III]. Although ovarian cancer is likely, pelvic inflammatory disease and metastases from other sites could give this appearance. Pelvic inflammatory disease spares the ovaries, so it is important to perform an endovaginal examination to determine if the **ovaries are part of the mass.** *Gut involvement* is not easy to assess with ultrasound. With this extent of disease, it is unlikely that pelvic structures would be *mobile. Para-aortic nodes* and *hydronephrosis* would not be visible with the endovaginal probe.

117. **C** [15,II F]. The image provided is a side view of a **normal foot.** If *clubfoot* were present, both long bones in the leg would most likely be seen at the same time. If this were a *rocker-bottom foot,* the heel would be unduly prominent.

118. **D** [29,VI]. A cystic mass with an irregular border can be seen adjacent to, but outside of, the ovary and uterus. Of the entities mentioned, only **hydrosalpinx** is extraovarian and extrauterine.

119. **A** [26,IV]. The diagnosis of ambiguous genitalia should be made early to assign sex and avoid psychologic disorders. **Defining the internal anatomy** via sonography is a way to ascertain the presence or absence of a uterus, a cervix, and ovaries. In addition, the kidneys and adrenal glands should be scanned to exclude anomalies of the kidneys and adrenal hyperplasia. The physician should also order chromosomal and hormonal studies. *Hermaphroditism* (see Appendix B) is suspected based on external properties. *Labioscrotal fusion, micropenis,* and *clitoral hypertrophy* are external features, not sonographic findings.

120. **B** [24,V]. The **obturator muscles** line the lateral aspects of the pelvis.

121. **E** [21,II]. This image shows overlapping of the skull bones (i.e., Spalding's sign) and skin thickening around the skull. These findings are most often consistent with **fetal death.** Overlapping skull bones are not associated with *thanatophoric dwarfism, osteogenesis imperfecta, diabetes mellitus,* or *hydrops.*

122. **E** [21,II]. Because there is no flow in the umbilical cord with fetal death, **resistance in the umbilical cord will not be increased on Doppler.** As the contents of the fetus become *macerated, amniotic fluid echoes* appear. The fetal position assumes

that of gravity, and there is *loss of visualization of the internal structures. Absence of fetal heart motion* is the earliest and best way of making the diagnosis of fetal death.

123. **C** [17,III]. The **cerebral peduncles** may easily be mistaken by an inexperienced sonographer for the thalamus on an axial view of the fetal brain. However, the peduncles lie inferior and slightly posterior to the thalamus. The *interhemispheric fissure* and *cavum septum pellucidum* should be found on a biparietal diameter measurement. The *choroid plexus* is best seen on a higher level. The *temporal horns of the lateral ventricle* are not normally visualized, unless the ventricular system is dilated.

124. **A** [15,II E]. The arrowhead is pointing to the fetal **kidneys.** There is often so little fat in the renal sinuses *in utero* that no echogenic area is seen in the center of the fetal kidney.

125. **A** [16,V]. The arrow is pointing to the **cord insertion,** which appears normal with no *omphalocele* or *allantoic cyst* (both of these entities involve the cord insertion). No *gastroschisis* is seen on this transverse image, and the portal vein would not be seen at the skin surface.

126. **C** [18,II]. Because there is a thick intervening membrane showing the twin peak sign, this is an example of **dichorionic diamniotic twins.** *Monochorionic diamniotic twins* would have a thin membrane between the two sacs. *Monochorionic monoamniotic twins* would have no membrane at all. Two gestational sacs and fetuses can be seen, so this is not a *singleton pregnancy.* A diagnosis of *fetal death* cannot be made unless an M-mode tracing is obtained through the heart showing no cardiac motion or one of the signs of fetal death develops, such as Spalding's sign, maceration, or severe skin thickening.

127. **C** [18,II]. Identification of **different fetal genitalia** is the most definitive way of confirming the diagnosis of dichorionic diamniotic twins (i.e., fraternal twins) if the fetuses are of opposite sex. *First trimester* detection of a thick intervening membrane is the next most accurate method, followed by detection of the *twin peak sign. Counting the components of the membrane* is difficult and of questionable accuracy. The least accurate method is identification of *two placentas* because the second placenta often lies adjacent to the first, or a succenturiate lobe can suggest dichorionicity.

128. **C** [29,VII]. The image using color flow shows that **vessels extend from the uterus to the mass, indicating a fibroid** rather than an ovarian mass.

129. **C** [14,VI]. A **fetal heart rate of 50,** which is usually associated with impending fetal death, is the worst of these bad prognostic signs.

130. **A** [16,VII]. In most early cases of partial placenta previa, the **placenta will move toward the fundus within 6–8 weeks** and will cease to be an apparent placenta previa. This movement occurs because the placenta lies adjacent to the internal os, but is not attached at this site. In a few cases, the placenta will remain a placenta previa. In asymptomatic patients, no special management is necessary except for the performance of a later sonogram. Placental tissue over or near the os is never considered a *normal variant. Vaginal bleeding* does not usually occur with symptomatic placenta previa in this location early in pregnancy. If it does, it is much more likely that persistent placenta previa will occur and that the placenta will not change position.

131. **C** [15,II]. The mass indicated by the thick black arrow is a **pelvic kidney;** note the central echogenic sinus echoes. The kidney is clearly separate from the uterus and from the left ovary, which lies adjacent to the uterus.

132. **C** [29,I]. The endometrial echoes are **much thicker than normal.**

133. **B** [29,I]. Of the options listed, only a **decidual reaction** results in a thick endometrium. A thick endometrial reaction measuring over 1 cm in a possibly pregnant woman is suspicious for **ectopic pregnancy.** Some women have this thickness in the normal secretory phase of the menstrual cycle, not the *proliferative phase. Heavy menstruation* may result in blood in the endometrial cavity, but does not look evenly echogenic. *Intracavitary fibroids* look hypoechoic with an echogenic rim rather than densely echogenic.

134. **E** [31,VI]. The appearances on this image are suggestive of an ectopic pregnancy. **Using an endovaginal probe to look for heart motion** is diagnostic of this condition if heart motion is detected. Local *tenderness* would be of some help, but is not diagnostic of an ectopic pregnancy. *Color flow* is not helpful, but pulsed Doppler would be of some value if it showed a low-resistance pattern.

135. **A** [17,V]. The **umbilical artery** is not seen when measuring the abdominal circumference at the proper level. Structures that are seen include the *aorta, stomach, fetal adrenal glands,* and *transverse spine.* The portal sinus (i.e., *umbilical vein*) is another helpful landmark.

136. **E** [15,II A]. This profile view is **normal.** A portion of a limb lies close to the forehead suggesting a *proboscis;* however, it is not attached to the skull and contains a small portion of bone and so does

not represent a proboscis. Because the orbit is not visible and the chin can be seen, this is a technically satisfactory (not *unsatisfactory*) view on which *micrognathia* and *frontal bossing* can be assessed; neither is present.

137. **C** [22,VI]. On this image, the heart is displaced to the right and a cystic mass (i.e., the stomach) is seen on the left, making a **diaphragmatic hernia** the most likely diagnosis. *Type III cystic adenomatoid malformations* create so many specular reflectors that they do not actually appear cystic, but echogenic instead. A *mediastinal teratoma* would not appear as a simple cyst but would have a complex appearance. If this were a *vascular malformation,* it would be extremely large and the heart would also be enlarged with evidence of hydrops. The abnormal cystic area would not be a feature of *situs inversus.*

138. **A** [22,VI]. The **stomach** is almost always located in the chest with left-sided diaphragmatic hernias, in which case it **would not appear on a view of the abdomen.** Diaphragmatic hernias are usually associated with a small fetal abdomen, not a *large fetal abdomen. Large bowel dilation* almost never occurs *in utero.* However, small bowel dilation may be present and would be a helpful supporting sign. *Cardiac abnormalities* are quite common in association with diaphragmatic hernias but are difficult to recognize because the position of the heart is so distorted.

139. **A** [29,VI]. There is nothing except fluid in the dilated tube, so no **shadowing artifact** would be expected.

140. **B** [18,II]. A second trimester demise with maceration is a **fetus papyraceous.** *Vanishing twin* refers to visualization of the gestational sac with our without an embryo in the first trimester that subsequently disappears. *Acardiac twins* share a blood supply with reversed circulation. *Twin-to-twin transfusion syndrome* (i.e., placental steal) occurs in monochorionic monoamniotic twins with a shared placenta. *Conjoined twins* are the result of a late division with the fetuses joined most commonly at the thorax.

141. **B** [18,I]. A fetus cannot be **overactive;** activity is one of the features of a normal biophysical profile. *Fetal hiccups* make it difficult to assess fetal breathing, and *premature rupture of membranes* can result in absent amniotic fluid, which limits fetal movement. Movement usually increases after the mother has eaten and is no longer *fasting. Resting* (i.e., sleeping) fetuses can give a spuriously inactive biophysical profile.

142. **B** [26,III]. The internal echoes in the endometrial cavity indicate that it is full of fluid, which is most likely blood. At 17 years of age, it is still possible for the patient not to have had menstrual bleeding from her vagina (i.e., **amenorrhea**). Her episodes of lower abdominal pain most likely occur when she menstruates into the blocked uterus.

143. **D** [26,III]. The obstruction is at the **internal os.** Note that the cervix is closed. Thus, this condition is hematometra, in which only the uterus is distended with blood. If the vagina were also distended, it would be hematocolpometra.

144. **C** [14,II]. A **normal yolk sac** is present on this image. It is located somewhat unusually superior to the head. An *intrasac bleed* would be adjacent to the sac, *nuchal edema* would be along the posterior surface of the embryo, a *large yolk sac* would be over 5 mm in size, and a *halo* is not a medical term.

145. **C** [28,III]. Providing the endometrial cavity is smooth when it is less than 5 mm thick, **endometrial atrophy** can be diagnosed, eliminating the need to perform further procedures. Normally, postmenopausal bleeding is followed by endometrial biopsy. If most of the cavity is 1–2 mm thick but there is a local bulge, a *polyp* or *neoplasm* can still be present in a thin cavity.

146. **B** [15,II C]. The arrow is pointing to a normal **right ventricular outflow tract.** The choices indicate that this question relates to the fetal heart, and the only structure that crosses transversely without showing other cardiac anatomy is the right ventricular outflow tract (i.e., the pulmonary artery).

147. **D** [18,III A]. **Maternal diabetes** can result in polyhydramnios and macrosomia. *Preeclampsia* is pregnancy-induced hypertension with proteinuria and is associated with intrauterine growth restriction. *Maternal hypertension* typically results in oligohydramnios and intrauterine growth restriction. *Placental insufficiency* causes the placenta, and usually the fetus, to be too small. Fetal blood pressure cannot be measured, so fetal hypertension would not be discovered.

148. **D** [17,IV]. The femur in the **near field** will afford the best measurement. In addition, the ultrasound beam needs to be **perpendicular** to the object being evaluated to obtain the best image. **Either the medial or the lateral border** of the femur can be measured. Near field measurements may be distorted when using a *sector scanner.* The *epiphysis* should not be included in a femur measurement.

149. **D** [22,VII]. The measured structures are **bilateral distended renal pelves.** Note that the fluid-filled areas lie alongside the spine and so are too far posterior to be any of the other entities mentioned.

150. **E** [22,VII]. Renal conditions do not affect the **liver.** However, when renal pelvic dilation is found, consider the rest of the genitourinary system. The *renal parenchyma, ureters,* and *bladder* all should be examined in detail. If there are abnormalities in addition to pelvic dilation, the prognosis or diagnosis may change. *Gender* should be determined because posterior urethral valves, the most serious potential differential diagnosis, affects only males.

151. **E** [23,IV]. The placenta is greatly enlarged and contains many small hypoechoic areas, which is an appearance typical of a **partial mole.** *Placental infarct, diabetes mellitus, intraplacental bleed,* and *TORCH infection* do not cause enlargement and cystic changes in the placenta.

152. **A** [20,II]. The findings on this image strongly suggest triploidy, so karyotyping the amniotic fluid from an **amniocentesis** is the next logical step. The serum β-human chorionic gonadotropin (β-HCG) levels will most likely be elevated but do not give a definitive answer on the nature of the process; a *urinary β-HCG* would be even less helpful, only indicating that a pregnancy is present. *Serum estriol levels* are part of the triple screen test performed to detect Down syndrome. *Serum α-fetoprotein analysis* is a test performed to screen for spina bifida and is a component of the triple screen. A *dilation and curettage* is a surgical procedure to abort the pregnancy, but before it is performed a more definitive diagnosis would be needed.

153. **C** [23,III]. **Thecalutein cysts** are found in about 40% of moles and may also be seen with partial moles. Multiple large cysts are seen in greatly enlarged ovaries. *Corpus luteum cysts* develop in the secretory phase of the menstrual cycle and in association with normal early pregnancies. *Follicular cysts* are unruptured follicles, and *endometriomas* are blood collections associated with endometriosis. A *hydrosalpinx* is a blocked fallopian tube dilated with fluid and is usually a consequence of pelvic inflammatory disease.

154. **C** [29,III]. The echogenic mass that is hard to distinguish from bowel and mesentery is a large **ovarian dermoid.** Ovarian dermoids are easy to miss because they are often confused with *bowel.* The high-level echoes in the mass are related to the contents (i.e., a mixture of fat and hair). Color flow would show ovarian vessels supplying the mass.

155. **E** [29,III]. Dermoids come in several different forms, which include *echo-free cysts, cysts containing areas of shadowing,* masses with unusual *fluid levels,* and *cysts with multiple thick septa.* A **hypoechoic, solid mass** is almost unheard of with dermoids.

156. **B** [31,II]. At 70 years of age, this patient is inevitably menopausal, so the **date of her last normal menstrual period** is irrelevant to the examination. *Abdominal surgery* (e.g., appendicitis) can be of importance because secondary infection and adhesions are possible. Both *tuberculosis and diabetes mellitus* can have pelvic manifestations. *Complaints of abdominal pain* will influence the way in which the sonogram is performed.

157. **A** [24,I]. The **fundus** is the superior portion of the uterus.

158. **A** [24,I]. The **cervix** is the inferior segment of the uterus.

159. **C** [24,I]. The **corpus** is the body of the uterus.

160. **E** [24,I]. The **endometrium** is the tissue that borders the endometrial cavity. It is more echogenic than the myometrium.

161. **D** [24,I]. The **internal os** is at the proximal end of the cervical canal.

162. **E** [24,I]. The **external os** is at the distal end of the cervical canal.

163. **D** [18,II]. In twin-to-twin transfusion syndrome, blood is shunted through the *large intraplacental arterioarterial anastamoses anastomosis,* causing the *donor twin to become small and anemic* and the *recipient twin to become large and edematous.* Therefore, there is not a **small recipient twin.**

164. **B** [26,II]. **Precocious puberty** is the term used to describe the development of female sexual characteristics before 8 years of age. *Pseudoprecocious puberty* is not affected by pituitary gonadotropins, but is due to ovarian or adrenal dysfunction.

165. **C** [29,II]. Nabothian cysts are a **normal variant finding.**

166. **E** [26,III]. A **bicornuate uterus** is not associated with fluid in the endometrial cavity. An *imperforate hymen* causes retained menstrual fluid at puberty. With *menstruation,* fluid may be seen in the endometrial cavity if a partially obstructing process, such as a fibroid, is present. When performing a *hysterosonogram,* fluid is placed in the endometrial cavity. *Radiation to cervical cancer* may cause cervical stenosis, with subsequent fluid backup in the endometrial cavity.

167. **C** [15,II E]. There is a **small hydrocele** surrounding the left testicle.

168. **C** [22,VII]. Small hydroceles are a **common normal variant,** occasionally associated with *hydrops*

because the *processus vaginalis* normally connects the scrotal and peritoneal contents *in utero*.

169. **C** [16,V]. The structure indicated by the arrow is most likely an **umbilical artery,** but a *urachal remnant* is also possible. A patent urachus may communicate with the fetal bladder as well as the abdominal wall, creating a cystic tract between the abdominal wall and the fetal bladder. However, both urachal remnants and *abdominal masses* are uncommon.

170. **C** [16,V]. **Color flow analysis** will confirm that the structure is a normal umbilical artery. *Harmonics* is a technique for analyzing the frequency of the returning signal, which is helpful in obese patients but would not help in this case because the image is of adequate quality.

171. **E** [22,I]. **Cerebellar hypoplasia** is not a sonographic feature of isolated agenesis of the corpus callosum. Because the corpus callosum is absent, the midline structures are affected, the third ventricle is pulled up into the space that is normally occupied by the cavum septi pellucidi (i.e., *high-riding third ventricle*), and the *gyri are vertically aligned*. *Colpocephaly* (i.e., selective dilation of the posterior part of the lateral ventricles) is often associated with agenesis of the corpus callosum.

172. **E** [14,II]. The **chorionic membrane** is not normally visible during the first trimester unless there is a subchorionic bleed. The amnion and the chorion are not fused in the first trimester, so the *amniotic membrane* is normally visible between the amniotic fluid and the extracelomic space. The *vitelline duct* is a small, normal structure leading to the yolk sac that can sometimes be seen in the first trimester. The *yolk sac* is normally visible from 5 weeks until about 12 weeks. A *nuchal line less than 3 mm thick* is a normal finding late in the first trimester.

173. **C** [15,II C]. The arrow is pointing to an **echogenic focus in the heart** in the right ventricle. The cardiac configuration is otherwise normal.

174. **B** [22,XI]. There is a weak but fairly convincing association between chromosomal abnormalities such as **trisomy 21** (Down syndrome) and echogenic foci in the heart. However, most clinicians feel that this finding in isolation is not enough to warrant an amniocentesis. Therefore, the sonographer should search carefully for other signs of trisomy 21; if any are found, an amniocentesis will be advised.

175. **C** [29,III]. The images suggest an adnexal mass other than the ovary and raise the question of ectopic pregnancy; therefore, it is important to determine the **date of the patient's last period.** In fact, the date of the last menstrual period is always an appropriate question for a patient of childbearing age. If you answered "E"—does she have *pain with intercourse*—you are on the right track; this certainly could be pelvic inflammatory disease. However, it is more important to rule out ectopic pregnancy first.

176. **D** [25,I]. Follicle-stimulating hormone and luteinizing hormone are gonadotropic hormones released by the **anterior lobe of the pituitary gland.** These hormones are carried to the *ovaries* where they cause follicular development and ovulation. The *corpus albicans* is the remnant of the corpus luteum. *Proliferation of the endometrial lining* occurs after menses and before ovulation. *Graafian follicles* do not secrete follicle-stimulating hormone or luteinizing hormone.

177. **D** [15,II A]. This is a view of a **fetal ear** with the cranium below.

178. **D** [18,I]. A **two-vessel cord** does not cause intrauterine growth restriction (IUGR) when it is the only finding. Pregnancies with mothers who are older (e.g., *40 years*) or young (e.g., *15 years*), who have a poor diet for the fetus (e.g., *fast food, vegan*), or who live at *high altitudes* are all at risk for IUGR.

179. **D** [27,III]. A **luteinized, unruptured follicle** is a common cause of infertility that results when a follicle develops but does not ovulate. The follicle continues to grow and eventually atrophies. A normal, unstimulated dominant follicle ovulates when it reaches a size of 1.5–2.6 cm. Ovulation may occur from day 9 on, but has usually occurred by day 18 in a normal 28-day cycle. If ovulation has occurred by day 18, a *corpus luteum* should have developed, but a corpus luteum generally contains internal echoes. An *endometrioma* develops during menstruation rather than late in the cycle and is not echo-free.

180. **D** [18,IV A]. Over the course of 5 minutes the fluid entered the cervical canal and the cervical length changed from 4.6 to 1.94 cm. These changes can be caused by uterine contractions associated with **premature labor** (i.e., premature rupture of membranes) **or cervical incompetence.** Associated contraction pain makes premature labor more likely.

 Read ALL of the choices before deciding on the correct answer. One choice may be right, but another choice may be even more right.

181. **C** [16,VII]. A **partial placenta previa** appears to be present because the placenta is partially covering the internal os. As a myometrial contraction occurs, fluid enters the internal os and it is apparent that the placenta does not cover it. These two images show why it is important to spend some time watching before deciding that a placenta previa is present.

182. **D** [28,III]. A large, echogenic mass, which is **choriocarcinoma,** occupies most of the uterus. *Multiple fibroids* would show several distinct, homogeneous masses. *Hematocolpos* implies a vagina full of blood. *Adenomyosis* gives a more subtle, "moth-eaten" appearance with small, hypoechoic, discrete masses in the central myometrium, almost like tiny, ill-defined fibroids. In the case of a *partial mole,* there would be a fetus and amniotic fluid in addition to the mass.

183. **B** [28,III]. With choriocarcinoma, the **liver,** brain, and chest are the common sites for metastases. However, the chest and brain cannot be adequately examined with ultrasound.

184. **D** [29,IV]. The appearances on this image suggest an endometrioma with even, high-level echoes in the mass. Therefore, it is likely that the patient will have a history of **pelvic pain and infertility.** *Cervical tenderness and vaginal discharge* are symptoms of pelvic inflammatory disease; in this condition, the walls of the fallopian tube would be visible and the contents would be more heterogeneous. It would be highly unlikely for this patient to be *asymptomatic.*

185. **B** [22,IV]. Both of these images show **spina bifida.** Note the skin defect on the prone view and the widened posterior elements on the transverse view. No meningocele is present. A normal empty bladder is seen on the sagittal image. There is no *midabdominal mass* present.

186. **D** [20,II]. In spina bifida, the **acetylcholinesterase** level is typically elevated in the amniotic fluid. Maternal blood, not amniotic fluid, is used to evaluate *maternal serum α-fetoprotein* (MSAFP) levels. However, in spina bifida the amniotic fluid α-fetoprotein (MAAFP) level is also elevated. *Triglyceride* is a blood level associated with cholesterol elevation, not used in the detection of pregnancy abnormalities; *estriol* and *human chorionic gonadotropin* are both components of the triple screen used in detecting trisomies 18 and 21.

187. **D** [22,IV]. The spine curves slightly posteriorly at about L5. A skin defect can be seen two vertebral levels above L5, so the approximate level at which this spina bifida begins is **L3.**

188. **B** [29,IX]. The white arrow is pointing to a **para-ovarian cyst.** Both the ovary and the neighboring cyst can be seen; therefore, this is not a *dominant follicle* or *dermoid,* which are intraovarian processes. The *iliac artery* and vein can be seen alongside the ovary and cyst. The *bladder* is not visible on this image.

189. **A** [25,I]. Estrogen is secreted by developing **graafian follicles.** The *corpus luteum* produces progesterone. The *anterior lobe of the pituitary gland* produces luteinizing hormone and follicle-stimulating hormone.

190. **C** [18,I]. In **symmetrical intrauterine growth restriction,** the entire fetus is abnormally small; therefore, the head:abdomen ratio is normal. In *microcephaly,* the head is abnormally small, and in *macrosomia,* the abdomen is abnormally large, both of which change the head:abdomen ratio. In *hydrocephalus,* the head is abnormally large, which also changes the head:abdomen ratio. In *gastroschisis,* because the bowel is outside of the abdomen, the abdominal measurement may be small or inaccurate.

191. **B** [16,IV]. Low-level echoes in an area enclosed by a membrane are indicative of blood. The location of this bleed alongside the placenta is typical of a **marginal bleed.** An *amniotic sheet* would have clear amniotic fluid on both sides of it and a broad base where it attaches to the uterine wall. Amniotic sheets do not adhere to the fetus and, unlike *amniotic bands,* do not cause fetal malformations. The amniotic cavity remaining following a *resorbed twin* would not have a linear shape alongside the uterine wall and would not contain internal echoes.

192. **B** [16,VI]. The echoes in the measured area are not easy to see. **Increasing the gain** would demonstrate the evidence of blood in this area much better. Because there is no flow, *Doppler* and *color flow* would not help. *Increasing transducer frequency* might show internal echoes better but is less effective and more time-consuming than increasing the gain. *Placing the patient in the decubitus position* would not improve the image because the suspect area is already close to the transducer.

193. **C** [22,V]. **Gastroschisis** is seen on this image. Note that the cord enters to one side of the mass rather than through the center. There is no membrane around this mass of small bowel as would be seen with an *omphalocele. Sacrococcygeal teratoma* arises from the coccyx rather than the anterior abdominal wall. *Umbilical hernias* are similar to omphaloceles, occurring at the cord insertion and surrounded by a membrane; they are much smaller than this mass.

194. **D** [22,V]. Only **bowel distention** is a complication of gastroschisis. *Cardiac abnormalities, pentalogy of Cantrell, karyotypic abnormalities,* and *hydronephrosis* are all complications of omphaloceles.

195. **D** [28,III]. The mass indicated by the arrow is **partially cystic and partially solid.** Note the acoustic enhancement.

196. **E** [28,III]. The mass is located **superior to the uterus.**

197. **C** [28,III]. **Ovarian cancer** seems more likely than *ovarian cystadenoma* because there are both cystic and sizable solid components. A *uterine fibroid* would be more solid, and an *endometrioma* would have more homogeneous contents. An *inflammatory mass* would be unlikely to be so large and singular.

198. **E** [31,VI]. **Looking in the endometrial cavity for polyps** would not help in the diagnosis of this adnexal mass. All of the other techniques would be appropriate with a mass of this complexity, which proved to be an ovarian cancer.

199. **B** [31,II]. This patient's history is mostly of little relevance to the gynecologic sonogram. The two important items are the foul-smelling discharge and the **history of amenorrhea** at this young age.

200. **A** [15,II B]. This is a normal prone view of the **iliac crests and the spine** (i.e., the lumbosacral vertebrae). *Spina bifida* is not present. The *bladder* is not shown—the apparent bladder distension suggestive of *posterior urethral valves* is shadowing created by the iliac crest and spine.

201. **E** [15,II B]. **Cord tethering** cannot be diagnosed on a transverse view of the distal spine. Widening of the normal right angle between the iliac crests is seen in *bladder extrophy, Down syndrome,* and *spina bifida.* In fact, the widening of the posterior elements of the spine associated with spina bifida is best seen on this type of view and is most common at this level. The mass associated with myelomeningocele and *sacrococcygeal teratoma* could also be seen on this image.

202. **D** [22,IV]. Identification of the uppermost level of spina bifida *in utero* can be used to **predict the chance of limited leg motion**—the higher the level, the greater the chance of poor leg motion. Myelomeningoceles above T12 are always associated with absence of leg motion. *Hydrocephalus* correlates better with ventricular appearance than spinal level. The severity of *urinary* and *rectal mal-*

function is hard to predict from spinal appearances.

203. **A** [18,II]. There is little or no fluid around the twin from which the Doppler signals are obtained, making it likely that **absent diastolic flow is due to the stuck twin syndrome.** Absent diastolic flow is considered evidence of fetal compromise, and sometimes triggers emergency cesarean section. It is often seen in stuck twin syndrome. The affected fetus can survive once therapeutic maneuvers are performed. There is a sizable diastolic component to *normal umbilical artery flow;* normal umbilical vein flow does not differentiate between systole and diastole. *Oligohydramnios* is often associated with absent diastolic flow but does not cause it.

204. **C** [21,II]. The structure being measured is most likely a **dead twin.** The small, distorted twin is definitely dead because the cranium is so deformed. A *rudimentary twin* is a miniature live twin.

205. **A** [20,I]. The α-fetoprotein level is elevated with twins and fetal death. Therefore, in this case it would be expected to be high, and is most likely to be **8 multiples of the mean (MoM).** The normal α-fetoprotein level with twins is *4 MoM,* which is double the upper limits of normal in singletons (i.e., *2 MoM*).

206. **B** [22,I]. The lateral ventricle is dilated, consistent with **ventriculomegaly.** A *choroid plexus cyst* is not present because the normal choroid plexus is visible within the dilated lateral ventricle.

207. **A** [22,I]. The posterior horn of the lateral ventricle is dilated but not the anterior horn; this is known as **colpocephaly.** All of the other findings are also features of agenesis of the corpus callosum.

208. **E** [22,I]. A **sagittal view** is invaluable in showing the radiating gyri and demonstrating that the corpus callosum is absent. It is often best obtained with the endovaginal probe if the fetus is vertex. *Coronal views* are helpful in seeing the relative position of the third ventricle.

209. **B** [29,III]. Two cysts are present on the image: **a complex cyst and a simple cyst.** Note the subtle low-level echoes in the larger cyst, which is too large to be a *follicle. Dermoids* and *neoplasms* would most likely contain more material, and the fat or hair in the dermoid would cause some attenuation of the sound.

210. **C** [31,VI]. The second image shown here shows all of the internal structures that were visible after **increasing the gain.** This was the most helpful of the techniques mentioned.

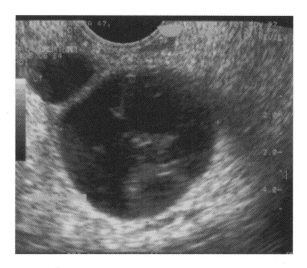

211. **D** [16,IX]. Grade 3 placentas represent intraplacental calcification and are a natural part of the maturation process. A grade 3 placenta is an acceptable normal variant from **36 weeks** on; however, at *45 weeks* the patient should have been delivered and is grossly postmature. A grade 3 placenta occurring *earlier than 36 weeks* may be associated with intrauterine growth restriction and may not be a normal variant.

212. **D** [22,VII,VIII]. **Pericardial cysts** do not lie in the peritoneum; they are located in the chest. *Duplication cysts, mesenteric cysts, meconium cysts,* and *ovarian cysts* are all intraperitoneal.

213. **B** [15,II A]. The arrow is pointing to the **forehead.** The lips can be seen below the nose.

214. **A** [28,III]. The mass is **submucosal** because it lies adjacent to the cavity, which is slightly dilated adjacent to the mass. The mass extends to the myometrium; therefore, it is not *intracavitary.* The mass is clearly not within the myometrium (*intramural*) or distorting the surface of the uterus (*subserosal*), and it is not *pedunculated* (i.e., lying away from the uterus on a stalk).

215. **D** [28,III]. The complex mass contains **many interfaces.** It is most likely a polyp, although lipoleiomyomas, (a type of fibroid that contains fat) occasionally occur in the uterus. There is not much acoustic shadowing, so the mass does not contain *gas* or *calcium.* A mass that contains *fat* only is echo-free. Masses that contain fat with other material (such as hair) are frequently very echogenic. *Pus* is not this echogenic.

216. **E** [18,I]. Pulsed Doppler can be used to assess the **physiologic status** of the fetus by identifying the direction of blood flow, flow disturbance, abnormal flow patterns, and blood velocity through sampling of the umbilical cord artery. Sampling can also be done using the fetal middle cerebral artery. Neoplasms (e.g., *chorioangioma*) and *placenta abruptio* occur in the placenta and do not cause intrauterine growth restriction. *Fetal breathing* and *fetal tone* are visual observations made during the biophysical profile.

217. **B** [22,I]. A width of approximately 11 mm is considered the threshold for the diagnosis of ventriculomegaly.

218. **C** [23,II]. This sonogram reveals a large **cyst superior to the uterus.** Note the excellent through transmission, ruling out a *fibroid.*

219. **C** [23,II]. **Corpus luteum cysts** are seen in a number of pregnancies in the first trimester and usually disappear spontaneously by 16–18 weeks. Therefore, a follow-up sonogram is often done at 16–18 weeks. Corpus luteum cysts are by far the most common cysts with pregnancy. *Dermoid cysts* come next in frequency, are more common than *cystadenomas,* and may be echo-free. *Mesenteric and liver cysts* are very rare.

220. **E** [22;VII]. Both of the cysts seen on this sonogram are too anterior to the spine to be *renal cysts.* The cyst with a more irregular outline is the stomach. At this low level (i.e., where no liver can be seen) an intraperitoneal mass in a female is most likely an **ovarian cyst.** Therefore, determining the gender of the fetus becomes important.

221. **B** [25,I]. A graafian follicle, usually known as a dominant follicle, secretes estrogen and **supports the growth of the ovum** until it matures at ovulation. A *primary follicle* is one of many follicles that begin to grow in the follicular stage. The *corpus luteum* develops after ovulation where the dominant follicle was previously. It supplies estrogen and progesterone to prepare the endometrium for the fertilized ovum. If fertilization does not occur, the corpus luteum regresses into the corpus albicans.

222. **A** [29,III]. Note that ovarian tissue surrounds the echogenic mass like a claw, confirming that it is intraovarian. Because the echogenic mass is in the ovary, an *intrauterine contraceptive device,* a *portion of gut containing gas,* and *tubal ligation clips* are not logical considerations. The acoustic shadowing on this image is consistent with **calcification in the ovary.** A *fat- and hair-filled dermoid* appears as a densely echogenic mass with shadowing, but does not have the bright, discrete, echogenic foci of calcification.

223. **A** [29,III]. Most calcifications in the ovary are thought to be the result of old calcifications from a *corpus luteum* with *hemorrhage* (corpus albi-

cans), but some are **dermoids** (i.e., benign cystic teratomas). Calcification does not occur with *recent hemorrhage from a corpus luteum.* Neither *ovarian cancer* nor *hydrosalpinx* present with isolated calcification.

224. **C** [22,VII]. These kidneys are large for a fetus at term and much too large for a fetus at 28 weeks. Very large echogenic kidneys are typical of **infantile polycystic kidney disease** (known more correctly as autosomal recessive polycystic kidney disease). *Medical renal disease* is almost unknown *in utero* and is not characterized by renal enlargement. In the initial phase of *dysplastic kidney disease,* the kidneys are echogenic and mildly enlarged. Later, small cysts are seen in the periphery of the kidney.

 When more than one choice is factually correct (e.g., the second and third choices of question #224), choose the one that is the most specific (e.g., infantile polycystic disease rather than medical renal disease or masses).

225. **B** [22,VII]. Infantile polycystic kidney disease is an **autosomal recessive** condition. It is usually, but not always, *lethal in utero.* Adult polycystic kidney disease is *autosomal dominant* and associated with *intracranial aneurysms* and *cysts in the pancreas and liver.*

226. **D** [29,III]. **Ovarian dermoids** are benign lesions that do not spread. A rare similar entity, known as teratocarcinoma of the ovary, can metastasize to the liver. *Breast cancer, ovarian cancer,* and *choriocarcinoma* can all metastasize to the liver. *Pelvic inflammatory disease* can occasionally spread to the region around the liver, giving rise to the Fitz-Hugh–Curtis syndrome.

227. **A** [14,III]. The first recognizable structure is the **heart** because one can see motion. Embryos that are less than 3 mm long do not normally show cardiac motion.

228. **C** [22,I]. A **lemon-shaped skull** is seen on this sonogram. Note the frontal flattening.

229. **A** [22,I]. There is a **banana-shaped cerebellum** in the fetal brain. This finding, along with an absent *cisterna magna,* is diagnostic of the Arnold-Chiari II malformation.

 Although the sonogram with question #229 is not a great example of a banana-shaped cerebellum, none of the other answers work with this entity. Do not be afraid to rely on knowledge and logic even if the picture is not obvious.

230. **B** [22,I]. Arnold-Chiari II malformation characterized by a lemon-shaped skull, a banana-shaped cerebellum, and an absent cisterna magna is associated with spinal cord neural crest anomalies, most often **myelomeningocele.** *Klippel-Feil syndrome* is a condition in which the neck is very short because of congenital fusion or less than the usual number of cervical vertebrae. None of the other conditions listed are related to intracranial pathology.

231. **B** [22,I]. Based on the findings on this sonogram, there will almost certainly be a spina bifida present. Clubfeet and absence of leg movement may accompany spina bifida and are important in predicting prognosis, so it is necessary to look in detail at the **lower extremities.**

232. **A** [24,IV]. The **fimbriae** are the peritoneal outlet of the fallopian tubes.

233. **C** [24,IV]. The letter "B" marks the **ampullary** portion of the fallopian tube.

234. **B** [24,IV]. The letter "C" marks the **isthmic** portion of the fallopian tube.

235. **E** [24,IV]. The **cornu** of the fallopian tube is the mouth of the fallopian tube as it joins the endometrial cavity.

236. **D** [24,IV]. The letter "E" marks the **ovary.**

237. **A** [24,IV]. The letter "F" marks the **endometrial cavity.**

238. **B** [28,II]. It is best to perform endovaginal sonography at the **beginning of the hormonal cycle,** when the endometrium is thinnest.

239. **D** [16,III]. The most likely diagnosis is a **venous lake.** The venous flow is so slow that no flow is detected with a typical color flow system. *Chorioangiomas* contain arterial flow, which is obvious on color flow Doppler. There may be a few random movements in a *marginal bleed,* but this is not a typical location; marginal bleeds are usually located at the lateral margin of the placenta rather than on the surface. There will be no movement in *Wharton's jelly,* which normally coats the umbilical cord, or in a *placental cyst.*

240. **A** [15,II A]. The arrowhead is pointing to the **anterior (frontal) horn of the lateral ventricle.** The *cavum septum pellucidum* can be seen medial and to the left of the lateral ventricle. The *temporal horn of the lateral ventricle* would be more laterally placed and at a more inferior level. The thalamus is not fluid filled, and a third ventricular cyst would be midline and posterior to the arrowed location.

241. **A** [15,II A]. The question mark lies in the lateral recess of the **cisterna magna,** posterior to the *cerebellum.* The *tentorium* is seen as the border between the cerebellum and the cerebrum. The *ambient cistern,* which is not in the posterior fossa, appears echogenic on ultrasound. The *vermis* is the echogenic central portion of the cerebellum.

242. **D** [15,II A]. The arrow is pointing to the area just deep to the skull where the **dura mater,** which surrounds the brain, lies. The *cavum septum pellucidum, lateral ventricles, third ventricle,* and *thalamus* are not adjacent to the skull.

243. **C** [22,I]. This sonogram shows an **arachnoid cyst.** The cyst lies medial to the lateral ventricle, so *dilated lateral ventricles* can be excluded. A *dilated third ventricle* can be ruled out because the cyst is posterior and inferior to the thalamus, which surrounds the third ventricle. The lateral ventricle, which would contain a *choroid plexus cyst,* is displaced laterally by the cyst.

244. **D** [16,VIII]. A portion of the placenta is separate from the main placenta; therefore, a **succenturiate lobe** is present. *Placenta previa* cannot be diagnosed from this transverse image—note that the cervix is not visible. The placenta does not have the texture of a *molar pregnancy* or a *grade 3 placenta. Venous lakes* are located on the amniotic aspect of the placenta just below the chorionic plate.

245. **D** [16,VIII]. **Color flow Doppler** is invaluable in showing the connecting vessel linking the sequestrated lobe with the main placental component. The *endovaginal probe* would not be of help because the pathology is not adjacent to the cervix.

246. **E** [16,VIII]. A succenturiate lobe does not cause **premature labor.**

247. **E** [31,II]. The **number of adoptions** is irrelevant because the patient's personal health history is not involved. When recording parity, "para 4112" represents four pregnancies, one miscarriage or abortion, one premature birth, and two full-term deliveries.

248. **E** [28,II]. Tamoxifen is used to prevent breast cancer, not for **hormone replacement therapy.** The *increased risk of endometrial cancer* is slight and can be monitored with endovaginal ultrasound, whereas the *decrease in the risk of breast cancer recurrence* is great. Both *endometrial polyps* and *subendometrial endometriosis deposits* are side effects of tamoxifen use.

249. **E** [22,I]. No brain or cranium is present above the orbits; therefore, **anencephaly** is present. The distance between the orbits is not too wide as in *hypertelorism.* The lens cannot be seen within the orbit, so a *cataract* cannot be assessed. The outline of the process above the orbits is too irregular to be a *proboscis,* which is a single projecting structure usually associated with hypotelorism (orbits too close together).

250. **E** [22,I]. **Hydrocephalus** cannot be present because there is no ventricular system. Anencephaly may inhibit swallowing, so *polyhydramnios* is common. All of the other neural crest anomalies (i.e., *iniencephaly, myelomeningocele, meningocele*) may be seen in addition to anencephaly.

251. **C** [30,III]. The hydronephrosis is bilateral, so the responsible pathology is obstructing the urethra or both ureters. The only process mentioned that can be multifocal and affect both ureters is **pelvic lymphoma.** The lymphatic chains in the pelvis run roughly parallel to the iliac vessels and are in a good position to obstruct the ureters when enlarged.

252. **C** [15,II C]. The arrow is pointing to the **interventricular septum.**

253. **B** [15,II C]. This is a standard **four-chamber view.** All four chambers of the heart can be seen, but not the *outlet tracts* or the *arch of ductus.*

254. **D** [22,VII]. A **pelvic kidney** that is markedly **hydronephrotic** is seen. It is clear that the arrowed process is renal by the shape of the dilated calyces. The narrow rim of renal parenchyma rules out a *multicystic kidney.* No convincing *ureterocele* can be seen. The mass is not an *ovarian cyst* or *hydrometrocolpos* because a renal pelvis is seen, there is a rim of renal parenchyma, and the mass has a complex internal structure.

255. **C** [22,VII]. The normally located kidney is too large for a 30-week pregnancy; the normal kidney at birth is 4.5 cm long. The severely hydronephrotic pelvic kidney seen in the right flank does not have normal renal function, so the other kidney has taken over part of its role and has grown large to compensate. This phenomenon is called **compensatory hypertrophy.** There is **mild hydronephrosis** in addition. Such mild pelvicalyceal dilation is common when there are multicystic dysplastic or hydronephrotic changes in the contralateral kidney.

256. **D** [18,III]. **Spina bifida** is not associated with skin thickening. *Macrosomia* is a common cause of skin thickening caused by fat deposition in the third trimester, and is often associated with diabetes. In *fetal death* and *cystic hygroma,* skin thickening is associated with pleural effusion and the other features of *hydrops.*

257. **C** [15,I]. Structures that should be seen on a good-quality image taken for measuring the biparietal diameter include the **thalamus, third ventricle, and cavum septum pellucidum.** Most of the other choices mention anatomy that is in the posterior fossa (e.g., *cisterna magna, cerebellum*) or is located at too superior a level (e.g., *cavum vergae*). Angling too obliquely, which shows the posterior fossa, or putting the transducer at too superior a level both give inaccurate biparietal diameter measurements.

258. **C** [25,I]. The letter "A" represents the **proliferative** or follicular phase of the menstrual cycle.

259. **A** [25,I]. The letter "B" represents the **secretory** or luteal phase of the menstrual cycle.

260. **A** [25,I]. The letter "C" represents **follicle-stimulating hormone.**

261. **B** [25,I]. The letter "D" represents **luteinizing hormone.** The surge of luteinizing hormone induces ovulation.

262. **C** [25,I]. The letter "E" represents **estrogen,** which is produced throughout the cycle. Increases in estrogen occur in the middle of the secretory and proliferative phases.

263. **D** [25,I]. The letter "F" represents **progesterone.** It is produced in the secretory or luteal phase of the cycle when the corpus luteum is present, preparing the endometrium to accept a zygote.

264. **D** [22,I]. In **Arnold-Chiari II malformation,** which is seen with spina bifida, the brain is pulled toward the occiput, presumably by spinal cord tethering at the site of the spina bifida. The cisterna magna may be obliterated, and the cerebellum often lies in the upper cervical spinal canal. Arnold-Chiari II malformation is a finding usually associated with ventriculomegaly. In *Dandy-Walker syndrome*, the cisterna magna is enlarged. *Hydranencephaly, holoprosencephaly,* and *anencephaly* do not affect the cisterna magna.

265. **B** [15,II A]. The arrow is pointing to the **cavum septum pellucidum.** This cystic space is in the midline and is anterior to the thalamus.

266. **D** [15,II A]. The star is placed on the **thalamus.** This hypoechoic structure is centrally located in the cerebrum and surrounds the *third ventricle*.

267. **C** [31,IV]. Prolonged use of pulsed or continuous wave Doppler induces **tissue heating**—a slight increase in body temperature—at the target site. Tissue cavitation producing *tissue explosions* occurs at higher levels of ultrasound power than are cur-

rently used in diagnostic medicine. A decrease in fetal body weight has been reported in studies in rats, but increased weight (i.e., *macrosomia*) has not been seen with the use of diagnostic ultrasound. *Induced abortions* resulting from the use of diagnostic Doppler ultrasound have not been reported in humans.

268. **D** [27,III]. The mass does not lie in the uterus and does not have the shape of an ovary. Because it is extraovarian, possible explanations include a pelvic abscess, a *paraovarian cyst*, an *endometrioma,* and **hydrosalpinx;** the shape is highly suggestive of hydrosalpinx. In the case of hydrosalpinx, the fimbriated end is always larger than the cornual end and the dilated tube often turns on itself to form a serpiginous shape.

269. **C** [22,IX]. The sonogram shows a large extra digit arising proximal to the thumb and the four fingers, which is typical of **polydactyly of the hand.** There are two types of polydactyly: preaxial is an extra digit arising before the extremity, as seen in this case, and postaxial is an extra digit at the normal digit site. The clear presence of phalanges makes it evident we are not looking at a nose, ruling out the presence of a *proboscis*. The other options relate to forms of dwarfism; the phalanges are of normal length and structure without fractures.

270. **C** [14,I]. The **extracelomic** fluid, which lies outside the amnion, is slightly more echogenic than the amniotic fluid. It is surrounded by the chorion.

271. **B** [14,III]. The **embryo** is indicated by the letter "B" in this diagram of a 7-week pregnancy.

272. **E** [14,II]. Note the **yolk sac** (letter "C") lying in the extracelomic space.

273. **D** [14,I]. A potential space, the **endometrial cavity** (letter "D"), may be difficult to see on an actual sonogram.

274. **A** [14,I]. The **chorion frondosum** (letter "E") is shown in black on the diagram.

275. **E** [14,I]. The **decidua basalis** (letter "F") surrounds the gestational sac.

276. **B** [14,I]. The embryo is surrounded by amniotic fluid, which is enclosed in the **amniotic membrane** (letter "G").

277. **A** [17,II]. The **crown-rump length** is the most accurate way of estimating gestational age in the first trimester. *Biparietal diameter* and *femur length* are usable from about 12 weeks on and are equally accurate at the end of the first trimester. *Gestational sac size* has a much wider range of mea-

surements for a given gestational age; however, it may be of value if the fetal pole has not yet developed. *Head circumference* cannot be used in the first trimester.

278. **D** [29,IV]. The history suggests endometriosis involving the colon because the patient bleeds at monthly intervals and has been infertile. Typical sonographic findings with endometriosis are **masses containing evenly echogenic material both within and outside of the ovaries.** Bilateral hydrosalpinx appears as *bilateral dilated tubular structures* and is associated with infertility but not rectal bleeding. Dermoids (i.e., *masses with calcification and high-level echoes*), fibroma with Meigs' syndrome (i.e., a *solid ovarian mass with ascites*), and *hydronephrotic pelvic kidneys* are not associated with infertility or rectal bleeding.

279. **E** [30,I]. Uncomplicated **dermoids** do not cause fluid in the cul-de-sac. The internal echoes suggest pus or blood, such as might be seen in a *ruptured ectopic pregnancy*. A small amount of blood is released into the cul-de-sac with *normal ovulation*. A *solid mass in the ovary* (such as a fibroma) is associated with ascites in Meigs' syndrome.

280. **E** [24,III]. Ovaries have a dual arterial supply from the **uterine and ovarian arteries.**

281. **A** [23,V]. A **myometrial contraction** is the most likely explanation for the appearance of this sonogram. The placenta can be seen separate from the mass, so *chorioangioma* can be excluded. The texture of the mass area is the same as the rest of the myometrium, making *leiomyoma* unlikely. Because the thickened area is posterior rather than lateral, this is not a *bicornuate uterus.*

282. **C** [23,V]. Because the likely diagnosis is a myometrial contraction, **reexamination after 20 minutes** is appropriate. Myometrial contractions last about 20 minutes and may move slowly around the uterine wall. The area is too far superior for an *endovaginal probe* to be of any value. If done immediately, reexamination with the *patient in the erect position* would show little change. *Reexamination the next day* might show a similar appearance because a uterus prone to contractions could have a similar contraction another day.

283. **A** [22,I]. Neural crest anomalies are abnormalities that involve the nervous system. Therefore, a **cleft lip** is not a neural crest anomaly.

284. **B** [29,I]. The mass on the left has a smooth border and contains an echogenic line, which represents the **decidual reaction in a uterus didelphys.** No gestational sac is seen on the left, so a *twin ectopic pregnancy* can be ruled out. The mass is connected to the uterus, so it is not an *ovarian mass.* The mass is solid, so it is not a *dilated ureter.* Because there is no strong echo with acoustic shadowing, the mass is not a *fibroid with calcific degeneration.*

285. **C** [22,I]. This sonogram shows an empty cranium above the brainstem, and the appearances are consistent with **hydranencephaly.** With other abnormalities (e.g., *anencephaly, holoprosencephaly, acrania, severe hydrocephalus*) a small rim of brain mantle would be visible.

286. **C** [14,III]. The rhombencephalon, which is the precursor of the **fourth ventricle,** is visible as a large cystic area in the cranium of a 9-week pregnancy and is sometimes mistaken for a pathologic structure.

287. **D** [24,VIII]. The ovarian artery Doppler flow pattern in the secretory phase of the menstrual cycle is **low resistance,** with a high diastolic flow pattern.

288. **A** [30,I]. The shape of the fluid-filled structure alongside and posterior to the uterus is most suggestive of free **fluid in the cul-de-sac.** A *fluid-filled loop of colon* is less likely because of the small finger of fluid extending to the right posterior to the uterus. A *dilated fallopian tube* is unlikely because such tubes are more tortuous. *Paraovarian cysts* and *ovarian cysts* are round.

289. **D** [30,I]. **Color flow Doppler** would not help in this situation because one would not expect fluid in the cul-de-sac or gut to show any color flow changes. A *history* might reveal the source of pelvic fluid (e.g., ectopic pregnancy). A *water enema* could be used to determine if the tubular structure is gut. Placing the patient in the *Trendelenburg position* might confirm that the area is fluid, if it moves. Performing a *culdocentesis* (i.e., putting a needle into the pelvis through the vagina) might yield blood.

290. **C** [26,III]. The arrowhead is pointing to a hypoechoic area in the center of the uterus, which is most likely **fluid in the endometrial cavity.**

291. **C** [25,II]. **Radioimmune assay of β-human chorionic gonadotropin (β-HCG)** in a blood sample is the most accurate pregnancy test. Pregnancy tests using urine (e.g., *monoclonal enzyme-linked assay of urine* β-HCG) are improving rapidly, but are not as reliable. α-*Fetoprotein* is measured in amniotic fluid to test for neural tube defects. *Carcinoembryonic antigen* increases in certain malignancies with metastases to the liver.

292. **D** [14,VII]. This sonogram shows a uterus to the left, so this is clearly a female patient. The mass

process is only seen on the right, so this is unlikely to be pelvic inflammatory disease in a woman with *multiple sexual partners;* pelvic inflammatory disease is usually bilateral. A probable gestational sac is seen on the right, so this is most likely an *ectopic pregnancy* in a woman with a history of **a positive pregnancy test and abdominal pain.** Although *ovarian cancer* is still possible, it is unusual in a 25-year-old woman and is generally bilateral in its advanced stages. The uterus is too large for *a 90-year-old woman.*

293. **B** [14,VII]. **β-Human chorionic gonadotropin levels** are used to follow presumed ectopic pregnancies. Many ectopic pregnancies in which there is no free fluid are treated with methotrexate rather than surgical removal. Surgical removal is usually performed via laparoscopy, not *laparotomy.* A *transrectal sonogram* would not be as helpful as an endovaginal sonogram, which would certainly be performed. α-*Fetoprotein levels* would not be helpful. A *CAT scan* would be contraindicated because of radiation hazard.

294. **C** [23,II]. The structure on the left is a pregnancy, which appears to be intrauterine. A cyst is seen on the right. A **corpus luteum cyst** larger than 3 cm is common in pregnancy, so it is the most likely entity being measured. The cystic structure does not have a thick wall, so it is unlikely to be the *bladder.* Because this is a transverse view at the level of the uterus, the entity is unlikely to be a *renal cyst. Mesenteric cysts* are rare, although this is a possible location. Because there is no trophoblastic reaction around the cyst, this is not an *ectopic pregnancy.* In addition, intrauterine pregnancies coexisting with extrauterine pregnancies are rare (about 1 in 9000).

295. **B** [25,III]. Maternal serum β-human chorionic gonadotropin (β-HCG) **gradually increases throughout the first trimester in a normal pregnancy,** doubling every 2 days. Within 2 months of a pregnancy ending at any stage, the level falls to zero; therefore, β-HCG is not *greatest 1 month after conception.* Because levels do not continue to rise in the second trimester, β-HCG cannot be used to *monitor fetal health in the second trimester.* With most *ectopic pregnancies,* the level is less than the normal intrauterine pregnancy, but if the ectopic pregnancy is viable, levels continue to rise.

296. **D** [27,II]. **Membership in a Catholic order of nuns** may limit opportunity for intercourse, but does not impair fertility. A *submucosal fibroid* may prevent implantation of the fertilized egg. *Pelvic inflammatory disease, endometrial implants in the adnexa,* and *a burst appendix* all induce adhesions, which may prevent the ovum from reaching the uterine cavity to be fertilized.

297. **C** [24,II]. An apparent **vaginal mass** is present on this image. It is actually a tampon used during menstruation. Note that the mass is adjacent to the *bladder* and is therefore anterior to the *rectum.* The uterus is normal for a menstruating patient, not for a *prepubertal* patient.

298. **C** [18,II]. The visible twin has not fallen into a dependent position, as would be expected with the mother in a right lateral decubitus position. This is a finding only seen in **stuck twin syndrome,** which is also indicated by the large amount of amniotic fluid around one twin and none around the "stuck" twin. This rare syndrome is an obstetric emergency that greatly improves with the removal of the excess amniotic fluid.

299. **E** [14,VI]. The ultrasound study shows an empty uterus, so a **blighted ovum** is not possible because an empty sac would be visible in the uterine cavity. *Ectopic pregnancy, early intrauterine pregnancy,* and *complete spontaneous abortion* are all possible diagnoses under these circumstances. However, complete spontaneous abortion is only in the differential if there has been vaginal bleeding. *False-positive pregnancy tests* are rare with current testing equipment, but can occur in the presence of coincident diseases (e.g., systemic lupus erythematosis).

300. **C** [19,V]. Amniotic fluid volume at 13 weeks is under the control of the mother rather than the fetus, so decreased amniotic fluid at this early stage is almost certainly caused by **premature rupture of membranes.** The well-trained sonographer will take the opportunity to look at the cervix. Renal causes of decreased fluid such as *hydronephrosis, infantile polycystic kidney disease,* and *renal agenesis* do not cause oligohydramnios until 15–16 weeks. *Intrauterine growth restriction* at this early gestational age is very rare, usually accompanies a chromosomal anomaly, and is not usually associated with oligohydramnios at 13 weeks gestational age.

301. **C** [24,V]. An echogenic shadowing structure typical of a **loop of bowel** is being measured on this image. The *right ovary* can be seen adjacent to the mass. The mass is not cystic, so it is not an *extraovarian paraovarian cyst.* It does not have features of an *endometrioma* or a *dermoid,* which are complex masses.

302. **D** [31,VI]. **Real-time imaging** is the simplest way of pursuing the diagnosis. Eventually, it is likely that peristalsis would be seen. *Doppler* techniques would not be useful.

303. **A** [17,I]. The pregnancy is **intrauterine** because a double decidual reaction can be seen. Pregnancies are ordinarily dated by ultrasound since the

last menstrual period. This is known as *gestational age* and is different from *conceptual age,* which is the age since conception. This pregnancy is about 5 weeks gestational age because there is a yolk sac, but no fetal pole can be seen. Therefore, it is **3 weeks postconceptual age.**

304. **D** [14,I]. The sonogram shows a gestational sac with a double decidual reaction that results from an intrauterine pregnancy. The large white arrow is pointing to a **decidual reaction of the endometrium.**

305. **C** [14,II]. Because no fetal pole is visible, the structure indicated by the small white arrow is the **secondary yolk sac.** The secondary yolk sac forms adjacent to the fetal abdomen and is associated with formation of the gut. Only two lines can be seen rather than a circle, because ultrasound is reflected principally by structures at right angles to it. The *chorionic membrane* is never seen and the *amniotic membrane* may not be seen at this early stage. *Intrasac bleeds* do not appear as linear structures.

306. **C** [14,I]. The black arrow is pointing to the **decidua basalis.** The *chorion frondosum* (i.e., the beginning of the placenta) is the thicker area adjacent to the arrow. A *decidual reaction of the endometrium* is not part of the trophoblastic reaction around the gestational sac; rather, it refers to the proliferation of the endometrium seen in early pregnancy.

307. **A** [23,III]. With the positive pregnancy test, the multiple cysts in both ovaries are most likely to be theca-lutein cysts. They are induced by excess human chorionic gonadotropin (HCG) and are seen in about 40% of *hydatidiform moles,* with *hyperstimulation syndrome* when excess HCG is given, sometimes with *partial moles,* and occasionally with *twins.* **Intraovarian endometrioma** in both ovaries would indicate severe endometriosis, and with endometriosis it is extremely unlikely that the patient would be pregnant and that these cysts would all be echo-free.

308. **C** [26,II]. The normal shape of the uterus at puberty is **pear shaped with a thick endometrial lining.** The uterus is normally *tubular* before puberty with a thin endometrial lining. Small ovarian cysts (e.g., a *1-cm cyst*) are common before puberty. An *echogenic* rather than cystic area in the ovary is suggestive of a dermoid. *Height* is not directly related to puberty.

309. **B** [29,VIII B]. The mass indicated by the arrow arises from the **bladder wall.** It is not *sediment* because it is not in a dependent position. Only low-level echoes are seen in the mass, so it is not a *stone.*

310. **C** [29,VIII B]. The mass indicated by the arrow is

most likely a **bladder wall endometrioma.** *Fungal infections* are not known to spread from the adnexa to the bladder or vice versa. *Ovarian cancer* rarely metastasizes to the bladder. *Trauma to the bladder wall and left adnexa* would be most unlikely to cause a small bladder wall mass.

311. **C** [24,V]. The echogenic focus in the laterally placed muscle is typical of the **sciatic nerve in the psoas muscle.** The ovary, measured with the calipers, is in its typical location between the psoas muscle and the uterus.

312. **E** [30,I]. **Urinary tract infections** do not induce fluid in the cul-de-sac. Normal *ovulation* creates a small amount of fluid in the cul-de-sac.

313. **D** [14,I]. This sonogram shows a **bleed between the gestational sac and endometrial lining.** The absence of a yolk sac and embryo indicates that this is an early pregnancy or a blighted ovum (anembryonic pregnancy). One sac is round and echo-free and the second apparent "sac" is eccentrically shaped with internal echoes. A *normal twin pregnancy* would not show such a discrepancy in sac appearance. No bleed is visible in the well-seen sac, so an *intrasac bleed* can be ruled out. The border of the probable bleed is thick, so this is not a *subchorionic bleed.* The placenta has not formed at this time, so an *intraplacental bleed* is not possible.

314. **C** [23,III]. Hydatidiform moles are associated with nausea and vomiting (i.e., *hyperemesis gravidarum*), *vaginal bleeding,* and *early-onset hypertension.* **Human chorionic gonadotropin** levels are greatly increased rather than **decreased.** The incidence of moles in pregnancies in the United States is about 1 in 2000, whereas it is as high as 1 in 80 in some parts of *Asia.*

315. **E** [25,I]. Pregnancy is most likely to occur midcycle, when the **three-line pattern is seen in the endometrium.** In an unstimulated patient, a dominant follicle measuring 1.5 cm or more is also seen. The *corpus luteum* does not develop until after the follicle ruptures. In the luteal or secretory phase, the *endometrium can be 10 mm thick.* Early in the cycle, during the proliferative stage, the *endometrium is 3 mm thick* or less.

316. **B** [29,II]. This image shows an **intracavitary fibroid** pushing into the endometrial cavity; it is not in a *subserosal* or *pedunculated* location. The fibroid has the same acoustic consistency as the rest of the uterus, which is typical of a fibroid without *degeneration. Endometrial cancer* is echogenic rather than hypoechoic and starts in the endometrium.

317. **A** [14,III]. Organogenesis (i.e., development of all the major organs) takes place from **4–10 weeks.**

This is the most dangerous time for the mother to have an infection or to take drugs of any type.

318. **D** [15,I]. A profile view is used to obtain information about the **chin,** the nose shape, and the forehead. In fact, it is the best way to assess a small chin. The *eyes* are not seen on a properly performed profile view because they are not midline. The *nostrils,* as opposed to the nose, are also not midline structures. The *ears* and the *cheeks* are far from the midline.

319. **C** [18,I]. Abdominal circumference is the most sensitive indicator of **intrauterine growth retardation** (IUGR), and in this case it is 4 weeks less than expected. Note that this is asymmetrical IUGR, as opposed to symmetrical IUGR. The circumference measurement could be technically suboptimal, so be certain it is a technically satisfactory image.

320. **A** [18;I]. With intrauterine growth retardation, the amniotic fluid index (AFI) will be decreased and consistent with oligohydramnios, unless a malformation such as a chromosomal anomaly is present. The normal range at 32 weeks is approximately 8–16, so an **AFI of 5** is expected with poor growth.

321. **A** [22,I]. Of the anomalies listed, only anencephaly can be diagnosed in the first trimester. Absence of the skull is responsible for **acrania anencephaly complex.** The skull first forms at 10 weeks, so the earliest this malformation can be detected is at about 11 weeks when the irregularly outlined brain will be seen, but will not be surrounded by the skull. *Duodenal stenosis, achondroplasia,* and *osteogenesis imperfecta* all develop later in pregnancy.

322. **A** [14,I]. The arrow is pointing to the **amniotic membrane,** which is separate from the chorionic membrane until about 14 weeks. The *chorionic membrane* is not normally separated from the trophoblastic reaction, and so is not visible. The *vitelline duct* is a small linear structure leading to the yolk sac and is not visible on this sonogram. *Nuchal thickening* is not visible in this embryo. No *intra-amniotic bleed* is seen in the amniotic fluid.

323. **C** [24,I]. The uterus on the image is **retroverted and retroflexed.** Note the acute posterior angulation of the body of the uterus, whereas the cervical region is only slightly tilted backward.

324. **A** [19,III]. Of the fluids listed, the least echogenic is **amniotic fluid in the first trimester.** *Extracelomic fluid* (i.e., fluid between the chorionic and amniotic membranes) is noticeably more echogenic than first trimester fluid. *Amniotic fluid in the third trimester* contains vernix, which is visible. *Intra-am-*

niotic blood contains internal echoes to a varying degree. *Fluid in the yolk sac* is difficult to assess because reverberation artifact makes it difficult to see.

325. **C** [28,I]. The postmenopausal uterus retains the adult **pear shape** and usually shrinks to approximately **6 × 4 × 3 cm.** Before puberty, the uterus is *tube shaped.*

326. **E** [14,VI]. The prognosis with a **perisac bleed and a viable embryo** is good, with at least a 95% survival rate. A *small, calcified yolk sac;* a *large yolk sac;* an *embryo pulse rate of less than 80;* and *good 5.5 weeks dates with no embryo visible* are all findings that make a poor outcome likely.

327. **E** [16,VI]. First trimester bleeds are most common in the *amniotic cavity* and in a subchorionic location. They can also occur in the *extracelomic space* and *around the gestational sac in the uterine cavity.* Bleeds are not known to occur in the **yolk sac.**

328. **C** [23,III]. The sonographic appearances and β-human chorionic gonadotropin level are typical of a **hydatidiform mole.** No fetus can be seen, so *placenta previa, placenta accreta,* and *missed abortion* are not good options. Unless there had been a complete spontaneous abortion, a *fibroid* would not account for the positive pregnancy test.

329. **A** [23,III]. Typical symptoms of a hydatidiform mole include **vaginal bleeding,** nausea, and vomiting.

330. **C** [23,III]. Hydatidiform moles are much more common in Asian women (e.g., **Japanese** women) than in women from other parts of the world.

331. **D** [28,II]. The effect of estrogen, the principal component of hormone replacement therapy, is to **thicken the endometrium to a variable degree.** Because the amount of thickening is variable, a single measurement cannot be given.

332. **C** [25,IV]. A **zygote** is the result of the successful fertilization of the sperm and ovum. A *morula* is the result of the mitotic change that the zygote undergoes. A *blastocyst* is the resultant structure, which implants in the uterus. An *oocyte* is an incompletely developed ovum. A *fimbria* are the finger-like projections on the end of the fallopian tube.

333. **E** [14,VII]. Although a **missed abortion** is common with an eccentric gestational sac location, it is the consequence, not the cause, of this abnormal position. Because a *cornual pregnancy* occurs in the tube near the uterus, it can look like an eccentric intrauterine pregnancy. *Fibroids* may displace the sac position. With a *bicornuate uterus,* the sac implants in one horn, where it appears eccentric, and the

other horn has a decidual reaction. On some occasions, the sac is eccentric with an empty bladder but looks more centrally located with a full bladder; therefore, this finding can be a *normal variant.*

334. **A** [28,II]. Prolonged estrogen administration **decreases the risk of heart disease and osteoporosis,** but slightly increases the risk of uterine *cancer.* Estrogen administration does not effect *infection* rates. Although there may be an improvement in *hot flashes* and *sexual drive,* these benefits are not the main reason for prolonged administration of estrogen.

335. **C** [18,IV B]. The findings are suggestive of hydrops. The components of hydrops are **pleural effusion,** pericardial effusion, ascites, skin thickening, and placentomegaly. Polyhydramnios is often seen as well. If any one feature of hydrops is seen, search immediately for the other signs.

336. **C** [18,IV B]. The history is suggestive of **Rh incompatibility,** providing the father's blood group is Rh positive. Hydrops is not seen with *neural crest anomalies.* Although isolated fetal ascites is seen with *prune-belly syndrome,* it is not usually a recurrent syndrome and is not associated with placentomegaly. *Down syndrome* is not recurrent, although hydrops may be present. Hydrops is not a typical feature of *rubella* infection.

337. **E** [14,VII]. When no embryo is visible and the sac is less than 1.8 cm on a transabdominal sonogram, it is not possible to distinguish between an *early, normal pregnancy* and a *blighted ovum,* or *anembryonic pregnancy.* Because no mention is made of the adnexa, it is possible that a *heterotopic pregnancy* (i.e., ectopic and intrauterine pregnancy) is present. *Demise of the second twin* may take place at any time, but is especially common in the first trimester, and a second empty sac is seen. By definition, a **missed abortion** means that an embryonic remnant is visible.

338. **D** [20,IV]. **Chorionic villi sampling** requires that a catheter be introduced into the developing placenta to draw off villi for karyotyping. *Amniocentesis* is performed in the second trimester. *Gamete intrafallopian transfer* and *zygote intrafallopian tube transfer* are methods of assisted reproductive technology. *Percutaneous umbilical blood sampling* (cordocentesis) is a method of rapid karyotyping for the evaluation of fetal anemia and for the performance of fetal blood transfusions. A needle is inserted into the cord in the second or third trimester.

339. **C** [17,VII]. The transcerebellar diameter only equals gestational age up to **20 weeks.**

340. **A** [28,II]. Progesterone is administered in addi-

tion to estrogen because it **diminishes the side effects** caused by estrogen when given alone.

341. **B** [24,I]. The uterus is **anteverted.** The cervical region, body, and fundus of the uterus are positioned in the same direction—anteriorly. If the cervical region is pointing anteriorly but the fundus is tilted posteriorly, the uterus is said to be anteverted and *retroflexed.*

342. **C** [24,I]. The large, pear-shaped uterus suggests a multiparous woman who is still menstruating; therefore, she is most likely between **30 and 40 years of age.**

343. **C** [31,VII]. The sagittal view shows a single gestational sac in the endometrial cavity, but on the transverse view it appears to be doubled. This is the result of the **rectus muscle artifact.** If the transducer is placed directly over the rectus abdominis muscle, the sound waves can refract to give a double image of an intrauterine structure (e.g., intrauterine contraceptive device, gestational sac).

344. **E** [15,II D]. Because the diaphragm is normally seen with ultrasound, only the fetal **heart** is expected to be seen in the fetal chest. The *gallbladder, stomach, liver,* and *spleen* are all intra-abdominal organs.

345. **B** [18,I]. The biophysical profile scoring system normally used allocates 2 points for each of the following: fetal breathing, an amniotic fluid–filled space greater than 2 cm, fetal movement, good fetal tone, and a satisfactory nonstress test. In this case, there was good fetal breathing (2 points) and normal fluid volume (2 points), but no fetal movement (0 points), and therefore no fetal tone (0 points). Therefore, the biophysical profile score is **4** out of 8 because a nonstress test was not performed.

346. **C** [29,IX]. **Gartner's duct cysts** are congenital cysts seen on the anterolateral vaginal wall. *Nabothian cysts* are cervical cysts. A *ureterocele* is a bulge at the distal end of the ureter. *Paraovarian cysts* lie in the broad ligament, which is superior to the middle of the vagina.

347. **C** [16,VII]. A full bladder elongates the cervix and may create a false-positive placenta previa. All examinations for placental location should be performed with an empty bladder. A **marginal placenta previa with an empty bladder** will probably move toward the fundus, but should be followed up to be sure it is no longer a previa later in the pregnancy.

348. **B** [25,I]. *Menses* occurs from day 1 through approximately days 4–5 of the cycle. Menses is fol-

lowed by the **proliferative phase.** The *follicular phase* of the ovarian cycle occurs simultaneously with the proliferative phase of the endometrium.

349. **C** [29,I]. The uterus can be seen on this image, but the **cervix and vagina are absent.** In the case of an *imperforate hymen* or *transverse vaginal septum,* a buildup of blood would be seen in the obstructed vagina and uterus.

 Okay, we know what you are thinking—"the cervix and vagina are probably 1 cm to the left or right of here. How can we tell without a transverse of the affected area?" Because if the registry shows you only one image, all the pertinent information has to be there, that is why. Do not waste time fuming about it, just accept that idea and go on; then you will see that only one answer works.

350. **B** [29,I]. When the uterus is obstructed, blood accumulates in the endometrial cavity. With complete obstruction, the uterine cavity eventually fills and blood refluxes into the adnexa through the fallopian tubes, forming a **hematoma** alongside the ovaries.

 Do not be alarmed if a question addresses a bizarre entity you have never encountered. The question would not be asked if you could not figure it out with common sense. Don't waste time on panic. The process of elimination will give you the correct answer.

351. **C** [15,II G]. A **breech presentation at 38 weeks** (i.e., a term breech presentation) is normally treated by cesarean section. *Vertex, cephalic,* and *occiput* presentations occur when the fetus presents headfirst, in which case the fetus is delivered vaginally. A *breech presentation at 22 weeks* would not be viable if delivered that early, so cesarean section would not be considered.

352. **B** [17,IV]. The **distal femoral epiphysis** should not be included in a femoral length measurement. However, it is a useful dating feature because it is only seen after 32 weeks. Both the *lateral femoral shaft* and the *medial femoral shaft* can be used for measurement, even though the medial aspect is curved. The *femoral head* is not ossified *in utero* and so is not visible.

353. **E** [16,XII]. **An avascular area between the placenta and the uterine wall** does not suggest placenta accreta because the area between the placenta and the uterine wall is vascularized, especially at the site of the placenta accreta. Pla-

centa accreta is a difficult diagnosis, but *history of a previous cesarean section* is almost always the case. A *thinned uterine wall, vertically aligned intraplacental vessels,* and a *history of intrauterine surgery* are also typical findings with placenta accreta.

354. **C** [24,II]. The arrow is pointing to the normal **urethra,** which is lying anterior to the vagina. It looks surprisingly like the prostate in the male.

355. **B** [24,II]. The arrowhead is pointing to the normal **vagina.**

356. **C** [31,VII]. With a **full bladder,** sound can be bounced around the curved edge of the bladder so there is a delay before the sound wave returns to the transducer, creating the appearance of a fluid-filled mass posterior to the bladder.

357. **C** [18,I]. **Opening and closing the hand** is one of the indications of good fetal tone. Rolling movements and extension and flexion of a limb are additional indicators.

358. **D** [17,VI]. The **cavum septum pellucidum** belongs on a head circumference measurement. The *orbits, cerebellum,* and *tentorium* do not belong on a head circumference measurement because they are all at too inferior a level. (The tentorium is the extension of the falx cerebri that separates the cerebrum from the cerebellum.) The ideal head circumference measurement should include the thalami, cavum septum pellucidum, and third ventricle, and it should be symmetrical. *Symmetry of the hemispheres* is ensured by the midline structures being placed truly in the midline.

359. **A** [22,XI]. The angle of the iliac wings should measure **slightly less than 90°.** A widened hip angle may be indicative of a neural tube defect, Down syndrome, or bladder extrophy.

360. **B** [26,III]. Both an imperforate hymen and a transverse vaginal septum will obstruct menstruation, leading to **hematocolpos** (i.e., blood in the vagina) or hematocolpometra (i.e., blood in the uterus and vagina). A *leiomyoma* is a benign muscle tumor of the uterus seen in adult women. *Diethylstilbestrol exposure anomalies* typically present with a T-shaped uterus and can lead to infertility and cervical cancer. A *unicornuate uterus* and *uterus didelphys* are both congenital uterine anomalies that would not prevent menses.

361. **D** [19,III]. The uterus is divided into four quadrants. To obtain the amniotic fluid index, measure the **anteroposterior measurement of the largest fluid pocket in each quadrant.** Take the measurements in a vertical axis, and add together the findings from each quadrant.

362. **B** [16;III]. **Maternal hypertension** does not result in an abnormally thick placenta. However, placentomegaly is one of the features of *nonimmune hydrops,* and it is occasionally a feature of *maternal diabetes.* Infections such as *syphilis* and cytomegalovirus may cause an enlarged placenta. *Triploidy* is associated with a thick placenta containing hypoechoic areas.

363. **D** [29,II]. Because there is no border between the mass and the uterus, a large **cervical fibroid** is most likely pushing anteriorly on the vagina, which can be seen as a linear structure behind the bladder. A *rectal neoplasm* is unlikely because it would typically have an echogenic center. The posterior aspect of the mass can be seen separate from the rectum, and *fecal material* would contain more echoes with shadowing.

364. **B** [24,V]. The apparent mass is the **normal urethra** and surrounding muscles. The central line in the mass is the urethral opening. The area indicated by the arrow is too low to be related to the ureteral opening and is not cystic, so it is not a *ureteral diverticulum* or a *Foley catheter.*

365. **D** [18,IV]. A normal-sized, pregnant, **retroverted uterus** usually becomes anteverted during the first trimester of pregnancy and may appear smaller or larger than it really is because of its position; however, by the third trimester it is no longer a problem. *Fetal renal anomalies* and *premature rupture of membranes* are likely to cause oligohydramnios, which would explain the small uterine size. *Maternal hypertension* and *chromosomal anomalies* (other than Down syndrome) are associated with intrauterine growth restriction and may present as small for dates.

366. **A** [20,IV]. The procedure described is **chorionic villi sampling.** *Amniocentesis* is a procedure in which a small amount of amniotic fluid is removed transabdominally and analyzed. *Percutaneous umbilical vein sampling* and *cordocentesis* both involve sampling blood from the umbilical cord of the fetus. *Uterine biopsy* is rarely performed, and never in a gravid uterus.

367. **A** [29,I]. **Diethylstilbestrol** was given from the 1940s to the 1960s to help prevent miscarriage. It has caused infertility problems in the male and female offspring of women who took the drug. A T-shaped uterus is the typical appearance in the offspring of women with diethylstilbestrol exposure. Having multiple sex partners (e.g., *prostitution*) does not change the shape of the uterus; however, other risks of promiscuity include pelvic inflammatory disease and cervical cancer. *Syphilis* and *chemical poisoning* do not affect the uterus. *Radiation therapy* can damage the uterus,

but does not cause a T-shaped change in appearance.

368. **D** [18,IV B]. **Exchange transfusion** by means of cordocentesis is the normal method of treatment at the relatively early gestational age of 26 weeks. At a gestational age of more than 32 weeks, *early delivery* is preferred. *Pigtail catheter insertion* is occasionally used in the treatment of posterior urethral valves. *Amniocentesis* and *chorionic villi sampling* are diagnostic tests not generally used for treatment.

369. **C** [16,VII]. Painless vaginal bleeding is a typical feature of **placenta previa.** With a *placental abruption* there is usually abdominal pain. Bleeding may occur with an *incompetent cervix,* but it is usually associated with pain and amniotic fluid loss. *Ectopic pregnancy* does not occur in the second or third trimesters. *Trauma* is a rare and painful cause of bleeding.

370. **C** [27,I]. The alignment of the series of strong echoes with visible shadowing is typical of a **Lippes loop intrauterine contraceptive device (IUCD).** A *Dalkon shield IUCD* has only two echoes because it is circular. *Retained bony products of conception* would not give rise to five separate, evenly spaced echoes. *Endometrial neoplasms* rarely calcify and would not be so regular in appearance. The *arcuate artery* is located in the periphery of the uterus.

371. **E** [24,II]. The bladder wall is well maintained and there is good through transmission through the mass, suggesting it is a cystic area and not any of the solid masses listed (i.e., *solid vaginal* mass, *rectal neoplasm,* or *bladder wall mass*). The fluid-filled mass is open-ended inferiorly and is consistent with a **fluid-filled vagina.** Urine from a distended bladder may fill the vagina when a patient is incontinent and lying supine.

372. **C** [29,II]. **Adenomyosis** is a condition in which endometrial tissue implants in the myometrium. The implants bleed, causing uterine enlargement and pelvic pain. *Endometriosis* refers to endometrial tissue implanted outside of the uterus. *Hypermenorrhea* is excessive bleeding. *Pelvic inflammatory disease* is inflammation of the fallopian tubes, uterus, cervix, and peritoneal surfaces.

373. **C** [28,III]. Endometrial thickening does not occur with **pedunculated fibroids,** which protrude from the exterior of the uterus rather than into the uterine cavity.

374. **C** [16,VII]. The **transvaginal** (or endovaginal) approach gives the most accurate diagnosis of placenta previa. The fetal head often obscures a *transabdominal* approach and the procedure has

to be done with an empty bladder so visualization is often poor. The *translabial* approach, also known as the *transperineal* approach, is sometimes obscured by rectal gas. A *transrectal* approach is probably as accurate as a transvaginal approach, but it is not regularly performed because of discomfort.

 Whenever you see two answers that have an identical meaning, such as transperineal and traslabial, you can eliminate those options. Fortunately for the test taker, there is only one right answer allowed.

---

375. **B** [17,X]. The **lecithin:sphingomyelin ratio from the amniotic fluid** is the only accurate way to predict lung maturity. A *grade 3 placenta* and *meconium in the fetal colon* are signs that favor lung maturity, but are not sufficiently accurate to be reliable. A *proximal humeral epiphysis*, which does not appear sonographically until the fetus is 39 weeks gestational age, is a good indicator of age but does not relate to lung maturity. *Echogenic lungs* do not accurately predict lung maturity.

376. **B** [15,II A]. The large arrow is pointing to the **anterior (frontal) horn of the lateral ventricle.**

377. **D** [15,II A]. The question mark is placed in the **third ventricle.**

378. **D** [15,II A]. The small arrow is pointing to the enlarged **temporal horn of the lateral ventricle.**

379. **B** [15,II A]. The asterisk is placed in the **fourth ventricle.**

380. **A** [15,II A]. The pound sign is placed in the **cisterna magna.**

381. **C** [22,I]. Because the lateral ventricles, the third ventricle, and the fourth ventricle are all enlarged there are two possible explanations for the ventricular enlargement: **Dandy-Walker syndrome** and cranial atrophy. In *Arnold-Chiari malformation*, the cisterna magna would not be visible. In *hydranencephalus*, no cortical mantle would be present. In *aqueduct stenosis*, the fourth ventricle would not be enlarged. Because both ventricles are enlarged, *unilateral ventriculomegaly* is not an option.

382. **D** [18,I]. A biophysical profile is a study of fetal well-being in the third trimester. **Antiepileptic drug administration** is not an indication for a biophysical profile. Although these drugs can affect organogenesis early in pregnancy, they would not be responsible for an abnormal biophysical profile. *Intrauterine growth restriction, post-term gestation, maternal diabetes,* and *pregnancy-induced hypertension* all put the fetus at risk for problems that can be evaluated with a biophysical profile.

383. **B** [27,I]. Currently, **Paragard** is the intrauterine contraceptive device (IUCD) most commonly inserted in the United States. *Lippes loop, Dalkon shield,* and *Copper 7* are no longer inserted. However, patients may still have IUCDs that were never removed, or they may be from other countries that still use the Lippes loop or Copper 7.

384. **A** [25,IV]. The sperm swims upstream. It takes approximately **24 hours** from the time of ovulation for the sperm to reach its target, the ovum.

385. **D** [17,VII]. The **cerebellum** lies posterior to the cerebrum.

386. **C** [29,II]. The cystic area lies in the lower part of the cervix and does not have echogenic walls; therefore, it is a **nabothian cyst.** A second nabothian cyst is also present. Nabothian cysts are often multiple. Both a *cervical pregnancy* and an *aborting gestational sac* would have echogenic walls. *Urine in the vagina* would pool posteriorly. The cyst is not contiguous with the bladder wall, so it is not a *bladder neoplasm.*

387. **B** [18,I]. Fetal tone refers to both the *extension and flexion of an extremity or the spine.* **Movement of the tongue** is not one of the criteria for a biophysical profile.

388. **B** [17,XI]. The upper limit of normal for the cisterna magna is **10 mm.** A larger cystic space in the posterior fossa raises the question of a Dandy-Walker malformation or an extra-axial arachnoid cyst.

389. **B** [28,III]. **Anorexia** does not increase the risk of endometrial cancer. *Tamoxifen* is administered to patients with a history of breast cancer to prevent another breast cancer; however, it increases the risk of endometrial cancer. *Diabetes, hypertension,* and *obesity* are also risk factors for endometrial cancer.

390. **A** [25,I]. Estrogen levels **increase** with follicular growth.

391. **D** [18,III A]. **Increased placental transfer of glucose** causes the placenta to become enlarged. *Overeating* and *obesity* do not affect the placenta. *Trisomy anomalies* do not cause enlarged placentas. Triploidy, a chromosomal disorder in which all chromosomes are triplicated, causes an enlarged placenta. *VACTERL syndrome* occurs in diabetics but does not cause placental enlargement.

392. **D** [29,IX]. **Hysterosalpingography** involves watch-

ing the infusion of saline or contrast into the fallopian tubes with ultrasound. Visualization of the uterus only is called *hysterosonography.* A *hysterectomy* refers to the surgical removal of the uterus. *Hysterography* is a radiographic technique in which radiographic contrast is inserted to visualize the endometrium. *Hysteroscopy* involves visually examining the endometrium through a small tube.

393. **E** [27,II]. A **history of cesarean section** has no effect on fertility.

394. **D** [28,III]. There is a **small endometrial mass** on this image. The focal thickening of the endometrial echo makes the cavity too irregular to be normal in any phase of menstruation (e.g., *secretory phase, proliferative phase*). There is no shadowing, so an *intrauterine contraceptive device* is not an acceptable option.

395. **D** [31,VI]. **A procedure in which saline is infused into the endometrial cavity** would be the most helpful because the mass is not well seen. This type of procedure has several names, including hysterosonography, sonohysterography, and saline infusion sonography.

396. **C** [28,II]. An endometrial cavity size of **8–10 mm** is considered the upper limit of normal in a postmenopausal patient taking hormone replacement therapy. It does not require further investigation if the patient is on hormone replacement therapy.

397. **C** [25,I]. **Menorrhagia** means heavy periods. *Dysmenorrhea* means painful periods. *Menometrorrhagia* means frequent, heavy periods; because only an isolated incidence was described, menorrhagia is a better answer choice. Neither *metrorider* nor *mennonite* are known syndromes.

Note: The numerals in brackets following each set of answer choices indicate the topic area of the question. Refer to the Self-Evaluation Charts in this section.

1. Ⓐ Ⓑ Ⓒ Ⓓ Ⓔ [13, II]	41. Ⓐ Ⓑ Ⓒ Ⓓ Ⓔ [3, VI]	81. Ⓐ Ⓑ Ⓒ Ⓓ Ⓔ [1, V]
2. Ⓐ Ⓑ Ⓒ Ⓓ Ⓔ [8, VI]	42. Ⓐ Ⓑ Ⓒ Ⓓ Ⓔ [4, III]	82. Ⓐ Ⓑ Ⓒ Ⓓ Ⓔ [1, V]
3. Ⓐ Ⓑ Ⓒ Ⓓ Ⓔ [8, II]	43. Ⓐ Ⓑ Ⓒ Ⓓ Ⓔ [4, VII]	83. Ⓐ Ⓑ Ⓒ Ⓓ Ⓔ [1, III]
4. Ⓐ Ⓑ Ⓒ Ⓓ Ⓔ [8, IV]	44. Ⓐ Ⓑ Ⓒ Ⓓ Ⓔ [4, VI]	84. Ⓐ Ⓑ Ⓒ Ⓓ Ⓔ [1, IX]
5. Ⓐ Ⓑ Ⓒ Ⓓ Ⓔ [10, V]	45. Ⓐ Ⓑ Ⓒ Ⓓ Ⓔ [4, VI]	85. Ⓐ Ⓑ Ⓒ Ⓓ Ⓔ [2, I]
6. Ⓐ Ⓑ Ⓒ Ⓓ Ⓔ [6, V]	46. Ⓐ Ⓑ Ⓒ Ⓓ Ⓔ 4, VII]	86. Ⓐ Ⓑ Ⓒ Ⓓ Ⓔ [2, IV]
7. Ⓐ Ⓑ Ⓒ Ⓓ Ⓔ [6, IV]	47. Ⓐ Ⓑ Ⓒ Ⓓ Ⓔ [4, XI]	87. Ⓐ Ⓑ Ⓒ Ⓓ Ⓔ [2, VII]
8. Ⓐ Ⓑ Ⓒ Ⓓ Ⓔ [11, IV]	48. Ⓐ Ⓑ Ⓒ Ⓓ Ⓔ [4, XI]	88. Ⓐ Ⓑ Ⓒ Ⓓ Ⓔ [3, I]
9. Ⓐ Ⓑ Ⓒ Ⓓ Ⓔ [11, I]	49. Ⓐ Ⓑ Ⓒ Ⓓ Ⓔ [4, XIV]	89. Ⓐ Ⓑ Ⓒ Ⓓ Ⓔ [2, I]
10. Ⓐ Ⓑ Ⓒ Ⓓ Ⓔ [11, II]	50. Ⓐ Ⓑ Ⓒ Ⓓ Ⓔ [4, XIV]	90. Ⓐ Ⓑ Ⓒ Ⓓ Ⓔ [4, I]
11. Ⓐ Ⓑ Ⓒ Ⓓ Ⓔ [11, VII]	51. Ⓐ Ⓑ Ⓒ Ⓓ Ⓔ [4, XIV]	91. Ⓐ Ⓑ Ⓒ Ⓓ Ⓔ [4, III]
12. Ⓐ Ⓑ Ⓒ Ⓓ Ⓔ [11, VIII]	52. Ⓐ Ⓑ Ⓒ Ⓓ Ⓔ [4, IV]	92. Ⓐ Ⓑ Ⓒ Ⓓ Ⓔ [4, XIII]
13. Ⓐ Ⓑ Ⓒ Ⓓ Ⓔ [11, II]	53. Ⓐ Ⓑ Ⓒ Ⓓ Ⓔ [5, V]	93. Ⓐ Ⓑ Ⓒ Ⓓ Ⓔ [4, XIII]
14. Ⓐ Ⓑ Ⓒ Ⓓ Ⓔ [11, IV]	54. Ⓐ Ⓑ Ⓒ Ⓓ Ⓔ [5, IV]	94. Ⓐ Ⓑ Ⓒ Ⓓ Ⓔ [4, VIII]
15. Ⓐ Ⓑ Ⓒ Ⓓ Ⓔ [11, I]	55. Ⓐ Ⓑ Ⓒ Ⓓ Ⓔ [7, X]	95. Ⓐ Ⓑ Ⓒ Ⓓ Ⓔ [4, VIII]
16. Ⓐ Ⓑ Ⓒ Ⓓ Ⓔ [11, II]	56. Ⓐ Ⓑ Ⓒ Ⓓ Ⓔ [7, IX]	96. Ⓐ Ⓑ Ⓒ Ⓓ Ⓔ [4, I]
17. Ⓐ Ⓑ Ⓒ Ⓓ Ⓔ [11, X]	57. Ⓐ Ⓑ Ⓒ Ⓓ Ⓔ [12, V]	97. Ⓐ Ⓑ Ⓒ Ⓓ Ⓔ [6, I]
18. Ⓐ Ⓑ Ⓒ Ⓓ Ⓔ [11, III]	58. Ⓐ Ⓑ Ⓒ Ⓓ Ⓔ [12, V]	98. Ⓐ Ⓑ Ⓒ Ⓓ Ⓔ [6, III]
19. Ⓐ Ⓑ Ⓒ Ⓓ Ⓔ [9, I]	59. Ⓐ Ⓑ Ⓒ Ⓓ Ⓔ [9, VII]	99. Ⓐ Ⓑ Ⓒ Ⓓ Ⓔ [5, VII]
20. Ⓐ Ⓑ Ⓒ Ⓓ Ⓔ [8, I]	60. Ⓐ Ⓑ Ⓒ Ⓓ Ⓔ [1, VII]	100. Ⓐ Ⓑ Ⓒ Ⓓ Ⓔ [4, III]
21. Ⓐ Ⓑ Ⓒ Ⓓ Ⓔ [1, I]	61. Ⓐ Ⓑ Ⓒ Ⓓ Ⓔ [10, I]	101. Ⓐ Ⓑ Ⓒ Ⓓ Ⓔ [4, III]
22. Ⓐ Ⓑ Ⓒ Ⓓ Ⓔ [1, I]	62. Ⓐ Ⓑ Ⓒ Ⓓ Ⓔ [10, V]	102. Ⓐ Ⓑ Ⓒ Ⓓ Ⓔ [7, I]
23. Ⓐ Ⓑ Ⓒ Ⓓ Ⓔ [1, I]	63. Ⓐ Ⓑ Ⓒ Ⓓ Ⓔ [10, V]	103. Ⓐ Ⓑ Ⓒ Ⓓ Ⓔ [7, X]
24. Ⓐ Ⓑ Ⓒ Ⓓ Ⓔ [9, IX]	64. Ⓐ Ⓑ Ⓒ Ⓓ Ⓔ [11, V]	104. Ⓐ Ⓑ Ⓒ Ⓓ Ⓔ [9, V]
25. Ⓐ Ⓑ Ⓒ Ⓓ Ⓔ [2, I]	65. Ⓐ Ⓑ Ⓒ Ⓓ Ⓔ [9, V]	105. Ⓐ Ⓑ Ⓒ Ⓓ Ⓔ [1, VI]
26. Ⓐ Ⓑ Ⓒ Ⓓ Ⓔ [1, III]	66. Ⓐ Ⓑ Ⓒ Ⓓ Ⓔ [1, I]	106. Ⓐ Ⓑ Ⓒ Ⓓ Ⓔ [2, I]
27. Ⓐ Ⓑ Ⓒ Ⓓ Ⓔ [1, III]	67. Ⓐ Ⓑ Ⓒ Ⓓ Ⓔ [9, IX]	107. Ⓐ Ⓑ Ⓒ Ⓓ Ⓔ [2, III]
28. Ⓐ Ⓑ Ⓒ Ⓓ Ⓔ [1, III]	68. Ⓐ Ⓑ Ⓒ Ⓓ Ⓔ [13, III]	108. Ⓐ Ⓑ Ⓒ Ⓓ Ⓔ [2, V]
29. Ⓐ Ⓑ Ⓒ Ⓓ Ⓔ [1, V]	69. Ⓐ Ⓑ Ⓒ Ⓓ Ⓔ [2, VI]	109. Ⓐ Ⓑ Ⓒ Ⓓ Ⓔ [5, VI]
30. Ⓐ Ⓑ Ⓒ Ⓓ Ⓔ [2, I]	70. Ⓐ Ⓑ Ⓒ Ⓓ Ⓔ [2, VIII]	110. Ⓐ Ⓑ Ⓒ Ⓓ Ⓔ [5, VI]
31. Ⓐ Ⓑ Ⓒ Ⓓ Ⓔ [9, IX]	71. Ⓐ Ⓑ Ⓒ Ⓓ Ⓔ [2, V]	111. Ⓐ Ⓑ Ⓒ Ⓓ Ⓔ [5, VI]
32. Ⓐ Ⓑ Ⓒ Ⓓ Ⓔ [9, IX]	72. Ⓐ Ⓑ Ⓒ Ⓓ Ⓔ [4, XIII]	112. Ⓐ Ⓑ Ⓒ Ⓓ Ⓔ [5, VI]
33. Ⓐ Ⓑ Ⓒ Ⓓ Ⓔ [4, XIV]	73. Ⓐ Ⓑ Ⓒ Ⓓ Ⓔ [12, I]	113. Ⓐ Ⓑ Ⓒ Ⓓ Ⓔ [5, VII]
34. Ⓐ Ⓑ Ⓒ Ⓓ Ⓔ [4, XV]	74. Ⓐ Ⓑ Ⓒ Ⓓ Ⓔ [8, I]	114. Ⓐ Ⓑ Ⓒ Ⓓ Ⓔ [5, VII]
35. Ⓐ Ⓑ Ⓒ Ⓓ Ⓔ [1, VIII]	75. Ⓐ Ⓑ Ⓒ Ⓓ Ⓔ [7, II]	115. Ⓐ Ⓑ Ⓒ Ⓓ Ⓔ [8, V]
36. Ⓐ Ⓑ Ⓒ Ⓓ Ⓔ [1, VI]	76. Ⓐ Ⓑ Ⓒ Ⓓ Ⓔ [1, V]	116. Ⓐ Ⓑ Ⓒ Ⓓ Ⓔ [8, V]
37. Ⓐ Ⓑ Ⓒ Ⓓ Ⓔ [2, V]	77. Ⓐ Ⓑ Ⓒ Ⓓ Ⓔ [9, V]	117. Ⓐ Ⓑ Ⓒ Ⓓ Ⓔ [12, I]
38. Ⓐ Ⓑ Ⓒ Ⓓ Ⓔ [2, VI]	78. Ⓐ Ⓑ Ⓒ Ⓓ Ⓔ [11, XI]	118. Ⓐ Ⓑ Ⓒ Ⓓ Ⓔ [12, II]
39. Ⓐ Ⓑ Ⓒ Ⓓ Ⓔ [3, I]	79. Ⓐ Ⓑ Ⓒ Ⓓ Ⓔ [4, XII]	119. Ⓐ Ⓑ Ⓒ Ⓓ Ⓔ [12, VI]
40. Ⓐ Ⓑ Ⓒ Ⓓ Ⓔ [3, III]	80. Ⓐ Ⓑ Ⓒ Ⓓ Ⓔ [4, XII]	120. Ⓐ Ⓑ Ⓒ Ⓓ Ⓔ [9, I]

121. Ⓐ Ⓑ Ⓒ Ⓓ Ⓔ [9, I]
122. Ⓐ Ⓑ Ⓒ Ⓓ Ⓔ [9, I]
123. Ⓐ Ⓑ Ⓒ Ⓓ Ⓔ [9, I]
124. Ⓐ Ⓑ Ⓒ Ⓓ Ⓔ [9, I]
125. Ⓐ Ⓑ Ⓒ Ⓓ Ⓔ [9, I]
126. Ⓐ Ⓑ Ⓒ Ⓓ Ⓔ [1, II]
127. Ⓐ Ⓑ Ⓒ Ⓓ Ⓔ [1, I]
128. Ⓐ Ⓑ Ⓒ Ⓓ Ⓔ [3, I]
129. Ⓐ Ⓑ Ⓒ Ⓓ Ⓔ [1, I]
130. Ⓐ Ⓑ Ⓒ Ⓓ Ⓔ [9, I]
131. Ⓐ Ⓑ Ⓒ Ⓓ Ⓔ [9, I]
132. Ⓐ Ⓑ Ⓒ Ⓓ Ⓔ [3, I]
133. Ⓐ Ⓑ Ⓒ Ⓓ Ⓔ [9, I]
134. Ⓐ Ⓑ Ⓒ Ⓓ Ⓔ [1, II]
135. Ⓐ Ⓑ Ⓒ Ⓓ Ⓔ [1, I]
136. Ⓐ Ⓑ Ⓒ Ⓓ Ⓔ [9, I]
137. Ⓐ Ⓑ Ⓒ Ⓓ Ⓔ [1, V]
138. Ⓐ Ⓑ Ⓒ Ⓓ Ⓔ [1, V]
139. Ⓐ Ⓑ Ⓒ Ⓓ Ⓔ [1, V]
140. Ⓐ Ⓑ Ⓒ Ⓓ Ⓔ [9, IX]
141. Ⓐ Ⓑ Ⓒ Ⓓ Ⓔ [9, IX]
142. Ⓐ Ⓑ Ⓒ Ⓓ Ⓔ [3, I]
143. Ⓐ Ⓑ Ⓒ Ⓓ Ⓔ [9, IX]
144. Ⓐ Ⓑ Ⓒ Ⓓ Ⓔ [4, VI]
145. Ⓐ Ⓑ Ⓒ Ⓓ Ⓔ [4, XI]
146. Ⓐ Ⓑ Ⓒ Ⓓ Ⓔ [4, XI]
147. Ⓐ Ⓑ Ⓒ Ⓓ Ⓔ [8, VIII]
148. Ⓐ Ⓑ Ⓒ Ⓓ Ⓔ [4, VII]
149. Ⓐ Ⓑ Ⓒ Ⓓ Ⓔ [4, I]
150. Ⓐ Ⓑ Ⓒ Ⓓ Ⓔ [4, XIII]
151. Ⓐ Ⓑ Ⓒ Ⓓ Ⓔ [4, XI]
152. Ⓐ Ⓑ Ⓒ Ⓓ Ⓔ [4, XI]
153. Ⓐ Ⓑ Ⓒ Ⓓ Ⓔ [4, I]
154. Ⓐ Ⓑ Ⓒ Ⓓ Ⓔ [4, II]
155. Ⓐ Ⓑ Ⓒ Ⓓ Ⓔ [4, I]
156. Ⓐ Ⓑ Ⓒ Ⓓ Ⓔ [4, XIII]
157. Ⓐ Ⓑ Ⓒ Ⓓ Ⓔ [4, VII]
158. Ⓐ Ⓑ Ⓒ Ⓓ Ⓔ [4, VII]
159. Ⓐ Ⓑ Ⓒ Ⓓ Ⓔ [4, II]
160. Ⓐ Ⓑ Ⓒ Ⓓ Ⓔ [4, XI]
161. Ⓐ Ⓑ Ⓒ Ⓓ Ⓔ [4, VII]
162. Ⓐ Ⓑ Ⓒ Ⓓ Ⓔ [4, XIII]
163. Ⓐ Ⓑ Ⓒ Ⓓ Ⓔ [4, X]
164. Ⓐ Ⓑ Ⓒ Ⓓ Ⓔ [4, II]
165. Ⓐ Ⓑ Ⓒ Ⓓ Ⓔ [4, IV]
166. Ⓐ Ⓑ Ⓒ Ⓓ Ⓔ [4, VIII]
167. Ⓐ Ⓑ Ⓒ Ⓓ Ⓔ [3, I]
168. Ⓐ Ⓑ Ⓒ Ⓓ Ⓔ [3, I]
169. Ⓐ Ⓑ Ⓒ Ⓓ Ⓔ [3, III]
170. Ⓐ Ⓑ Ⓒ Ⓓ Ⓔ [3, V]
171. Ⓐ Ⓑ Ⓒ Ⓓ Ⓔ [10, I]

172. Ⓐ Ⓑ Ⓒ Ⓓ Ⓔ [3, II]
173. Ⓐ Ⓑ Ⓒ Ⓓ Ⓔ [3, VI]
174. Ⓐ Ⓑ Ⓒ Ⓓ Ⓔ [3, III]
175. Ⓐ Ⓑ Ⓒ Ⓓ Ⓔ [3, II]
176. Ⓐ Ⓑ Ⓒ Ⓓ Ⓔ [3, V]
177. Ⓐ Ⓑ Ⓒ Ⓓ Ⓔ [2, II]
178. Ⓐ Ⓑ Ⓒ Ⓓ Ⓔ [3, I]
179. Ⓐ Ⓑ Ⓒ Ⓓ Ⓔ [3, II]
180. Ⓐ Ⓑ Ⓒ Ⓓ Ⓔ [3, VII]
181. Ⓐ Ⓑ Ⓒ Ⓓ Ⓔ [3, II]
182. Ⓐ Ⓑ Ⓒ Ⓓ Ⓔ [3, I]
183. Ⓐ Ⓑ Ⓒ Ⓓ Ⓔ [3, IV]
184. Ⓐ Ⓑ Ⓒ Ⓓ Ⓔ [3, IV]
185. Ⓐ Ⓑ Ⓒ Ⓓ Ⓔ [2, V]
186. Ⓐ Ⓑ Ⓒ Ⓓ Ⓔ [10, VII]
187. Ⓐ Ⓑ Ⓒ Ⓓ Ⓔ [10, VII]
188. Ⓐ Ⓑ Ⓒ Ⓓ Ⓔ [11, I]
189. Ⓐ Ⓑ Ⓒ Ⓓ Ⓔ [11, I]
190. Ⓐ Ⓑ Ⓒ Ⓓ Ⓔ [11, I]
191. Ⓐ Ⓑ Ⓒ Ⓓ Ⓔ [11, VII]
192. Ⓐ Ⓑ Ⓒ Ⓓ Ⓔ [6, I]
193. Ⓐ Ⓑ Ⓒ Ⓓ Ⓔ [6, I]
194. Ⓐ Ⓑ Ⓒ Ⓓ Ⓔ [6, VI]
195. Ⓐ Ⓑ Ⓒ Ⓓ Ⓔ [12, III]
196. Ⓐ Ⓑ Ⓒ Ⓓ Ⓔ [12, II]
197. Ⓐ Ⓑ Ⓒ Ⓓ Ⓔ [9, IX]
198. Ⓐ Ⓑ Ⓒ Ⓓ Ⓔ [1, V]
199. Ⓐ Ⓑ Ⓒ Ⓓ Ⓔ [1, VII]
200. Ⓐ Ⓑ Ⓒ Ⓓ Ⓔ [3, VII]
201. Ⓐ Ⓑ Ⓒ Ⓓ Ⓔ [3, II]
202. Ⓐ Ⓑ Ⓒ Ⓓ Ⓔ [4, XV]
203. Ⓐ Ⓑ Ⓒ Ⓓ Ⓔ [4, II]
204. Ⓐ Ⓑ Ⓒ Ⓓ Ⓔ [2, V]
205. Ⓐ Ⓑ Ⓒ Ⓓ Ⓔ [2, I]
206. Ⓐ Ⓑ Ⓒ Ⓓ Ⓔ [2, VII]
207. Ⓐ Ⓑ Ⓒ Ⓓ Ⓔ [9, I]
208. Ⓐ Ⓑ Ⓒ Ⓓ Ⓔ [2, VI]
209. Ⓐ Ⓑ Ⓒ Ⓓ Ⓔ [2, VIII]
210. Ⓐ Ⓑ Ⓒ Ⓓ Ⓔ [8, V]
211. Ⓐ Ⓑ Ⓒ Ⓓ Ⓔ [8, VII]
212. Ⓐ Ⓑ Ⓒ Ⓓ Ⓔ [4, XI]
213. Ⓐ Ⓑ Ⓒ Ⓓ Ⓔ [4, X]
214. Ⓐ Ⓑ Ⓒ Ⓓ Ⓔ [13, II]
215. Ⓐ Ⓑ Ⓒ Ⓓ Ⓔ [4, X]
216. Ⓐ Ⓑ Ⓒ Ⓓ Ⓔ [11, VIII]
217. Ⓐ Ⓑ Ⓒ Ⓓ Ⓔ [5, I]
218. Ⓐ Ⓑ Ⓒ Ⓓ Ⓔ [5, VII]
219. Ⓐ Ⓑ Ⓒ Ⓓ Ⓔ [5, VII]
220. Ⓐ Ⓑ Ⓒ Ⓓ Ⓔ [4, VIII]
221. Ⓐ Ⓑ Ⓒ Ⓓ Ⓔ [4, VIII]
222. Ⓐ Ⓑ Ⓒ Ⓓ Ⓔ [4, XV]

223. Ⓐ Ⓑ Ⓒ Ⓓ Ⓔ [4, XV]
224. Ⓐ Ⓑ Ⓒ Ⓓ Ⓔ [1, VI]
225. Ⓐ Ⓑ Ⓒ Ⓓ Ⓔ [4, V]
226. Ⓐ Ⓑ Ⓒ Ⓓ Ⓔ [12, II]
227. Ⓐ Ⓑ Ⓒ Ⓓ Ⓔ [9, I]
228. Ⓐ Ⓑ Ⓒ Ⓓ Ⓔ [3, VII]
229. Ⓐ Ⓑ Ⓒ Ⓓ Ⓔ [7, VIII]
230. Ⓐ Ⓑ Ⓒ Ⓓ Ⓔ [7, VIII]
231. Ⓐ Ⓑ Ⓒ Ⓓ Ⓔ [7, I]
232. Ⓐ Ⓑ Ⓒ Ⓓ Ⓔ [7, II]
233. Ⓐ Ⓑ Ⓒ Ⓓ Ⓔ [4, I]
234. Ⓐ Ⓑ Ⓒ Ⓓ Ⓔ [4, IV]
235. Ⓐ Ⓑ Ⓒ Ⓓ Ⓔ [7, VIII]
236. Ⓐ Ⓑ Ⓒ Ⓓ Ⓔ [2, I]
237. Ⓐ Ⓑ Ⓒ Ⓓ Ⓔ [4, XI]
238. Ⓐ Ⓑ Ⓒ Ⓓ Ⓔ [4, II]
239. Ⓐ Ⓑ Ⓒ Ⓓ Ⓔ [1, V]
240. Ⓐ Ⓑ Ⓒ Ⓓ Ⓔ [2, VIII]
241. Ⓐ Ⓑ Ⓒ Ⓓ Ⓔ [2, VIII]
242. Ⓐ Ⓑ Ⓒ Ⓓ Ⓔ [5, VIII]
243. Ⓐ Ⓑ Ⓒ Ⓓ Ⓔ [7, IX]
244. Ⓐ Ⓑ Ⓒ Ⓓ Ⓔ [12, II]
245. Ⓐ Ⓑ Ⓒ Ⓓ Ⓔ [12, II]
246. Ⓐ Ⓑ Ⓒ Ⓓ Ⓔ [7, IX]
247. Ⓐ Ⓑ Ⓒ Ⓓ Ⓔ [7, I]
248. Ⓐ Ⓑ Ⓒ Ⓓ Ⓔ [2, V]
249. Ⓐ Ⓑ Ⓒ Ⓓ Ⓔ [1, IX]
250. Ⓐ Ⓑ Ⓒ Ⓓ Ⓔ [9, VI]
251. Ⓐ Ⓑ Ⓒ Ⓓ Ⓔ [10, IX]
252. Ⓐ Ⓑ Ⓒ Ⓓ Ⓔ [5, II]
253. Ⓐ Ⓑ Ⓒ Ⓓ Ⓔ [4, XIV]
254. Ⓐ Ⓑ Ⓒ Ⓓ Ⓔ [5, V]
255. Ⓐ Ⓑ Ⓒ Ⓓ Ⓔ [5, II]
256. Ⓐ Ⓑ Ⓒ Ⓓ Ⓔ [11, V]
257. Ⓐ Ⓑ Ⓒ Ⓓ Ⓔ [9, VI]
258. Ⓐ Ⓑ Ⓒ Ⓓ Ⓔ [9, II]
259. Ⓐ Ⓑ Ⓒ Ⓓ Ⓔ [4, XIV]
260. Ⓐ Ⓑ Ⓒ Ⓓ Ⓔ [1, VI]
261. Ⓐ Ⓑ Ⓒ Ⓓ Ⓔ [4, XIII]
262. Ⓐ Ⓑ Ⓒ Ⓓ Ⓔ [5, VI]
263. Ⓐ Ⓑ Ⓒ Ⓓ Ⓔ [8, VII]
264. Ⓐ Ⓑ Ⓒ Ⓓ Ⓔ [5, I]
265. Ⓐ Ⓑ Ⓒ Ⓓ Ⓔ [5, VII]
266. Ⓐ Ⓑ Ⓒ Ⓓ Ⓔ [5, II]
267. Ⓐ Ⓑ Ⓒ Ⓓ Ⓔ [5, V]
268. Ⓐ Ⓑ Ⓒ Ⓓ Ⓔ [5, VI]
269. Ⓐ Ⓑ Ⓒ Ⓓ Ⓔ [5, I]
270. Ⓐ Ⓑ Ⓒ Ⓓ Ⓔ [4, I]
271. Ⓐ Ⓑ Ⓒ Ⓓ Ⓔ [3, I]
272. Ⓐ Ⓑ Ⓒ Ⓓ Ⓔ [9, I]
273. Ⓐ Ⓑ Ⓒ Ⓓ Ⓔ [9, I]

274. Ⓐ Ⓑ Ⓒ Ⓓ Ⓔ [2, I]	**321.** Ⓐ Ⓑ Ⓒ Ⓓ Ⓔ [1, III]	**368.** Ⓐ Ⓑ Ⓒ Ⓓ Ⓔ [1, IX]
275. Ⓐ Ⓑ Ⓒ Ⓓ Ⓔ [3, I]	**322.** Ⓐ Ⓑ Ⓒ Ⓓ Ⓔ [4, VII]	**369.** Ⓐ Ⓑ Ⓒ Ⓓ Ⓔ [2, VII]
276. Ⓐ Ⓑ Ⓒ Ⓓ Ⓔ [3, VI]	**323.** Ⓐ Ⓑ Ⓒ Ⓓ Ⓔ [13, IV]	**370.** Ⓐ Ⓑ Ⓒ Ⓓ Ⓔ [2, VII]
277. Ⓐ Ⓑ Ⓒ Ⓓ Ⓔ [3, VI]	**324.** Ⓐ Ⓑ Ⓒ Ⓓ Ⓔ [4, VII]	**371.** Ⓐ Ⓑ Ⓒ Ⓓ Ⓔ [2, VII]
278. Ⓐ Ⓑ Ⓒ Ⓓ Ⓔ [3, IV]	**325.** Ⓐ Ⓑ Ⓒ Ⓓ Ⓔ [2, I]	**372.** Ⓐ Ⓑ Ⓒ Ⓓ Ⓔ [2, II]
279. Ⓐ Ⓑ Ⓒ Ⓓ Ⓔ [5, VIII]	**326.** Ⓐ Ⓑ Ⓒ Ⓓ Ⓔ [1, VI]	**373.** Ⓐ Ⓑ Ⓒ Ⓓ Ⓔ [5, III]
280. Ⓐ Ⓑ Ⓒ Ⓓ Ⓔ [5, VII]	**327.** Ⓐ Ⓑ Ⓒ Ⓓ Ⓔ [2, VI]	**374.** Ⓐ Ⓑ Ⓒ Ⓓ Ⓔ [6, I]
281. Ⓐ Ⓑ Ⓒ Ⓓ Ⓔ [5, VII]	**328.** Ⓐ Ⓑ Ⓒ Ⓓ Ⓔ [2, VI]	**375.** Ⓐ Ⓑ Ⓒ Ⓓ Ⓔ [13, III]
282. Ⓐ Ⓑ Ⓒ Ⓓ Ⓔ [5, IV]	**329.** Ⓐ Ⓑ Ⓒ Ⓓ Ⓔ [2, VI]	**376.** Ⓐ Ⓑ Ⓒ Ⓓ Ⓔ [10, VII]
283. Ⓐ Ⓑ Ⓒ Ⓓ Ⓔ [5, VII]	**330.** Ⓐ Ⓑ Ⓒ Ⓓ Ⓔ [2, VII]	**377.** Ⓐ Ⓑ Ⓒ Ⓓ Ⓔ [13, III]
284. Ⓐ Ⓑ Ⓒ Ⓓ Ⓔ [4, V]	**331.** Ⓐ Ⓑ Ⓒ Ⓓ Ⓔ [2, V]	**378.** Ⓐ Ⓑ Ⓒ Ⓓ Ⓔ [13, I]
285. Ⓐ Ⓑ Ⓒ Ⓓ Ⓔ [4, V]	**332.** Ⓐ Ⓑ Ⓒ Ⓓ Ⓔ [1, I]	**379.** Ⓐ Ⓑ Ⓒ Ⓓ Ⓔ [13, V]
286. Ⓐ Ⓑ Ⓒ Ⓓ Ⓔ [4, II]	**333.** Ⓐ Ⓑ Ⓒ Ⓓ Ⓔ [1, VI]	**380.** Ⓐ Ⓑ Ⓒ Ⓓ Ⓔ [1, V]
287. Ⓐ Ⓑ Ⓒ Ⓓ Ⓔ [4, XI]	**334.** Ⓐ Ⓑ Ⓒ Ⓓ Ⓔ [2, I]	**381.** Ⓐ Ⓑ Ⓒ Ⓓ Ⓔ [13, I]
288. Ⓐ Ⓑ Ⓒ Ⓓ Ⓔ [4, VIII]	**335.** Ⓐ Ⓑ Ⓒ Ⓓ Ⓔ [2, V]	**382.** Ⓐ Ⓑ Ⓒ Ⓓ Ⓔ [12, II]
289. Ⓐ Ⓑ Ⓒ Ⓓ Ⓔ [4, VI]	**336.** Ⓐ Ⓑ Ⓒ Ⓓ Ⓔ [2, VIII]	**383.** Ⓐ Ⓑ Ⓒ Ⓓ Ⓔ [12, II]
290. Ⓐ Ⓑ Ⓒ Ⓓ Ⓔ [4, I]	**337.** Ⓐ Ⓑ Ⓒ Ⓓ Ⓔ [7, IX]	**384.** Ⓐ Ⓑ Ⓒ Ⓓ Ⓔ [8, V]
291. Ⓐ Ⓑ Ⓒ Ⓓ Ⓔ [4, X]	**338.** Ⓐ Ⓑ Ⓒ Ⓓ Ⓔ [7, IX]	**385.** Ⓐ Ⓑ Ⓒ Ⓓ Ⓔ [8, VI]
292. Ⓐ Ⓑ Ⓒ Ⓓ Ⓔ [4, IV]	**339.** Ⓐ Ⓑ Ⓒ Ⓓ Ⓔ [7, VIII]	**386.** Ⓐ Ⓑ Ⓒ Ⓓ Ⓔ [10, V]
293. Ⓐ Ⓑ Ⓒ Ⓓ Ⓔ [3, I]	**340.** Ⓐ Ⓑ Ⓒ Ⓓ Ⓔ [7, VIII]	**387.** Ⓐ Ⓑ Ⓒ Ⓓ Ⓔ [2, V]
294. Ⓐ Ⓑ Ⓒ Ⓓ Ⓔ [3, II]	**341.** Ⓐ Ⓑ Ⓒ Ⓓ Ⓔ [7, I]	**388.** Ⓐ Ⓑ Ⓒ Ⓓ Ⓔ [9, V]
295. Ⓐ Ⓑ Ⓒ Ⓓ Ⓔ [3, V]	**342.** Ⓐ Ⓑ Ⓒ Ⓓ Ⓔ [7, I]	**389.** Ⓐ Ⓑ Ⓒ Ⓓ Ⓔ [1, VIII]
296. Ⓐ Ⓑ Ⓒ Ⓓ Ⓔ [3, II]	**343.** Ⓐ Ⓑ Ⓒ Ⓓ Ⓔ [1, V]	**390.** Ⓐ Ⓑ Ⓒ Ⓓ Ⓔ [8, VI]
297. Ⓐ Ⓑ Ⓒ Ⓓ Ⓔ [9, V]	**344.** Ⓐ Ⓑ Ⓒ Ⓓ Ⓔ [7, II]	**391.** Ⓐ Ⓑ Ⓒ Ⓓ Ⓔ [2, VI]
298. Ⓐ Ⓑ Ⓒ Ⓓ Ⓔ [9, V]	**345.** Ⓐ Ⓑ Ⓒ Ⓓ Ⓔ [1, V]	**392.** Ⓐ Ⓑ Ⓒ Ⓓ Ⓔ [1, V]
299. Ⓐ Ⓑ Ⓒ Ⓓ Ⓔ [9, V]	**346.** Ⓐ Ⓑ Ⓒ Ⓓ Ⓔ [7, VI]	**393.** Ⓐ Ⓑ Ⓒ Ⓓ Ⓔ [1, II]
300. Ⓐ Ⓑ Ⓒ Ⓓ Ⓔ [10, II]	**347.** Ⓐ Ⓑ Ⓒ Ⓓ Ⓔ [7, VI]	**394.** Ⓐ Ⓑ Ⓒ Ⓓ Ⓔ [1, I]
301. Ⓐ Ⓑ Ⓒ Ⓓ Ⓔ [10, I]	**348.** Ⓐ Ⓑ Ⓒ Ⓓ Ⓔ [9, I]	**395.** Ⓐ Ⓑ Ⓒ Ⓓ Ⓔ [1, I]
302. Ⓐ Ⓑ Ⓒ Ⓓ Ⓔ [10, VII]	**349.** Ⓐ Ⓑ Ⓒ Ⓓ Ⓔ [9, I]	**396.** Ⓐ Ⓑ Ⓒ Ⓓ Ⓔ [9, VII]
303. Ⓐ Ⓑ Ⓒ Ⓓ Ⓔ [10, VII]	**350.** Ⓐ Ⓑ Ⓒ Ⓓ Ⓔ [9, I]	**397.** Ⓐ Ⓑ Ⓒ Ⓓ Ⓔ [1, I]
304. Ⓐ Ⓑ Ⓒ Ⓓ Ⓔ [1, VIII]	**351.** Ⓐ Ⓑ Ⓒ Ⓓ Ⓔ [9, I]	**398.** Ⓐ Ⓑ Ⓒ Ⓓ Ⓔ [9, I]
305. Ⓐ Ⓑ Ⓒ Ⓓ Ⓔ [1, VIII]	**352.** Ⓐ Ⓑ Ⓒ Ⓓ Ⓔ [9, I]	**399.** Ⓐ Ⓑ Ⓒ Ⓓ Ⓔ [2, II]
306. Ⓐ Ⓑ Ⓒ Ⓓ Ⓔ [1, VIII]	**353.** Ⓐ Ⓑ Ⓒ Ⓓ Ⓔ [9, I]	**400.** Ⓐ Ⓑ Ⓒ Ⓓ Ⓔ [1, III]
307. Ⓐ Ⓑ Ⓒ Ⓓ Ⓔ [4, XI]	**354.** Ⓐ Ⓑ Ⓒ Ⓓ Ⓔ [2, V]	**401.** Ⓐ Ⓑ Ⓒ Ⓓ Ⓔ [1, III]
308. Ⓐ Ⓑ Ⓒ Ⓓ Ⓔ [4, I]	**355.** Ⓐ Ⓑ Ⓒ Ⓓ Ⓔ [2, V]	**402.** Ⓐ Ⓑ Ⓒ Ⓓ Ⓔ [2, II]
309. Ⓐ Ⓑ Ⓒ Ⓓ Ⓔ [6, III]	**356.** Ⓐ Ⓑ Ⓒ Ⓓ Ⓔ [2, II]	**403.** Ⓐ Ⓑ Ⓒ Ⓓ Ⓔ [1, I]
310. Ⓐ Ⓑ Ⓒ Ⓓ Ⓔ [6, II]	**357.** Ⓐ Ⓑ Ⓒ Ⓓ Ⓔ [1, V]	**404.** Ⓐ Ⓑ Ⓒ Ⓓ Ⓔ [2, IV]
311. Ⓐ Ⓑ Ⓒ Ⓓ Ⓔ [4, XI]	**358.** Ⓐ Ⓑ Ⓒ Ⓓ Ⓔ [1, V]	**405.** Ⓐ Ⓑ Ⓒ Ⓓ Ⓔ [2, I]
312. Ⓐ Ⓑ Ⓒ Ⓓ Ⓔ [4, XIII]	**359.** Ⓐ Ⓑ Ⓒ Ⓓ Ⓔ [1, V]	**406.** Ⓐ Ⓑ Ⓒ Ⓓ Ⓔ [2, V]
313. Ⓐ Ⓑ Ⓒ Ⓓ Ⓔ [4, VII]	**360.** Ⓐ Ⓑ Ⓒ Ⓓ Ⓔ [1, VI]	**407.** Ⓐ Ⓑ Ⓒ Ⓓ Ⓔ [2, VIII]
314. Ⓐ Ⓑ Ⓒ Ⓓ Ⓔ [4, VII]	**361.** Ⓐ Ⓑ Ⓒ Ⓓ Ⓔ [1, VI]	**408.** Ⓐ Ⓑ Ⓒ Ⓓ Ⓔ [1, VI]
315. Ⓐ Ⓑ Ⓒ Ⓓ Ⓔ [4, I]	**362.** Ⓐ Ⓑ Ⓒ Ⓓ Ⓔ [1, VI]	**409.** Ⓐ Ⓑ Ⓒ Ⓓ Ⓔ [1, VI]
316. Ⓐ Ⓑ Ⓒ Ⓓ Ⓔ [4, III]	**363.** Ⓐ Ⓑ Ⓒ Ⓓ Ⓔ [9, II]	**410.** Ⓐ Ⓑ Ⓒ Ⓓ Ⓔ [1, VI]
317. Ⓐ Ⓑ Ⓒ Ⓓ Ⓔ [4, X]	**364.** Ⓐ Ⓑ Ⓒ Ⓓ Ⓔ [9, VI]	**411.** Ⓐ Ⓑ Ⓒ Ⓓ Ⓔ [1, II]
318. Ⓐ Ⓑ Ⓒ Ⓓ Ⓔ [8, I]	**365.** Ⓐ Ⓑ Ⓒ Ⓓ Ⓔ [9, II]	**412.** Ⓐ Ⓑ Ⓒ Ⓓ Ⓔ [1, VII]
319. Ⓐ Ⓑ Ⓒ Ⓓ Ⓔ [1, II]	**366.** Ⓐ Ⓑ Ⓒ Ⓓ Ⓔ [1, IX]	
320. Ⓐ Ⓑ Ⓒ Ⓓ Ⓔ [4, VII]	**367.** Ⓐ Ⓑ Ⓒ Ⓓ Ⓔ [1, IX]	

ANSWER SHEET: OBSTETRICS AND GYNECOLOGY COMPREHENSIVE EXAMINATION

Note: The numerals in brackets following each set of answer choices indicate the topic area of the question. Refer to the Self-Evaluation Charts in this section.

1. Ⓐ Ⓑ Ⓒ Ⓓ Ⓔ [28, III]
2. Ⓐ Ⓑ Ⓒ Ⓓ Ⓔ [14, VII]
3. Ⓐ Ⓑ Ⓒ Ⓓ Ⓔ [18, III A]
4. Ⓐ Ⓑ Ⓒ Ⓓ Ⓔ [22, III]
5. Ⓐ Ⓑ Ⓒ Ⓓ Ⓔ [22, III]
6. Ⓐ Ⓑ Ⓒ Ⓓ Ⓔ [29, II]
7. Ⓐ Ⓑ Ⓒ Ⓓ Ⓔ [29, II]
8. Ⓐ Ⓑ Ⓒ Ⓓ Ⓔ [29, II]
9. Ⓐ Ⓑ Ⓒ Ⓓ Ⓔ [18, II]
10. Ⓐ Ⓑ Ⓒ Ⓓ Ⓔ [22, I]
11. Ⓐ Ⓑ Ⓒ Ⓓ Ⓔ [18, II]
12. Ⓐ Ⓑ Ⓒ Ⓓ Ⓔ [18, II]
13. Ⓐ Ⓑ Ⓒ Ⓓ Ⓔ [24, V]
14. Ⓐ Ⓑ Ⓒ Ⓓ Ⓔ [18, II]
15. Ⓐ Ⓑ Ⓒ Ⓓ Ⓔ [17, X]
16. Ⓐ Ⓑ Ⓒ Ⓓ Ⓔ [27, II]
17. Ⓐ Ⓑ Ⓒ Ⓓ Ⓔ [29, III]
18. Ⓐ Ⓑ Ⓒ Ⓓ Ⓔ [29, III]
19. Ⓐ Ⓑ Ⓒ Ⓓ Ⓔ [29, III]
20. Ⓐ Ⓑ Ⓒ Ⓓ Ⓔ [29, III]
21. Ⓐ Ⓑ Ⓒ Ⓓ Ⓔ [22, VI]
22. Ⓐ Ⓑ Ⓒ Ⓓ Ⓔ [20, III]
23. Ⓐ Ⓑ Ⓒ Ⓓ Ⓔ [15, II E]
24. Ⓐ Ⓑ Ⓒ Ⓓ Ⓔ [15, II E]
25. Ⓐ Ⓑ Ⓒ Ⓓ Ⓔ [17, V]
26. Ⓐ Ⓑ Ⓒ Ⓓ Ⓔ [25, I]
27. Ⓐ Ⓑ Ⓒ Ⓓ Ⓔ [21, II]
28. Ⓐ Ⓑ Ⓒ Ⓓ Ⓔ [14, I]
29. Ⓐ Ⓑ Ⓒ Ⓓ Ⓔ [14, I]
30. Ⓐ Ⓑ Ⓒ Ⓓ Ⓔ [31, III]
31. Ⓐ Ⓑ Ⓒ Ⓓ Ⓔ [29, III]
32. Ⓐ Ⓑ Ⓒ Ⓓ Ⓔ [25, III]
33. Ⓐ Ⓑ Ⓒ Ⓓ Ⓔ [22, VII]
34. Ⓐ Ⓑ Ⓒ Ⓓ Ⓔ [22, VII]
35. Ⓐ Ⓑ Ⓒ Ⓓ Ⓔ [24, V]
36. Ⓐ Ⓑ Ⓒ Ⓓ Ⓔ [27, IV]
37. Ⓐ Ⓑ Ⓒ Ⓓ Ⓔ [18, VI]
38. Ⓐ Ⓑ Ⓒ Ⓓ Ⓔ [17, III]
39. Ⓐ Ⓑ Ⓒ Ⓓ Ⓔ [28, III]
40. Ⓐ Ⓑ Ⓒ Ⓓ Ⓔ [28, III]

41. Ⓐ Ⓑ Ⓒ Ⓓ Ⓔ [28, III]
42. Ⓐ Ⓑ Ⓒ Ⓓ Ⓔ [29, II]
43. Ⓐ Ⓑ Ⓒ Ⓓ Ⓔ [17, III]
44. Ⓐ Ⓑ Ⓒ Ⓓ Ⓔ [17, IX]
45. Ⓐ Ⓑ Ⓒ Ⓓ Ⓔ [22, IX]
46. Ⓐ Ⓑ Ⓒ Ⓓ Ⓔ [22, IX]
47. Ⓐ Ⓑ Ⓒ Ⓓ Ⓔ [16, VI]
48. Ⓐ Ⓑ Ⓒ Ⓓ Ⓔ [14, VII]
49. Ⓐ Ⓑ Ⓒ Ⓓ Ⓔ [31, II]
50. Ⓐ Ⓑ Ⓒ Ⓓ Ⓔ [25, I]
51. Ⓐ Ⓑ Ⓒ Ⓓ Ⓔ [29, III]
52. Ⓐ Ⓑ Ⓒ Ⓓ Ⓔ [19, IV, V]
53. Ⓐ Ⓑ Ⓒ Ⓓ Ⓔ [22, II]
54. Ⓐ Ⓑ Ⓒ Ⓓ Ⓔ [18, I]
55. Ⓐ Ⓑ Ⓒ Ⓓ Ⓔ [24, II]
56. Ⓐ Ⓑ Ⓒ Ⓓ Ⓔ [29, IV]
57. Ⓐ Ⓑ Ⓒ Ⓓ Ⓔ [29, VII]
58. Ⓐ Ⓑ Ⓒ Ⓓ Ⓔ [22, II]
59. Ⓐ Ⓑ Ⓒ Ⓓ Ⓔ [17, VIII]
60. Ⓐ Ⓑ Ⓒ Ⓓ Ⓔ [22, I]
61. Ⓐ Ⓑ Ⓒ Ⓓ Ⓔ [18, I]
62. Ⓐ Ⓑ Ⓒ Ⓓ Ⓔ [29, I]
63. Ⓐ Ⓑ Ⓒ Ⓓ Ⓔ [14, I]
64. Ⓐ Ⓑ Ⓒ Ⓓ Ⓔ [15, II E]
65. Ⓐ Ⓑ Ⓒ Ⓓ Ⓔ [18, II]
66. Ⓐ Ⓑ Ⓒ Ⓓ Ⓔ [30, II]
67. Ⓐ Ⓑ Ⓒ Ⓓ Ⓔ [19, V]
68. Ⓐ Ⓑ Ⓒ Ⓓ Ⓔ [22, VII]
69. Ⓐ Ⓑ Ⓒ Ⓓ Ⓔ [24, V]
70. Ⓐ Ⓑ Ⓒ Ⓓ Ⓔ [24, V]
71. Ⓐ Ⓑ Ⓒ Ⓓ Ⓔ [16, V]
72. Ⓐ Ⓑ Ⓒ Ⓓ Ⓔ [15, II]
73. Ⓐ Ⓑ Ⓒ Ⓓ Ⓔ [22, IX]
74. Ⓐ Ⓑ Ⓒ Ⓓ Ⓔ [17, XI]
75. Ⓐ Ⓑ Ⓒ Ⓓ Ⓔ [22, I]
76. Ⓐ Ⓑ Ⓒ Ⓓ Ⓔ [22, I, V]
77. Ⓐ Ⓑ Ⓒ Ⓓ Ⓔ [27, IV]
78. Ⓐ Ⓑ Ⓒ Ⓓ Ⓔ [15, II A]
79. Ⓐ Ⓑ Ⓒ Ⓓ Ⓔ [22, V]
80. Ⓐ Ⓑ Ⓒ Ⓓ Ⓔ [22, V]

81. Ⓐ Ⓑ Ⓒ Ⓓ Ⓔ [22, V]
82. Ⓐ Ⓑ Ⓒ Ⓓ Ⓔ [22, V]
83. Ⓐ Ⓑ Ⓒ Ⓓ Ⓔ [29, IX]
84. Ⓐ Ⓑ Ⓒ Ⓓ Ⓔ [18, II]
85. Ⓐ Ⓑ Ⓒ Ⓓ Ⓔ [24, VI]
86. Ⓐ Ⓑ Ⓒ Ⓓ Ⓔ [17, III]
87. Ⓐ Ⓑ Ⓒ Ⓓ Ⓔ [18, I]
88. Ⓐ Ⓑ Ⓒ Ⓓ Ⓔ [28, III]
89. Ⓐ Ⓑ Ⓒ Ⓓ Ⓔ [29, II]
90. Ⓐ Ⓑ Ⓒ Ⓓ Ⓔ [31, VI]
91. Ⓐ Ⓑ Ⓒ Ⓓ Ⓔ [29, I]
92. Ⓐ Ⓑ Ⓒ Ⓓ Ⓔ [29, I]
93. Ⓐ Ⓑ Ⓒ Ⓓ Ⓔ [29, I]
94. Ⓐ Ⓑ Ⓒ Ⓓ Ⓔ [30, I]
95. Ⓐ Ⓑ Ⓒ Ⓓ Ⓔ [27, II]
96. Ⓐ Ⓑ Ⓒ Ⓓ Ⓔ [28, III]
97. Ⓐ Ⓑ Ⓒ Ⓓ Ⓔ [16, V]
98. Ⓐ Ⓑ Ⓒ Ⓓ Ⓔ [25, I]
99. Ⓐ Ⓑ Ⓒ Ⓓ Ⓔ [25, I]
100. Ⓐ Ⓑ Ⓒ Ⓓ Ⓔ [22, VI]
101. Ⓐ Ⓑ Ⓒ Ⓓ Ⓔ [22, VI]
102. Ⓐ Ⓑ Ⓒ Ⓓ Ⓔ [27, I]
103. Ⓐ Ⓑ Ⓒ Ⓓ Ⓔ [17, IX]
104. Ⓐ Ⓑ Ⓒ Ⓓ Ⓔ [15, II A]
105. Ⓐ Ⓑ Ⓒ Ⓓ Ⓔ [23, I]
106. Ⓐ Ⓑ Ⓒ Ⓓ Ⓔ [23, I]
107. Ⓐ Ⓑ Ⓒ Ⓓ Ⓔ [14, VII]
108. Ⓐ Ⓑ Ⓒ Ⓓ Ⓔ [14, VII]
109. Ⓐ Ⓑ Ⓒ Ⓓ Ⓔ [20, IV]
110. Ⓐ Ⓑ Ⓒ Ⓓ Ⓔ [18, VI C]
111. Ⓐ Ⓑ Ⓒ Ⓓ Ⓔ [29, III]
112. Ⓐ Ⓑ Ⓒ Ⓓ Ⓔ [29, V]
113. Ⓐ Ⓑ Ⓒ Ⓓ Ⓔ [29, V]
114. Ⓐ Ⓑ Ⓒ Ⓓ Ⓔ [18, II]
115. Ⓐ Ⓑ Ⓒ Ⓓ Ⓔ [28, III]
116. Ⓐ Ⓑ Ⓒ Ⓓ Ⓔ [28, III]
117. Ⓐ Ⓑ Ⓒ Ⓓ Ⓔ [15, II F]
118. Ⓐ Ⓑ Ⓒ Ⓓ Ⓔ [29, VI]
119. Ⓐ Ⓑ Ⓒ Ⓓ Ⓔ [26, IV]
120. Ⓐ Ⓑ Ⓒ Ⓓ Ⓔ [24, V]

#	A	B	C	D	E	Ref
121.	Ⓐ	Ⓑ	Ⓒ	Ⓓ	Ⓔ	[21, II]
122.	Ⓐ	Ⓑ	Ⓒ	Ⓓ	Ⓔ	[21, II]
123.	Ⓐ	Ⓑ	Ⓒ	Ⓓ	Ⓔ	[17, III]
124.	Ⓐ	Ⓑ	Ⓒ	Ⓓ	Ⓔ	[15, II E]
125.	Ⓐ	Ⓑ	Ⓒ	Ⓓ	Ⓔ	[16, V]
126.	Ⓐ	Ⓑ	Ⓒ	Ⓓ	Ⓔ	[18, II]
127.	Ⓐ	Ⓑ	Ⓒ	Ⓓ	Ⓔ	[18, II]
128.	Ⓐ	Ⓑ	Ⓒ	Ⓓ	Ⓔ	[29, VII]
129.	Ⓐ	Ⓑ	Ⓒ	Ⓓ	Ⓔ	[14, VI]
130.	Ⓐ	Ⓑ	Ⓒ	Ⓓ	Ⓔ	[16, VII]
131.	Ⓐ	Ⓑ	Ⓒ	Ⓓ	Ⓔ	[15, II]
132.	Ⓐ	Ⓑ	Ⓒ	Ⓓ	Ⓔ	[29, I]
133.	Ⓐ	Ⓑ	Ⓒ	Ⓓ	Ⓔ	[29, I]
134.	Ⓐ	Ⓑ	Ⓒ	Ⓓ	Ⓔ	[31, VI]
135.	Ⓐ	Ⓑ	Ⓒ	Ⓓ	Ⓔ	[17, V]
136.	Ⓐ	Ⓑ	Ⓒ	Ⓓ	Ⓔ	[15, II A]
137.	Ⓐ	Ⓑ	Ⓒ	Ⓓ	Ⓔ	[22, VI]
138.	Ⓐ	Ⓑ	Ⓒ	Ⓓ	Ⓔ	[22, VI]
139.	Ⓐ	Ⓑ	Ⓒ	Ⓓ	Ⓔ	[29, VI]
140.	Ⓐ	Ⓑ	Ⓒ	Ⓓ	Ⓔ	[18, II]
141.	Ⓐ	Ⓑ	Ⓒ	Ⓓ	Ⓔ	[18, I]
142.	Ⓐ	Ⓑ	Ⓒ	Ⓓ	Ⓔ	[26, III]
143.	Ⓐ	Ⓑ	Ⓒ	Ⓓ	Ⓔ	[26, III]
144.	Ⓐ	Ⓑ	Ⓒ	Ⓓ	Ⓔ	[14, II]
145.	Ⓐ	Ⓑ	Ⓒ	Ⓓ	Ⓔ	[28, III]
146.	Ⓐ	Ⓑ	Ⓒ	Ⓓ	Ⓔ	[15, II C]
147.	Ⓐ	Ⓑ	Ⓒ	Ⓓ	Ⓔ	[18, III A]
148.	Ⓐ	Ⓑ	Ⓒ	Ⓓ	Ⓔ	[17, IV]
149.	Ⓐ	Ⓑ	Ⓒ	Ⓓ	Ⓔ	[22, VII]
150.	Ⓐ	Ⓑ	Ⓒ	Ⓓ	Ⓔ	[22, VII]
151.	Ⓐ	Ⓑ	Ⓒ	Ⓓ	Ⓔ	[23, IV]
152.	Ⓐ	Ⓑ	Ⓒ	Ⓓ	Ⓔ	[20, II]
153.	Ⓐ	Ⓑ	Ⓒ	Ⓓ	Ⓔ	[23, III]
154.	Ⓐ	Ⓑ	Ⓒ	Ⓓ	Ⓔ	[29, III]
155.	Ⓐ	Ⓑ	Ⓒ	Ⓓ	Ⓔ	[29, III]
156.	Ⓐ	Ⓑ	Ⓒ	Ⓓ	Ⓔ	[31, II]
157.	Ⓐ	Ⓑ	Ⓒ	Ⓓ	Ⓔ	[24, I]
158.	Ⓐ	Ⓑ	Ⓒ	Ⓓ	Ⓔ	[24, I]
159.	Ⓐ	Ⓑ	Ⓒ	Ⓓ	Ⓔ	[24, I]
160.	Ⓐ	Ⓑ	Ⓒ	Ⓓ	Ⓔ	[24, I]
161.	Ⓐ	Ⓑ	Ⓒ	Ⓓ	Ⓔ	[24, I]
162.	Ⓐ	Ⓑ	Ⓒ	Ⓓ	Ⓔ	[24, I]
163.	Ⓐ	Ⓑ	Ⓒ	Ⓓ	Ⓔ	[18, II]
164.	Ⓐ	Ⓑ	Ⓒ	Ⓓ	Ⓔ	[26, II]
165.	Ⓐ	Ⓑ	Ⓒ	Ⓓ	Ⓔ	[29, II]
166.	Ⓐ	Ⓑ	Ⓒ	Ⓓ	Ⓔ	[26, III]
167.	Ⓐ	Ⓑ	Ⓒ	Ⓓ	Ⓔ	[15, II E]
168.	Ⓐ	Ⓑ	Ⓒ	Ⓓ	Ⓔ	[22, VII]
169.	Ⓐ	Ⓑ	Ⓒ	Ⓓ	Ⓔ	[16, V]
170.	Ⓐ	Ⓑ	Ⓒ	Ⓓ	Ⓔ	[16, V]
171.	Ⓐ	Ⓑ	Ⓒ	Ⓓ	Ⓔ	[22, I]
172.	Ⓐ	Ⓑ	Ⓒ	Ⓓ	Ⓔ	[14, II]
173.	Ⓐ	Ⓑ	Ⓒ	Ⓓ	Ⓔ	[15, II C]
174.	Ⓐ	Ⓑ	Ⓒ	Ⓓ	Ⓔ	[22, XI]
175.	Ⓐ	Ⓑ	Ⓒ	Ⓓ	Ⓔ	[29, III]
176.	Ⓐ	Ⓑ	Ⓒ	Ⓓ	Ⓔ	[25, I]
177.	Ⓐ	Ⓑ	Ⓒ	Ⓓ	Ⓔ	[15, II A]
178.	Ⓐ	Ⓑ	Ⓒ	Ⓓ	Ⓔ	[18, I]
179.	Ⓐ	Ⓑ	Ⓒ	Ⓓ	Ⓔ	[27, III]
180.	Ⓐ	Ⓑ	Ⓒ	Ⓓ	Ⓔ	[18, IV A]
181.	Ⓐ	Ⓑ	Ⓒ	Ⓓ	Ⓔ	[16, VII]
182.	Ⓐ	Ⓑ	Ⓒ	Ⓓ	Ⓔ	[28, III]
183.	Ⓐ	Ⓑ	Ⓒ	Ⓓ	Ⓔ	[28, III]
184.	Ⓐ	Ⓑ	Ⓒ	Ⓓ	Ⓔ	[29, IV]
185.	Ⓐ	Ⓑ	Ⓒ	Ⓓ	Ⓔ	[22, IV]
186.	Ⓐ	Ⓑ	Ⓒ	Ⓓ	Ⓔ	[20, II]
187.	Ⓐ	Ⓑ	Ⓒ	Ⓓ	Ⓔ	[22, IV]
188.	Ⓐ	Ⓑ	Ⓒ	Ⓓ	Ⓔ	[29, IX]
189.	Ⓐ	Ⓑ	Ⓒ	Ⓓ	Ⓔ	[25, I]
190.	Ⓐ	Ⓑ	Ⓒ	Ⓓ	Ⓔ	[18, I]
191.	Ⓐ	Ⓑ	Ⓒ	Ⓓ	Ⓔ	[16, IV]
192.	Ⓐ	Ⓑ	Ⓒ	Ⓓ	Ⓔ	[16, VI]
193.	Ⓐ	Ⓑ	Ⓒ	Ⓓ	Ⓔ	[22, V]
194.	Ⓐ	Ⓑ	Ⓒ	Ⓓ	Ⓔ	[22, V]
195.	Ⓐ	Ⓑ	Ⓒ	Ⓓ	Ⓔ	[28, III]
196.	Ⓐ	Ⓑ	Ⓒ	Ⓓ	Ⓔ	[28, III]
197.	Ⓐ	Ⓑ	Ⓒ	Ⓓ	Ⓔ	[28, III]
198.	Ⓐ	Ⓑ	Ⓒ	Ⓓ	Ⓔ	[31, VI]
199.	Ⓐ	Ⓑ	Ⓒ	Ⓓ	Ⓔ	[31, II]
200.	Ⓐ	Ⓑ	Ⓒ	Ⓓ	Ⓔ	[15, II B]
201.	Ⓐ	Ⓑ	Ⓒ	Ⓓ	Ⓔ	[15, II B]
202.	Ⓐ	Ⓑ	Ⓒ	Ⓓ	Ⓔ	[22, IV]
203.	Ⓐ	Ⓑ	Ⓒ	Ⓓ	Ⓔ	[18, II]
204.	Ⓐ	Ⓑ	Ⓒ	Ⓓ	Ⓔ	[21, II]
205.	Ⓐ	Ⓑ	Ⓒ	Ⓓ	Ⓔ	[20, I]
206.	Ⓐ	Ⓑ	Ⓒ	Ⓓ	Ⓔ	[22, I]
207.	Ⓐ	Ⓑ	Ⓒ	Ⓓ	Ⓔ	[22, I]
208.	Ⓐ	Ⓑ	Ⓒ	Ⓓ	Ⓔ	[22, I]
209.	Ⓐ	Ⓑ	Ⓒ	Ⓓ	Ⓔ	[29, III]
210.	Ⓐ	Ⓑ	Ⓒ	Ⓓ	Ⓔ	[31, VI]
211.	Ⓐ	Ⓑ	Ⓒ	Ⓓ	Ⓔ	[16, IX]
212.	Ⓐ	Ⓑ	Ⓒ	Ⓓ	Ⓔ	[22, VII, VIII]
213.	Ⓐ	Ⓑ	Ⓒ	Ⓓ	Ⓔ	[15, II A]
214.	Ⓐ	Ⓑ	Ⓒ	Ⓓ	Ⓔ	[28, III]
215.	Ⓐ	Ⓑ	Ⓒ	Ⓓ	Ⓔ	[28, III]
216.	Ⓐ	Ⓑ	Ⓒ	Ⓓ	Ⓔ	[18, I]
217.	Ⓐ	Ⓑ	Ⓒ	Ⓓ	Ⓔ	[22, I]
218.	Ⓐ	Ⓑ	Ⓒ	Ⓓ	Ⓔ	[23, II]
219.	Ⓐ	Ⓑ	Ⓒ	Ⓓ	Ⓔ	[23, II]
220.	Ⓐ	Ⓑ	Ⓒ	Ⓓ	Ⓔ	[22, VII]
221.	Ⓐ	Ⓑ	Ⓒ	Ⓓ	Ⓔ	[25, I]
222.	Ⓐ	Ⓑ	Ⓒ	Ⓓ	Ⓔ	[29, III]
223.	Ⓐ	Ⓑ	Ⓒ	Ⓓ	Ⓔ	[29, III]
224.	Ⓐ	Ⓑ	Ⓒ	Ⓓ	Ⓔ	[22, VII]
225.	Ⓐ	Ⓑ	Ⓒ	Ⓓ	Ⓔ	[22, VII]
226.	Ⓐ	Ⓑ	Ⓒ	Ⓓ	Ⓔ	[29, III]
227.	Ⓐ	Ⓑ	Ⓒ	Ⓓ	Ⓔ	[14, III]
228.	Ⓐ	Ⓑ	Ⓒ	Ⓓ	Ⓔ	[22, I]
229.	Ⓐ	Ⓑ	Ⓒ	Ⓓ	Ⓔ	[22, I]
230.	Ⓐ	Ⓑ	Ⓒ	Ⓓ	Ⓔ	[22, I]
231.	Ⓐ	Ⓑ	Ⓒ	Ⓓ	Ⓔ	[22, I]
232.	Ⓐ	Ⓑ	Ⓒ	Ⓓ	Ⓔ	[24, IV]
233.	Ⓐ	Ⓑ	Ⓒ	Ⓓ	Ⓔ	[24, IV]
234.	Ⓐ	Ⓑ	Ⓒ	Ⓓ	Ⓔ	[24, IV]
235.	Ⓐ	Ⓑ	Ⓒ	Ⓓ	Ⓔ	[24, IV]
236.	Ⓐ	Ⓑ	Ⓒ	Ⓓ	Ⓔ	[24, IV]
237.	Ⓐ	Ⓑ	Ⓒ	Ⓓ	Ⓔ	[24, IV]
238.	Ⓐ	Ⓑ	Ⓒ	Ⓓ	Ⓔ	[28, II]
239.	Ⓐ	Ⓑ	Ⓒ	Ⓓ	Ⓔ	[16, III]
240.	Ⓐ	Ⓑ	Ⓒ	Ⓓ	Ⓔ	[15, II A]
241.	Ⓐ	Ⓑ	Ⓒ	Ⓓ	Ⓔ	[15, II A]
242.	Ⓐ	Ⓑ	Ⓒ	Ⓓ	Ⓔ	[15, II A]
243.	Ⓐ	Ⓑ	Ⓒ	Ⓓ	Ⓔ	[22, I]
244.	Ⓐ	Ⓑ	Ⓒ	Ⓓ	Ⓔ	[16, VIII]
245.	Ⓐ	Ⓑ	Ⓒ	Ⓓ	Ⓔ	[16, VIII]
246.	Ⓐ	Ⓑ	Ⓒ	Ⓓ	Ⓔ	[16, VIII]
247.	Ⓐ	Ⓑ	Ⓒ	Ⓓ	Ⓔ	[31, II]
248.	Ⓐ	Ⓑ	Ⓒ	Ⓓ	Ⓔ	[28, II]
249.	Ⓐ	Ⓑ	Ⓒ	Ⓓ	Ⓔ	[22, I]
250.	Ⓐ	Ⓑ	Ⓒ	Ⓓ	Ⓔ	[22, I]
251.	Ⓐ	Ⓑ	Ⓒ	Ⓓ	Ⓔ	[30, III]
252.	Ⓐ	Ⓑ	Ⓒ	Ⓓ	Ⓔ	[15, II C]
253.	Ⓐ	Ⓑ	Ⓒ	Ⓓ	Ⓔ	[15, II C]
254.	Ⓐ	Ⓑ	Ⓒ	Ⓓ	Ⓔ	[22, VII]
255.	Ⓐ	Ⓑ	Ⓒ	Ⓓ	Ⓔ	[22, VII]
256.	Ⓐ	Ⓑ	Ⓒ	Ⓓ	Ⓔ	[18, III]
257.	Ⓐ	Ⓑ	Ⓒ	Ⓓ	Ⓔ	[15, I]
258.	Ⓐ	Ⓑ	Ⓒ	Ⓓ	Ⓔ	[25, I]
259.	Ⓐ	Ⓑ	Ⓒ	Ⓓ	Ⓔ	[25, I]
260.	Ⓐ	Ⓑ	Ⓒ	Ⓓ	Ⓔ	[25, I]
261.	Ⓐ	Ⓑ	Ⓒ	Ⓓ	Ⓔ	[25, I]
262.	Ⓐ	Ⓑ	Ⓒ	Ⓓ	Ⓔ	[25, I]
263.	Ⓐ	Ⓑ	Ⓒ	Ⓓ	Ⓔ	[25, I]
264.	Ⓐ	Ⓑ	Ⓒ	Ⓓ	Ⓔ	[22, I]
265.	Ⓐ	Ⓑ	Ⓒ	Ⓓ	Ⓔ	[15, II A]
266.	Ⓐ	Ⓑ	Ⓒ	Ⓓ	Ⓔ	[15, II A]
267.	Ⓐ	Ⓑ	Ⓒ	Ⓓ	Ⓔ	[31, IV]
268.	Ⓐ	Ⓑ	Ⓒ	Ⓓ	Ⓔ	[27, III]
269.	Ⓐ	Ⓑ	Ⓒ	Ⓓ	Ⓔ	[22, IX]
270.	Ⓐ	Ⓑ	Ⓒ	Ⓓ	Ⓔ	[14, I]
271.	Ⓐ	Ⓑ	Ⓒ	Ⓓ	Ⓔ	[14, III]
272.	Ⓐ	Ⓑ	Ⓒ	Ⓓ	Ⓔ	[14, II]

273. Ⓐ Ⓑ Ⓒ Ⓓ Ⓔ [14, I]
274. Ⓐ Ⓑ Ⓒ Ⓓ Ⓔ [14, I]
275. Ⓐ Ⓑ Ⓒ Ⓓ Ⓔ [14, I]
276. Ⓐ Ⓑ Ⓒ Ⓓ Ⓔ [14, I]
277. Ⓐ Ⓑ Ⓒ Ⓓ Ⓔ [17, II]
278. Ⓐ Ⓑ Ⓒ Ⓓ Ⓔ [29, IV]
279. Ⓐ Ⓑ Ⓒ Ⓓ Ⓔ [30, I]
280. Ⓐ Ⓑ Ⓒ Ⓓ Ⓔ [24, III]
281. Ⓐ Ⓑ Ⓒ Ⓓ Ⓔ [23, V]
282. Ⓐ Ⓑ Ⓒ Ⓓ Ⓔ [23, V]
283. Ⓐ Ⓑ Ⓒ Ⓓ Ⓔ [22, I]
284. Ⓐ Ⓑ Ⓒ Ⓓ Ⓔ [29, I]
285. Ⓐ Ⓑ Ⓒ Ⓓ Ⓔ [22, I]
286. Ⓐ Ⓑ Ⓒ Ⓓ Ⓔ [14, III]
287. Ⓐ Ⓑ Ⓒ Ⓓ Ⓔ [24, VIII]
288. Ⓐ Ⓑ Ⓒ Ⓓ Ⓔ [30, I]
289. Ⓐ Ⓑ Ⓒ Ⓓ Ⓔ [30, I]
290. Ⓐ Ⓑ Ⓒ Ⓓ Ⓔ [26, III]
291. Ⓐ Ⓑ Ⓒ Ⓓ Ⓔ [25, II]
292. Ⓐ Ⓑ Ⓒ Ⓓ Ⓔ [14, VII]
293. Ⓐ Ⓑ Ⓒ Ⓓ Ⓔ [14, VII]
294. Ⓐ Ⓑ Ⓒ Ⓓ Ⓔ [23, II]
295. Ⓐ Ⓑ Ⓒ Ⓓ Ⓔ [25, III]
296. Ⓐ Ⓑ Ⓒ Ⓓ Ⓔ [27, II]
297. Ⓐ Ⓑ Ⓒ Ⓓ Ⓔ [24, II]
298. Ⓐ Ⓑ Ⓒ Ⓓ Ⓔ [18, II]
299. Ⓐ Ⓑ Ⓒ Ⓓ Ⓔ [14, VI]
300. Ⓐ Ⓑ Ⓒ Ⓓ Ⓔ [19, V]
301. Ⓐ Ⓑ Ⓒ Ⓓ Ⓔ [24, V]
302. Ⓐ Ⓑ Ⓒ Ⓓ Ⓔ [31, VI]
303. Ⓐ Ⓑ Ⓒ Ⓓ Ⓔ [17, I]
304. Ⓐ Ⓑ Ⓒ Ⓓ Ⓔ [14, I]
305. Ⓐ Ⓑ Ⓒ Ⓓ Ⓔ [14, II]
306. Ⓐ Ⓑ Ⓒ Ⓓ Ⓔ [14, I]
307. Ⓐ Ⓑ Ⓒ Ⓓ Ⓔ [23, III]
308. Ⓐ Ⓑ Ⓒ Ⓓ Ⓔ [26, II]
309. Ⓐ Ⓑ Ⓒ Ⓓ Ⓔ [29, VIII B]
310. Ⓐ Ⓑ Ⓒ Ⓓ Ⓔ [29, VIII B]
311. Ⓐ Ⓑ Ⓒ Ⓓ Ⓔ [24, V]
312. Ⓐ Ⓑ Ⓒ Ⓓ Ⓔ [30, I]
313. Ⓐ Ⓑ Ⓒ Ⓓ Ⓔ [14, I]
314. Ⓐ Ⓑ Ⓒ Ⓓ Ⓔ [23, III]

315. Ⓐ Ⓑ Ⓒ Ⓓ Ⓔ [25, I]
316. Ⓐ Ⓑ Ⓒ Ⓓ Ⓔ [29, II]
317. Ⓐ Ⓑ Ⓒ Ⓓ Ⓔ [14, III]
318. Ⓐ Ⓑ Ⓒ Ⓓ Ⓔ [15, I]
319. Ⓐ Ⓑ Ⓒ Ⓓ Ⓔ [18, I]
320. Ⓐ Ⓑ Ⓒ Ⓓ Ⓔ [18, I]
321. Ⓐ Ⓑ Ⓒ Ⓓ Ⓔ [22, I]
322. Ⓐ Ⓑ Ⓒ Ⓓ Ⓔ [14, I]
323. Ⓐ Ⓑ Ⓒ Ⓓ Ⓔ [24, I]
324. Ⓐ Ⓑ Ⓒ Ⓓ Ⓔ [19, III]
325. Ⓐ Ⓑ Ⓒ Ⓓ Ⓔ [28, I]
326. Ⓐ Ⓑ Ⓒ Ⓓ Ⓔ [14, VI]
327. Ⓐ Ⓑ Ⓒ Ⓓ Ⓔ [16, VI]
328. Ⓐ Ⓑ Ⓒ Ⓓ Ⓔ [23, III]
329. Ⓐ Ⓑ Ⓒ Ⓓ Ⓔ [23, III]
330. Ⓐ Ⓑ Ⓒ Ⓓ Ⓔ [23, III]
331. Ⓐ Ⓑ Ⓒ Ⓓ Ⓔ [28, II]
332. Ⓐ Ⓑ Ⓒ Ⓓ Ⓔ [25, IV]
333. Ⓐ Ⓑ Ⓒ Ⓓ Ⓔ [14, VII]
334. Ⓐ Ⓑ Ⓒ Ⓓ Ⓔ [28, II]
335. Ⓐ Ⓑ Ⓒ Ⓓ Ⓔ [18, IV B]
336. Ⓐ Ⓑ Ⓒ Ⓓ Ⓔ [18, IV B]
337. Ⓐ Ⓑ Ⓒ Ⓓ Ⓔ [14, VII]
338. Ⓐ Ⓑ Ⓒ Ⓓ Ⓔ [20, IV]
339. Ⓐ Ⓑ Ⓒ Ⓓ Ⓔ [17, VII]
340. Ⓐ Ⓑ Ⓒ Ⓓ Ⓔ [28, II]
341. Ⓐ Ⓑ Ⓒ Ⓓ Ⓔ [24, I]
342. Ⓐ Ⓑ Ⓒ Ⓓ Ⓔ [24, I]
343. Ⓐ Ⓑ Ⓒ Ⓓ Ⓔ [31, VII]
344. Ⓐ Ⓑ Ⓒ Ⓓ Ⓔ [15, II D]
345. Ⓐ Ⓑ Ⓒ Ⓓ Ⓔ [18, I]
346. Ⓐ Ⓑ Ⓒ Ⓓ Ⓔ [29, IX]
347. Ⓐ Ⓑ Ⓒ Ⓓ Ⓔ [16, VII]
348. Ⓐ Ⓑ Ⓒ Ⓓ Ⓔ [25, I]
349. Ⓐ Ⓑ Ⓒ Ⓓ Ⓔ [29, I]
350. Ⓐ Ⓑ Ⓒ Ⓓ Ⓔ [29, I]
351. Ⓐ Ⓑ Ⓒ Ⓓ Ⓔ [15, II G]
352. Ⓐ Ⓑ Ⓒ Ⓓ Ⓔ [17, IV]
353. Ⓐ Ⓑ Ⓒ Ⓓ Ⓔ [16, XII]
354. Ⓐ Ⓑ Ⓒ Ⓓ Ⓔ [24, II]
355. Ⓐ Ⓑ Ⓒ Ⓓ Ⓔ [24, II]
356. Ⓐ Ⓑ Ⓒ Ⓓ Ⓔ [31, VII]

357. Ⓐ Ⓑ Ⓒ Ⓓ Ⓔ [18, I]
358. Ⓐ Ⓑ Ⓒ Ⓓ Ⓔ [17, VI]
359. Ⓐ Ⓑ Ⓒ Ⓓ Ⓔ [22, XI]
360. Ⓐ Ⓑ Ⓒ Ⓓ Ⓔ [26, III]
361. Ⓐ Ⓑ Ⓒ Ⓓ Ⓔ [19, III]
362. Ⓐ Ⓑ Ⓒ Ⓓ Ⓔ [16, III]
363. Ⓐ Ⓑ Ⓒ Ⓓ Ⓔ [29, II]
364. Ⓐ Ⓑ Ⓒ Ⓓ Ⓔ [24, V]
365. Ⓐ Ⓑ Ⓒ Ⓓ Ⓔ [18, IV]
366. Ⓐ Ⓑ Ⓒ Ⓓ Ⓔ [20, IV]
367. Ⓐ Ⓑ Ⓒ Ⓓ Ⓔ [29, I]
368. Ⓐ Ⓑ Ⓒ Ⓓ Ⓔ [18, IV B]
369. Ⓐ Ⓑ Ⓒ Ⓓ Ⓔ [16, VII]
370. Ⓐ Ⓑ Ⓒ Ⓓ Ⓔ [27, I]
371. Ⓐ Ⓑ Ⓒ Ⓓ Ⓔ [24, II]
372. Ⓐ Ⓑ Ⓒ Ⓓ Ⓔ [29, II]
373. Ⓐ Ⓑ Ⓒ Ⓓ Ⓔ [28, III]
374. Ⓐ Ⓑ Ⓒ Ⓓ Ⓔ [16, VII]
375. Ⓐ Ⓑ Ⓒ Ⓓ Ⓔ [17, X]
376. Ⓐ Ⓑ Ⓒ Ⓓ Ⓔ [15, II A]
377. Ⓐ Ⓑ Ⓒ Ⓓ Ⓔ [15, II A]
378. Ⓐ Ⓑ Ⓒ Ⓓ Ⓔ [15, II A]
379. Ⓐ Ⓑ Ⓒ Ⓓ Ⓔ [15, II A]
380. Ⓐ Ⓑ Ⓒ Ⓓ Ⓔ [15, II A]
381. Ⓐ Ⓑ Ⓒ Ⓓ Ⓔ [22, I]
382. Ⓐ Ⓑ Ⓒ Ⓓ Ⓔ [18, I]
383. Ⓐ Ⓑ Ⓒ Ⓓ Ⓔ [27, I]
384. Ⓐ Ⓑ Ⓒ Ⓓ Ⓔ [25, IV]
385. Ⓐ Ⓑ Ⓒ Ⓓ Ⓔ [17, VII]
386. Ⓐ Ⓑ Ⓒ Ⓓ Ⓔ [29, II]
387. Ⓐ Ⓑ Ⓒ Ⓓ Ⓔ [18, I]
388. Ⓐ Ⓑ Ⓒ Ⓓ Ⓔ [17, XI]
389. Ⓐ Ⓑ Ⓒ Ⓓ Ⓔ [28, III]
390. Ⓐ Ⓑ Ⓒ Ⓓ Ⓔ [25, I]
391. Ⓐ Ⓑ Ⓒ Ⓓ Ⓔ [18, III A]
392. Ⓐ Ⓑ Ⓒ Ⓓ Ⓔ [29, IX]
393. Ⓐ Ⓑ Ⓒ Ⓓ Ⓔ [27, II]
394. Ⓐ Ⓑ Ⓒ Ⓓ Ⓔ [28, III]
395. Ⓐ Ⓑ Ⓒ Ⓓ Ⓔ [31, VI]
396. Ⓐ Ⓑ Ⓒ Ⓓ Ⓔ [28, II]
397. Ⓐ Ⓑ Ⓒ Ⓓ Ⓔ [25, I]

Self-Evaluation Charts

There are two Self-Evaluation Charts: one for the Abdomen Comprehensive Examination and the other for the Obstetrics and Gynecology Comprehensive Examination. These charts will enable you to identify topic areas that you need to review further.

After you have completed one of the Comprehensive Examinations, check your answers against the Answers and Explanations section for that exam. The code within brackets next to each answer will refer you to a square in the Self-Evaluation Chart that indicates the general question topic, as well as the chapter and outline point in the book where the topic is covered. You may wish to keep track of *wrong answers only* on the chart, so that when you are finished you can see your weak areas at a glance.

For example: On the Obstetrics and Gynecology Comprehensive Examination, if you missed four "22, I"s, you should probably go back and review Chapter 22 (Fetal Abnormalities), outline point I (Cranial Abnormalities). You may also want to review your "weak" topics in other texts (see Appendix C, Suggested Readings).

SELF-EVALUATION CHART: ABDOMEN COMPREHENSIVE EXAMINATION

	1 Liver (16–24%)	2 Biliary Tree (10–18%)	3 Pancreas (6–14%)	4 Urinary Tract (16–24%)	5 Scrotum (3–7%)	6 Prostate (0–2%)	7 Spleen (1–5%)	8 Retro-peritoneum (3–7%)	9 Abdominal Vasculature (7–15%)	10 GI Tract (1–5%)	11 Neck (1–5%)	12 Superficial Structures (1–5%)	13 Instru-mentation (1–3%)
I	Anatomy	Anatomy	Anatomy	Anatomy	Anatomy	Anatomy	Anatomy	Anatomy	Anatomy	Anatomy	Anatomy	**Breast:** Anatomy **Musculoskeletal:** Anatomy **Noncardiac chest:** Normal chest appearance	Technique
II	Technique	Technique	Technique	Technique	Technique	Technique	Technique	Technique	Technique	Technique	Technique	**Breast:** technique **Musculoskeletal:** technique **Noncardiac chest:** pleural effusion	Transducers
III	Laboratory Values	Laboratory Values	Laboratory Values	Laboratory Values	Laboratory Values	Laboratory Values	Laboratory Values	Laboratory Values	Laboratory Values	Laboratory Values	Laboratory Values	**Breast:** Laboratory Values **Musculoskeletal:** Laboratory Values **Noncardiac Chest:** Peripheral Lung Masses	Image Recording

IV	Artifacts	**Breast:** Indications	**Musculoskeletal:** Indications	**Noncardiac Chest:** Lung Consolidation	Indications	Indications	Indications	Indications	Indications	Indications	Indications	Indications	Indications	Indications	Indications
V	Quality Assurance	**Breast:** Masses	**Musculoskeletal:** Masses—Soft Tissue or Bone Tumors		Thyroid Parenchymal Disease	Inflammatory Disease	Aneurysms	Masses—Adenopathy	Parenchymal Disease	Parenchymal Disease—Benign Prostatic Hypertrophy	Parenchymal Disease	Renal Parenchymal Disease	Parenchymal Disease	Dilation	Parenchymal Disease
VI	Invasive Procedures	**Breast:** Cysts and Fluid Collections	**Musculoskeletal:** Cysts and Fluid Collections		Thyroid Masses	Masses—Gut Cancer	Thrombus	Hematomas	Masses	Masses—Prostate Cancer	Masses	Masses	Masses	Masses	Masses
VII		**Breast:** Abscesses			Thyroid Cysts	Obstruction	Arteriovenous Shunts and Fistulas	Adrenal	Cysts	Cysts	Cysts and Fluid Collections	Cysts	Cysts and Pseudocysts	Cholelithiasis	Cysts

SELF-EVALUATION CHART: ABDOMEN COMPREHENSIVE EXAMINATION (CONTINUED)

	1 Liver (16–24%)	2 Biliary Tree (10–18%)	3 Pancreas (6–14%)	4 Urinary Tract (16–24%)	5 Scrotum (3–7%)	6 Prostate (0–2%)	7 Spleen (1–5%)	8 Retro-peritoneum (3–7%)	9 Abdominal Vasculature (7–15%)	10 GI Tract (1–5%)	11 Neck (1–5%)	12 Superficial Structures (1–5%)	13 Instru-mentation (1–3%)
												Musculoskeletal: Abscesses	
VIII	Abscesses	Cholecystitis		Abscesses	Inflammation	Abscesses	Abscesses		Pseudo-aneurysms	Hernia	Parathyroid Masses	Musculoskeletal: Hematomas and Other Trauma-Related Injuries	
IX	Hematomas			Hematomas	Hematomas		Hematomas		Doppler Waveforms	Peritoneal Fluid—Ascites	Abscesses		
X				Calculi			Infarctions				Lymph Nodes		
XI				Obstructive Disease							Carotid Arteries and Jugular Veins		
XII				Infarctions									
XIII				Anomalies									
XIV				Renal Transplants									
XV				Urinary Bladder									

SELF-EVALUTION CHART: OBSTETRICS AND GYNECOLOGY COMPREHENSIVE EXAMINATION

	14 First Trimester (6–8%)	15 Second and Third Trimester (8–12%)	16 Placenta (1–5%)	17 Assessment of Gestational Age (2–6%)	18 Complications (6–10%)	19 Amniotic Fluid (1–5%)	20 Genetic Studies (1–3%)	21 Fetal Demise (0–3%)	22 Fetal Abnormalities (10–15%)	23 Coexisting Disorders (0–3%)
I	Gestational Sac	Basic Guidelines for Obstetric Sonograms	Development	Gestational Sac	Intrauterine Growth Retardation	Characteristics	Maternal Serum Testing	Missed Abortion	Cranial Abnormalities	Leiomyomas (Fibroids)
II	Yolk Sac	Evaluation of Anatomy A. Cranium B. Spine C. Heart D. Thorax E. Abdomen F. Extremities G. Fetal Position	Position	Embryonic Size/Crown-Rump Length	Multiple Gestation	Functions	Amniotic Fluid Testing	Fetal Death	Facial Abnormalities	Cystic Disorders

SELF-EVALUATION CHART: OBSTETRICS AND GYNECOLOGY COMPREHENSIVE EXAMINATION

	14 First Trimester (6–8%)	15 Second and Third Trimester (8–12%)	16 Placenta (1–5%)	17 Assessment of Gestational Age (2–6%)	18 Complications (6–10%)	19 Amniotic Fluid (1–5%)	20 Genetic Studies (1–3%)	21 Fetal Demise (0–3%)	22 Fetal Abnormalities (10–15%)	23 Coexisting Disorders (0–3%)
III	Embryo		Anatomy	Biparietal Diameter	Maternal Illness A. Diabetes Mellitus B. Pregnancy-Induced Hypertension	Assessment	Amniocentesis		Neck Abnormalities	Gestational Trophoblastic Disease
IV	Ovaries		Membranes	Femur Length	Antepartum A. Preterm Labor, Cervical Incompetence, and Prom B. Rh Isoimmunization	Polyhydramnios	Chorionic Villi Sampling		Spinal Abnormalities—Spina Bifida	Partial Moles
V	Cul-De-Sac		Umbilical Cord	Abdominal Circumference	Fetal Therapy—Intrauterine Transfusion	Oligohydramnios	Dominant and Recessive Risk Occurrence		Abdominal Wall Abnormalities	Myometrial Contractions
VI	Pregnancy Failure		Abruption	Head Circumference	Postpartum A. Retained Products Of Conception		Teratogens		Thoracic Abnormalities	

VII	Ectopic Pregnancy	B. Cesarean Section	Previa	Transcerebellar Measurements	Genitourinary Abnormalities
VIII	Sonographic Examination in the First Trimester	C. Infections	Masses and Lesions	Ocular Measurements	Gastrointestinal Abnormalities
IX			Maturity and Grading	Cephalic Index	Skeletal Abnormalities
X			Doppler	Fetal Lung Maturity	Cardiac Abnormalities
XI			Physiology	Other	Syndromes
XII			Accreta		Other Abnormalities—Maternal Infections

SELF-EVALUATION CHART: OBSTETRICS AND GYNECOLOGY COMPREHENSIVE EXAMINATION

	24 Normal Pelvic Anatomy (10–15%)	25 Physiology (6–15%)	26 Pediatric Gynecology (1–5%)	27 Infertility and Endocrinology (2–6%)	28 Postmenopausal Gynecology (6–10%)	29 Pelvic Pathology (6–10%)	30 Extrapelvic Pathology Associated With Gynecology (1–3%)	31 OB/GYN Patient Care Preparation and Technique (1–5%)
I	Uterus	Menstrual Cycle	Normal Anatomy	Contraception—IUCDs	Anatomy and Physiology	Congenital Uterine Malformations	Ascites	Reviewing Charts
II	Vagina	Pregnancy Tests	Precocious Puberty	Causes of Infertility	Hormonal Replacement Therapy	Uterine Masses	Malignant Pelvic Masses	Explaining Examinations
III	Ovaries	Human Chorionic Gonadotropin	Hematometra and Hematocolpos	Sonographic Investigation of Infertility	Pathology	Ovarian Masses	Benign or Malignant Uterine or Ovarian Masses	Supine Hypotensive Syndrome
IV	Fallopian Tubes	Fertilization	Sexual Ambiguity	Medications and Treatment		Endometriosis		Biologic Effects
V	Supporting Structures					Polycystic Ovary Syndrome		Infectious Disease Control
VI	Potential Sites for Fluid Accumulation					Pelvic Inflammatory Disease		Scanning Techniques
VII	Vasculature					Doppler Flow Studies		Artifacts

	Physical Principles	
	Gynecology-Related Studies	Other Pathologies
	A. Gastrointestinal Studies	
	B. Genitourinary Studies	
VIII	Doppler	
IX		

INDEX